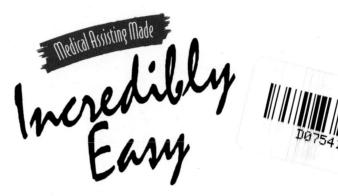

CLINICAL
COMPETENCIES

Medical Assisting Made

Incredibly Easy

CLINICAL COMPETENCIES

Michelle Buchman, RN, BSN, BC

Educational Support Services, LLC
St. John's Marian Center
Springfield, Missouri

 Wolters Kluwer | Lippincott Williams & Wilkins
Health

Philadelphia · Baltimore · New York · London
Buenos Aires · Hong Kong · Sydney · Tokyo

Executive Editor: John Goucher
Senior Managing Editor: Rebecca Kerins
Marketing Manager: Hilary Henderson
Production Editor: Eve Malakoff-Klein
Illustrator: Bot Roda
Designer: Joan Wendt
Compositor: Circle Graphics, Inc.
Printer: R.R. Donnelley & Sons—Crawfordsville

9 8 7 6 5 4 3 2 1

Library of Congress Cataloging-in-Publication Data

Buchman, Michelle.
   Clinical competencies / Michelle Buchman.
      p. ; cm. — (Medical assisting made incredibly easy)
   Includes index.
   ISBN-13: 978-0-7817-6345-5
   ISBN-10: 0-7817-6345-2
   1. Medical assistants. 2. Clinical medicine. I. Title. II. Series.
   [DNLM: 1. Clinical Medicine. 2. Allied Health Personnel. WB 102 B919c 2008]
   R728.8.B83 2008
   610.73'7069—dc22

                              2007001967

DISCLAIMER

PREFACE

Medical Assisting Made Incredibly Easy is an exciting new series designed to make learning enjoyable for medical assisting students. Each book in the series uses a light-hearted, humorous approach to presenting information. Maria, a Certified Medical Assistant, guides students through the books, offering helpful tips and insights along the way.

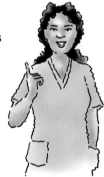

Medical Assisting Made Incredibly Easy takes a practical approach, providing students with the critical information that they need to know, including complete coverage of the core skills they must master in their studies. The series covers all competencies based on the standards and guidelines established for medical assisting by the Commission on Accreditation of Allied Health Educational Programs (CAAHEP) and the Accrediting Bureau of Health Education Schools (ABHES).

ABOUT THIS BOOK

Medical Assisting Made Incredibly Easy: Clinical Competencies provides instruction in CAAHEP's clinical competencies, as well as ABHES's competencies related to clinical duties and patient instruction. These are among the skills that students must master to pass the test required to become either a Certified Medical Assistant or a Registered Medical Assistant.

SPECIAL FEATURES

Medical Assisting Made Incredibly Easy: Clinical Competencies is designed to be enjoyable to read, as well as highly informative. Each chapter in this book includes special features designed to guide students in their study. These elements will help students to identify the most important information in the chapter and to understand all of it.

- 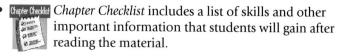 *Chapter Checklist* includes a list of skills and other important information that students will gain after reading the material.

- `Closer Look` *Closer Look* explores chapter information in more detail in a list or summary form.

- `Running Smoothly` *Running Smoothly* features situations that medical assistants may encounter in a medical office and shows how students can apply what they have learned to those situations.

- `Ask the Professional` *Ask the Professional* offers expert advice on how to handle difficult situations that medical assistants may face in the workplace.

- `Secrets for Success` *Secrets for Success* provides tips for studying, for remembering important material, and for success in a career as a medical assistant.

- `Legal Brief` *Legal Brief* provides important legal and ethical information, including how the Health Insurance Portability and Accountability Act (HIPAA) impacts medical assisting.

- `Word to the Wise` *Word to the Wise* covers terminology that students might find challenging, providing a definition and pronunciation for each term.

- `Your Turn to Teach` *Your Turn To Teach* provides students with valuable information regarding patient education.

- `Hands On` *Hands On* contains procedures for important skills and tasks.

- `Chapter Highlights` *Chapter Highlights* summarizes a chapter's key content.

In addition to the above features, this book also includes bolded key terms throughout each chapter and a Glossary in the back of the book, as well as many other boxed features and tables.

ADDITIONAL RESOURCES

In addition to the text, the following resources are available for students and instructors:

- *Study Guide for Medical Assisting Made Incredibly Easy: Clinical Competencies* includes learning activities and exercises, quizzes, puzzles, certification review questions, and competency evaluation forms so students can practice their skills and measure their success.

- An **Online Course** provides interactive exercises and review opportunities that support the text and classroom experience.

- An **Instructor's Resource CD-ROM** with test generator, PowerPoint slides, image bank, answers to study guide questions, and customizable competency evaluation forms helps instructors optimize their teaching. The Instructor's Resource CD-ROM also includes information on where in the book and Study Guide each ABHES and CAAHEP competency is covered.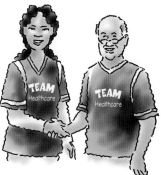

- A complete set of **Lesson Plans** is also available to instructors.

Medical Assisting Made Incredibly Easy: Clinical Competencies is designed to make the study of medical assisting fun and effective. The purpose of this book, and the entire *Medical Assisting Made Incredibly Easy* series, is student success!

USER'S GUIDE

Hello, my name is Maria. I'm a Certified Medical Assistant and educator, as well as your guide through this textbook. There are a number of features in this **Medical Assisting Made Incredibly Easy** text to help you learn everything you need to become a successful medical assistant. Read through this User's Guide to orient yourself to everything the text has to offer. Good luck in your medical assisting studies!

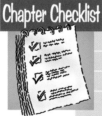

Chapter Checklist

- Identify the medical assistant's responsibilities before, during, and after the physical examination
- List the supplies typically needed in an examination room
- Prepare and maintain examination and treatment areas
- Explain the use of the common and specialized instruments used in a physical examination
- Describe the six basic techniques for examining patients
- Prepare patients for and assist with routine and specialty examinations
- Describe the basic examination positions and their uses
- Explain the typical procedures for examining different body structures
- List the basic sequence of the physical examination
- Explain how the physician tests posture, gait, and reflexes
- Teach patients how to recognize cancer warning signs
- List the guidelines for general physical examinations, immunizations, and cancer screening

Chapter Checklists orient you to the material that's covered in the current chapter.

Closer Look — RECORDING PATIENTS' TEMPERATURES

Temperature readings from different parts of the body shouldn't be taken as equal. A reading of 98.6°F is considered average for oral thermometers, but readings from other sites may be slightly different.

- Rectal temperatures are generally 1°F *higher* than oral temperatures. This is because of the blood supply and tightly closed environment of the rectum. A rectal temperature of 101°F is the equivalent to an oral temperature of 100°F.
- Axillary temperatures are usually 1°F *lower* than oral temperatures. It's difficult for patients to keep the axilla, or armpit, tightly closed. An axillary temperature of 101°F is the equivalent of an oral temperature of 102°F.
- Tympanic thermometers give similar readings to oral thermometers as long as they are used properly.

When you record a temperature in a patient's chart, you'll need to write where you took the measurement as well as the temperatu

Closer Look boxes explore topics in more detail.

Running Smoothly — USING THE HOLTER MONITOR CORRECTLY

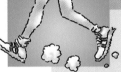

Running Smoothly boxes feature situations that you may encounter in a medical office and teach you to apply what you've learned to those situations.

A patient has returned to the office with the Holter monitor and his diary, but one of the leads isn't attached. What should I do?

Check to see if the patient has recorded in his diary when the lead became loose. You may need to check with the physician to see if enough time passed before the lead came loose to obtain sufficient information about the heart function. In some cases, the patient may not be aware the lead became loose. He may need to wear the Holter monitor for another period of time to collect more information.

Ask the Professional — PATHOGENS IN THE WAITING ROOM

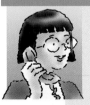

Q: *It's "flu season" again and some patients coming into the office show the symptoms of contagious respiratory illnesses. What can I do to protect the other patients and make the reception area a healthier place?*

A: You must manage the waiting room to protect patients who are waiting to be seen. When a patient arrives who shows signs of an upper respiratory infection, move him to an exam room as soon as one becomes available.

Make sure the reception area has tissues and trash cans for disposal of used tissues—and show the patient where to find them. Be sure to wash your own hands thoroughly after contact with the patient.

Ask the Professional boxes offer expert advice on how to handle difficult situations that you may face in the workplace.

Secrets for Success boxes provide tips for studying, for remembering important material, and for success in your career as a medical assistant.

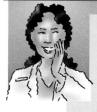

Secrets for Success

PRACTICE YOUR QUESTION-ASKING SKILLS

Asking good questions is critical for obtaining information. By becoming aware of the ways you use questions, you can improve your questioning skills. Here are some ways to practice using questions with friends and family.

- Think of three opportunities where you can use questions to probe for more information. Think about what kinds of questions you could ask.
- In a conversation, make it a point to ask a question to _____tion or to get another person's opin-_____peaker responds to your question.

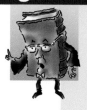

Legal Brief

DISPOSING OF INFECTIOUS WASTE

The Environmental Protection Agency (EPA) and OSHA set regulations and guidelines for disposing of hazardous materials. Individual states use these guidelines to determine their own policies.

Policies for disposing of infectious waste may be different in different states. You need to check your state and local regulations before making decisions about biohazardous waste.

Legal Briefs provide important legal and ethical information, including how the Health Insurance Portability and Accountability Act (HIPAA) affects your work in the medical office.

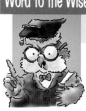

Word to the Wise

speculum (SPEK-yuh-luhm)

a medical tool that enlarges and separates the opening of a body cavity so the examiner can see the interior

Word to the Wise boxes cover terminology that you might find challenging, providing a definition and pronunciation for each term.

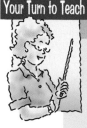

Your Turn to Teach

STOPPING THE SPREAD OF DISEASE AT HOME

As you work with patients, take time to teach them basic aseptic practices they can use at home.

- *Hand washing.* Remind patients that they can stop the spread of disease by washing their hands. Patients should wash their hands before and after meals; after sneezing, coughing, or blowing the nose; after using the bathroom; before and after changing a dressing; and after changing diapers.
- *Changing bandages.* Explain procedures to patients and family members who will need to change bandages. Take care to demonstrate how to apply sterile dressings and clean bandages. To check their understanding, ask the patients or family members to repeat what you showed them.

Your Turn to Teach boxes provide helpful information about patient education.

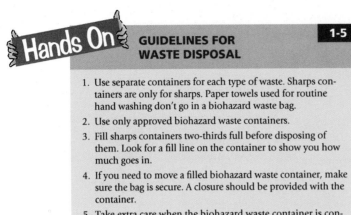

Hands On
GUIDELINES FOR WASTE DISPOSAL

1-5

1. Use separate containers for each type of waste. Sharps containers are only for sharps. Paper towels used for routine hand washing don't go in a biohazard waste bag.
2. Use only approved biohazard waste containers.
3. Fill sharps containers two-thirds full before disposing of them. Look for a fill line on the container to show you how much goes in.
4. If you need to move a filled biohazard waste container, make sure the bag is secure. A closure should be provided with the container.
5. Take extra care when the biohazard waste container is contaminated on the outside and wear gloves! Put the container inside another approved biohazard waste container. And be sure to wash your hands thoroughly afterward.
6. Place biohazard w
   designated area.

Hands On boxes contain step-by-step, easy-to-follow procedures for important skills and tasks.

Chapter Highlights

- Medical assistants use specific procedures and practices to prevent the spread of microorganisms that carry disease.
- The human body has natural barriers to protect itself. These barriers can be overpowered by virulent pathogens, especially in a susceptible host.
- By understanding what microorganisms need to survive and how they are transmitted, the medical assistant can break the chain of infection.
- The medical assistant follows guidelines from OSHA and the CDC. These standard precautions will control and prevent infections in the medical office.
- Medical asepsis keeps office areas free of microorganisms. The medical assistant also teaches patients basic aseptic practices to prevent the spread of microorganisms in their homes. Hand washing is critical.
- Different tools require different levels of infection control. The highest level of infection control is sterilization. It destroys all microorganisms and spores.
- It's important for the medical assistant to know when and how to use different disinfection methods. There are three different levels of disinfection.
- Specific policies and regulations protect medical assistants from biohazardous materials and infectious disease. Written policies in the medical office outline the exposure risk factor for each employee. They also provide an exposure control plan.
- Medical assistants protect themselves and their patients by following strict procedures for cleaning biohazardous waste. Improper disposal of biohazardous waste can lead to fines or imprisonment.
- Many medical assistants worry about exposure to HIV and HBV. Knowing how these viruses are transmitted helps reduce the risks. Medical assistants have a legal right to a vaccine for HBV at no cost. Exposure to HIV or HBV requires follow-up testing.

Chapter Highlights summarize a chapter's key content.

REVIEWERS

Julie Akason, BSN, MAEd
College of St. Catherine
St. Paul, Minnesota

Lori Andrews, MSEd
Ivy Tech Community College
Indianapolis, Indiana

Nina Beaman, MS, BA, AAS
Bryant and Stratton College
Richmond, Virginia

Bonnie Deister, RN, BSN, MS, MA, CMA, EdD
College of the Redwoods
Eureka, California

Tracie Fuqua, BS
Wallace State Community College
Hanceville, Alabama

Robyn Gohsman, AAS
Medical Careers Institute
Newport News, Virginia

Christine Golden, MS, MT (ASCP)
Waukesha County Technical College
Pewaukee, Wisconsin

Rebecca Hickey, RN, RMC, AHI, CHI, BA
Butler Technology and Career Development Schools
Fairfield Township, Ohio

Elizabeth Hoffman, MAEd, CMA, CPT
Baker College of Clinton Township
Clinton Township, Michigan

Joanna Holly, RN, BS, MS
Midstate College
Peoria, Illinois

Dorothy Kiel, BS
Rhodes State College
Lima, Ohio

Carol Lacy, RN, BSN, PHN
College of Marin
Novato, California

Maureen Messier, AS, BA
Branford Hall Career Institute
Southington, Connecticut

Lisa Nagle, BSEd, CMA
Augusta Technical College
Augusta, Georgia

Eva Oltman, MAEd
Jefferson Community and Technical College
Louisville, Kentucky

Jane Ryder, BA, CMA
Yakima Valley Community College
Yakima, Washington

Kathleen Schreiner, RN, MSHA
Montgomery County Community College
Pottstown, Pennsylvania

Cheryl Startzell, MA, BS, AAS
San Antonio College
San Antonio, Texas

Kathy Steinberg, RN, BSN
Midwest Technical Institute
Lincoln, Illinois

Nina Thierer, BS
Ivy Tech Community College
Fort Wayne, Indiana

Stacey Wilson, BS, MT/PBT, CMA
Cabarrus College of Health Sciences
Concord, North Carolina

CONTENTS

PREFACE   v

USER'S GUIDE   ix

REVIEWERS   xiii

Chapter 1
MEDICAL ASEPSIS AND INFECTION CONTROL   1

Chapter 2
MEDICAL HISTORY AND PATIENT ASSESSMENT   42

Chapter 3
ASSISTING WITH THE PHYSICAL EXAMINATION   105

Chapter 4
ASSISTING WITH MINOR OFFICE SURGERY   161

Chapter 5
PHARMACOLOGY AND
DRUG ADMINISTRATION   255

Chapter 6
DIAGNOSTIC TESTING   340

Chapter 7
PATIENT EDUCATION   392

Chapter 8
MEDICAL OFFICE EMERGENCIES   443

GLOSSARY   514

FIGURE CREDITS   532

INDEX   534

Chapter 1

MEDICAL ASEPSIS AND INFECTION CONTROL

Chapter Checklist

- Describe the conditions that help microorganisms live and grow

- Explain the chain of infection process

- List different ways that microorganisms are transmitted

- Describe how the immune system works to fight infection by microorganisms

- Compare the three levels of infection control and their effectiveness

- Explain the concept of medical asepsis

- Perform hand washing

- Demonstrate knowledge of OSHA guidelines for risk management in the medical office

- List the components of an exposure control plan

- Practice standard precautions

- Identify situations when personal protective equipment should be worn

- Demonstrate how to use and remove personal protective equipment

- Prepare and maintain examination and treatment areas

- Dispose of biohazardous materials

- Explain the facts about the transmission and prevention of HBV and HIV in the medical office

- Describe how to avoid becoming infected with HBV and HIV

Patients have different reasons for visiting a medical office. You're probably familiar with many of them. Some patients need physical examinations for their jobs. Others require follow-up care after surgery or care for an ongoing condition. But many patients visit the medical office because they have an illness.

When patients are ill, they can carry disease. **Contagious diseases** are diseases that can spread easily from one person to another. As a medical assistant, part of your job will be to prevent the spread of disease. You need to protect patients from contagious diseases. And you also need to protect yourself!

Disease and the Body

Many diseases spread through **microorganisms**—tiny living things that are too small to see without a microscope. Some people call them **microbes.** Many microbes are a normal part of the environment, but others can cause disease.

> By understanding how diseases are transmitted, you can protect your patients and yourself.

STOP DISEASE FROM SPREADING

Medical assistants help prevent disease from spreading in two ways:

- *Practicing medical asepsis.* **Medical asepsis** is a set of procedures for preventing the spread of disease. As a medical assistant, you'll use specific procedures to control the spread of disease in the medical office. Proper hand washing is one example of a medical aseptic procedure.

- *Teaching others.* Medical assistants show patients and their families how to prevent the spread of disease at home. Reminding a patient to cover his nose and mouth when coughing and sneezing is just one example of a teaching point.

BUGS AND GERMS

You may have heard people say, "I've caught a flu *bug,*" or "Sneezing spreads *germs.*" When people say these things, they are really talking about microbes that cause disease. In the medical office, such microbes are called **pathogens.** Most pathogens belong to one of four main groups—bacteria, viruses, fungi, or protozoa.

Bacteria

Bacteria are tiny one-celled creatures found in soil or water, or on other organisms. Thousands of different types of bacteria exist on earth. Many are harmless, and some are even helpful to humans. But some bacteria cause disease. For example, strep throat is caused by a kind of bacteria called streptococcus group A.

Bacteria also may form **spores.** Spores are protective protein capsules that some bacteria form around them. Then the bacteria rest until the conditions are right for growing.

Viruses

Viruses are tiny bits of protein-coated nucleic acid that invade and take over cells in other living organisms. They need living cells to reproduce. Most viruses cause disease. Influenza, commonly known as "the flu," is caused by a virus. So is the common cold.

Fungi

Fungi are a type of plant. They may be familiar to you as mushrooms or mold. Fungi live in the air, in the soil, on plants, and in water. Some tiny fungi also live in the human body. Only some of these fungi cause disease. An example of a disease caused by a fungus is ringworm, a disease of the skin.

Protozoa

Protozoa are tiny parasites—animals that live in or on another organism. They prefer to live in moist environments. In humans, protozoa often cause disease. One disease caused by protozoa is malaria, a disease with symptoms of high fever and chills.

Secrets for Success   WORKING WITH WORDS: PREFIXES

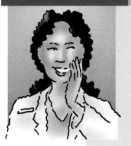

Learning medical terms can sometimes seem as difficult as learning a foreign language. Medical terms are often long and confusing. You can understand medical terms more easily if you break them into parts.

Some medical terms have a prefix, or word beginning. For example, *micro* means small, as in *micro*organism or *micro*scope. *Endo* means internal, as in *endo*crine and *endo*scopy.

WHEN GOOD BUGS TURN BAD

Most microbes are not pathogens. In fact, some microbes are necessary to stay healthy. These include some kinds of bacteria, fungi, and protozoa. They are referred to as **normal flora** or **resident flora** because they normally live in your body. Here are some places where normal flora are normally found:

- on your skin
- in your respiratory system
- in your gastrointestinal system
- in your genitourinary system

Normal flora usually don't cause disease. But they can sometimes become pathogens. This may happen if:

- they multiply until there are too many
- they move to a part of the body where they are not normally found

When microbes begin living in a part of the body where they usually aren't found, they're called **transient flora.** A key factor that affects whether transient flora become pathogens is resistance. **Resistance** refers to how well the human body fights disease. If a person's resistance is low, transient flora may become pathogens.

BODY PROTECTION

The human body has several ways to protect itself from disease.

Natural defenses help to keep pathogens out of body organs.

- *Skin.* Clean, unbroken skin acts as a barrier. It stops pathogens from getting into the body.
- *Eyes.* Eyelashes trap many microbes before they reach the eye. Some are destroyed by tears. Tears

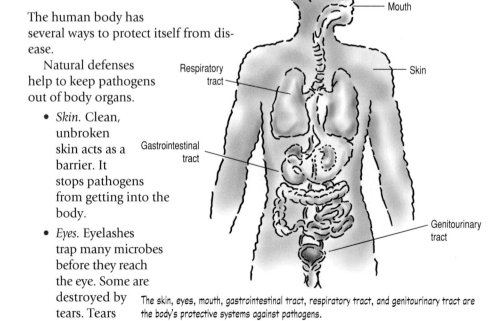

Eyes

Mouth

Respiratory tract

Skin

Gastrointestinal tract

Genitourinary tract

The skin, eyes, mouth, gastrointestinal tract, respiratory tract, and genitourinary tract are the body's protective systems against pathogens.

Secrets for Success   **WORKING WITH WORDS: ROOT WORDS**

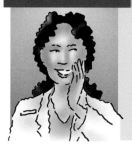

A long medical term can be easier to understand if you look for the root word. The root word gives you basic information about a word's meaning. For example, *cardio* is used in many terms relating to the heart, *osteo* refers to bones, and *gastro* refers to the stomach. When you see an unfamiliar medical term, try looking for the root word to gain clues about the word's meaning.

contain lysozyme, a substance found in the body that kills some kinds of bacteria.

- *Mouth.* More kinds of microbes are found in the mouth than anywhere else in the body. Luckily, saliva is slightly **bactericidal.** This means that it can destroy bacteria. Good oral hygiene can stop the growth of many pathogens in the mouth.

- *Gastrointestinal (GI) tract.* The stomach stops many microbes that enter the GI tract. Hydrochloric acid, an acid usually found in the stomach, destroys many pathogens.

- *Respiratory tract.* Hairs and cilia (fine hair-like structures) on membranes inside the nostrils stop microbes in the air from entering the nose. If these structures are unable to keep pathogens out, there's a second line of defense. Mucus membranes in the respiratory tract trap microorganisms. They help remove them from the body through sneezing, swallowing, or coughing.

- *Genitourinary tract.* Most microbes don't last long in the reproductive or the urinary systems because the environment is slightly acidic.

These protective systems often prevent pathogens from taking over in the human body. But the systems sometimes fail when they must deal with a virulent organism. A **virulent** organism is one that can overpower the body's defenses.

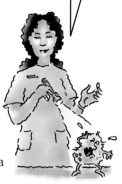

When you know what microbes need to survive, you can stop them from growing by changing their environment.

HOW MICROORGANISMS SURVIVE

Like other living things, microbes need certain things to live and grow.

- *Moisture.* Most microbes need water or moisture to live. Bacterial spores will not be active until they are moistened.

- *Nutrients.* All living things take in nutrients, or substances that help them grow and live. Humans get nutrients from food. Microbes find nutrients in the environment around them.

- *Temperature.* Some microbes grow best at the normal body temperature for humans (98.6°F). These are the ones most likely to become pathogens. Some microbes can survive even in freezing or boiling temperatures.

- *Darkness.* Many pathogenic bacteria can't survive in bright light, such as sunlight.

- *Neutral pH.* pH measures the acid-base balance of a solution on a scale from 1 to 14, where 7 is neutral. Many microbes that invade the body prefer pH levels like those in human blood (7.35 to 7.45).

- *Oxygen.* Microbes that need oxygen to survive are called **aerobes.** But a few types of microbes do not need oxygen to survive. They are called **anaerobes.**

THE PROCESS OF INFECTION

Many pathogens live in the environment, but they don't always cause disease. Infection occurs when pathogens invade the body and start growing. As a medical assistant, you must understand the process of infection. This process can damage body organs and tissues and can lead to disease.

Think of the process of infection as a chain. The chain of infection has five links.

Reservoir Host

The first link in the chain is the place where a microorganism lives and grows. A person or animal infected with a microorganism is a reservoir host. The host's body is a source of nutrients for the microbe. The reservoir host may or may not

POINT 1

Reservoir:
Place on which or in which organisms grow and reproduce. Examples include man and animals.

POINT 5

Susceptible host:
Person whose body cannot fight off organism once it enters the body and who therefore usually becomes ill.

POINT 2

Exit from reservoir:
Escape route for organisms. Examples include nose, throat, mouth, ear, intestinal tract, urinary tract, and wounds.

POINT 4

Portal of entry:
Part of body where organisms enter. Examples include any break in skin or mucous membrane, mouth, nose, and genitourinary tract.

POINT 3

Vehicle of transmission:
Means by which organisms are carried about. Examples include hands, equipment (e.g., bedpan), instruments, china and silverware, linens, and droplets.

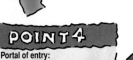

This diagram shows the infectious process cycle.

show signs of infection. But the reservoir host is a **carrier** of the pathogen with the potential to spread it to others.

Exiting the Reservoir

The reservoir host transmits disease if there is an escape route from the host's body. Some ways in which the microbe may exit the reservoir host are the mucous membranes of the nose and mouth, openings of the gastrointestinal system (mouth and rectum), or an open wound.

Vehicle of Transmission

The vehicle of transmission is the way the microbe is carried through the environment. For example, mucus or air droplets from the nose or mouth can be a vehicle of transmission. Coughing or sneezing can send microbes into the environment. Touching another person or object with an unclean hand also can transmit microbes.

Portal of Entry

Microbes that are loose in the environment need nutrients to survive. They can find these nutrients in a new host. The portal of entry is a place where microorganisms can enter the next host's body. Microbes in air droplets can enter through the nose and respiratory system. For microbes in food or drink, the portal of entry is the gastrointestinal system. For some microbes, a portal of entry can be a cut in the skin.

Breaking any link in the infection chain can stop pathogens from spreading.

Susceptible Host

Once a pathogen has entered a new host's body, that person is at risk for developing a disease. A susceptible host is a person who cannot fight the pathogen once it enters the body. It's the last link in the infection chain. If the body of the susceptible host provides the right conditions and nutrients, the microbes will grow and multiply. The susceptible host then becomes a carrier, or reservoir host, starting the infection chain again.

Fighting Infection and Disease

Skin, cough reflexes, tears, and stomach acid are some of the body's natural barriers to stop microbes from entering. But natural barriers don't always work. If pathogens get past the body's natural barriers, they can enter the body and start the process of infection. Then the body must fight back!

Inside the body, the **immune system** is a complex system of organs, tissues, and cells that work together to protect the body from infection and disease. The immune system works to:

- find invading pathogens
- attack pathogens before they start to reproduce
- minimize the damage caused by pathogens
- provide future protection from pathogens

RUSH TO THE SCENE

Inflammation is the first way the body responds to any outside attack. It's called a nonspecific response, because it occurs regardless of the kind of threat there is to the body. Some of these threats include:

- a foreign object, such as a splinter in the finger or a particle in the eye
- extreme temperatures
- trauma or injury
- pathogens entering the body

There are four main signs of inflammation:

- redness
- swelling
- heat
- pain

These signs are part of the body's natural response to infection or injury. Inflammation doesn't always mean the body is fighting infection caused by pathogens. But when infection occurs, inflammation will be part of the body's response.

The signs of inflammation occur when the body sends fluid into the damaged tissue. Swelling helps to keep invading pathogens away from other tissues. The fluid also contains cells from the immune system. They move into the damaged tissue to fight infection.

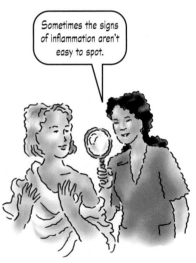

Sometimes the signs of inflammation aren't easy to spot.

DIRECTED ATTACK

The immune system produces several kinds of cells to fight infection. Some are white blood cells that attack and destroy any pathogens. In some cases, the immune system creates antibodies—structures that are designed to attack specific pathogens. Antibodies also can protect the body against future attacks by that type of pathogen.

The Immune System Remembers

A host's susceptibility to disease is related to the body's **immunity** to the disease. Immunity refers to the body's ability to fight specific pathogens. The immune system already may be able to produce antibodies for a specific pathogen. Immunity can result from:

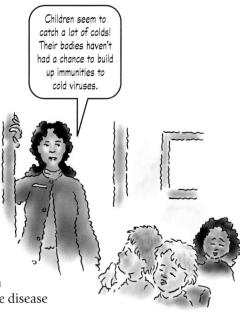

Children seem to catch a lot of colds! Their bodies haven't had a chance to build up immunities to cold viruses.

- previous infection by a specific pathogen
- **immunization** with a vaccine

Immunization is a way to protect the body from a specific pathogen. It involves the injection of a vaccine—a substance that signals the immune system to produce antibodies for the disease. Vaccination can provide permanent immunity from the disease caused by that pathogen.

Types of Immunity

There are different types of immunity. Some individuals are born with *natural immunity* to certain diseases. This type of immunity doesn't involve antibodies. It's already programmed into the person's DNA.

Another important type of immunity is called acquired immunity. Acquired immunity does involve antibodies. This type of immunity may be acquired either passively or actively. There are four different kinds of acquired immunity.

Passive Acquired Natural Immunity. *Passive acquired natural immunity* comes from another source, such as from the mother to the fetus across the placenta. It also can be passed from a nursing mother to her baby through breast milk.

Passive Acquired Artificial Immunity. *Passive acquired artificial immunity* is produced by injections of a special type of antibodies after possible exposure to an infectious pathogen. These antibodies are not a vaccine and only provide temporary protection.

For example, a patient with no tetanus immunization can have an injection to prevent tetanus after stepping on a rusty nail.

Active Acquired Natural Immunity. *Active acquired natural immunity* develops in a person who contracts a specific disease. It causes the body to produce antibodies and memory cells. For example, a person who gets chicken pox develops an active acquired natural immunity to the disease that should prevent him from getting chicken pox again in the future.

Active Acquired Artificial Immunity. *Active acquired artificial immunity* results from a vaccine. The vaccine stimulates the production of antibodies and memory cells to prevent specific diseases by killing the pathogen if it enters the body. Vaccines are available to prevent diseases such as measles, mumps, and rubella to name just a few.

When the Immune System Fails

Sometimes, the immune system can't control an infection. It may not stop pathogens from growing for one or both of two reasons:

- A virulent pathogen may be too powerful for the immune system to fight.
- The immune system may be **depleted.** That means it doesn't have the resources it normally possesses to fight infection or disease.

For example, in a person who is ill, the immune system may have already used up many cells fighting one illness. There may not be enough cells available to fight infection by another pathogen. This is why a person with a depleted immune system is more susceptible to infection and disease.

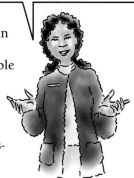

You need to understand how infections lead to disease so you can teach patients how to care for themselves and their families.

FROM INFECTION TO DISEASE

Infection occurs when pathogens enter a host and begin to multiply. Infection may or may not cause disease. Infection leads to disease if the immune system isn't able to stop the pathogen from damaging cells or tissues. Diseases that result from infections are called **infectious diseases.**

Symptoms are physical signs that the patient has a disease. There are many physical signs of infectious disease. Common symptoms include fever, weakness, fatigue, pain, and loss of appetite.

Closer Look   SPOTTING A SUSCEPTIBLE HOST

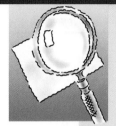

There are many reasons why a susceptible host can't fight off pathogens. Some of these include:

- *Age.* Body defenses against disease become less effective as you age. Elderly people may have weaker immune systems. At the other end of the spectrum, infants may not have fully developed immune systems. They are less able to fight pathogens.

- *Existing disease.* A person who already has an illness may have more trouble fighting off a pathogen. An ill person may have a depleted immune system.

- *Poor nutrition.* A diet lacking in nutrients (proteins, fats, carbohydrates, vitamins, and minerals) can harm the body's cells, making it difficult for the body to repair damage.

- *Poor hygiene.* Keeping the body clean will keep down the number of microorganisms on the skin. That means there are fewer microorganisms to spread disease.

Types of Infections

Some pathogens make you very sick for a short period of time. Others can leave you ill for a long time. There are three main types of infections—acute infections, chronic infections, and latent infections.

Acute Infections. *Acute infections* develop quickly and last only a short time. Influenza, or the flu, is an example of an acute infection. The immune system destroys the virus that causes the flu within two or three weeks and symptoms disappear.

Chronic Infections. *Chronic infections* last for long periods of time, possibly even a lifetime. Their symptoms may not always be noticeable. For example, hepatitis B is a chronic infection of the liver that is caused by a virus. People with hepatitis B may not show symptoms, but the virus can be detected in their blood.

Latent Infections. *Latent infections* have periods when the pathogen is **dormant,** or not active, for months or even years. Viruses often cause these kinds of infections. When the conditions are right for the virus to grow, the infection often reappears. During this active phase, the virus can be transmitted to other people. Cold sores and genital herpes are latent infections caused by viruses.

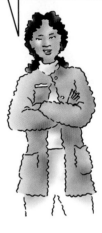

Hepatitis B is a serious health hazard. Infected people can spread it even when they show no symptoms. Make sure you're immunized against hepatitis B.

Stages of Infectious Disease

Different pathogens lead to different kinds of infectious disease. But many of these diseases develop in a similar way. They occur in five stages. Here's an explanation of each stage.

Stage One: Incubation Stage. After a person is exposed to a pathogen, some time passes before any symptoms appear. During this incubation stage, the pathogen grows and establishes itself in the body. For some diseases, the incubation stage lasts only a day or two before the first symptoms appear. For other diseases, it may take years before the person notices any symptoms.

Stage Two: Prodromal Stage. At the prodromal stage, the person may have only a general feeling of illness or fatigue. These general symptoms may suggest that an infectious disease might be developing.

Stage Three: Acute Stage. In the acute stage, specific symptoms become obvious. The infectious disease reaches its most severe point. The body's inflammatory process is at work. Medical treatments may be given to reduce pain or discomfort. Other treatments, such as **antibiotics,** may be prescribed to promote healing. Antibiotics fight infections caused by bacteria and other microorganisms.

Uh-oh! If patients stop taking medication too soon, microbes may become resistant to antibiotics. Explain to patients how to use antibiotics properly.

Stage Four: Declining Stage. During the declining stage, symptoms start to fade. However, the disease is still present. Because patients are feeling better, they sometimes stop taking their medications at this stage. They should be educated not to do this.

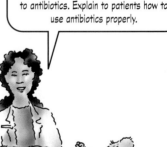

Stage Five: Convalescent Stage. At last, the disease is defeated! During the convalescent stage, the patient is recovering. The patient's body is working to return to its previous state of good health.

How Bugs Spread

Some patients in a medical office might be in one of the stages of infectious disease. This can expose you, other staff, and other patients to potential pathogens. By understanding their **vehicles,** or modes of transmission, you can break this link in the infection chain and prevent disease from spreading.

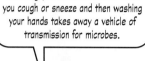

Covering your nose and mouth when you cough or sneeze and then washing your hands takes away a vehicle of transmission for microbes.

DIRECT TRANSMISSION

Direct transmission occurs when there is direct contact between the reservoir host and the susceptible host. Examples include:

- shaking hands
- touching the blood or body fluids of the reservoir host
- inhaling infected air droplets of the reservoir host
- intimate contact such as kissing or sexual intercourse

INDIRECT TRANSMISSION

Not all pathogens are spread through direct contact with an infected person. **Indirect transmission** occurs through a vector. A **vector** is an object that contains pathogens. Examples of indirect transmission include:

- eating food that is **contaminated** (Something that is contaminated has been touched by a source of pathogens.)
- drinking from an infected person's glass
- getting bitten by a disease-carrying insect
- using an improperly disinfected medical instrument
- touching a contaminated surface, such as a doorknob

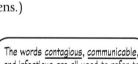

The words contagious, communicable, and infectious are all used to refer to diseases that can be transmitted from one person to another.

Sources of indirect transmission often aren't easy to see. Many microbes can stay **viable,** or alive, for long periods of time outside the human body. For example, a surface that once was in contact with saliva, blood, or pus from an infected wound can be full of pathogens even if it doesn't look contaminated.

WHO TRANSMITS PATHOGENS?

Most reservoir hosts are humans, animals, or insects.

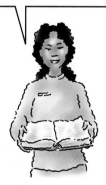

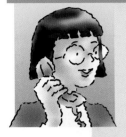

Ask the Professional — PATHOGENS IN THE WAITING ROOM

Q: *It's "flu season" again and some patients coming into the office show the symptoms of contagious respiratory illnesses. What can I do to protect the other patients and make the reception area a healthier place?*

A: You must manage the waiting room to protect patients who are waiting to be seen. When a patient arrives who shows signs of an upper respiratory infection, move him to an exam room as soon as one becomes available.

Make sure the reception area has tissues and trash cans for disposal of used tissues—and show the patient where to find them. Be sure to wash your own hands thoroughly after contact with the patient.

Human Hosts

The most common source of pathogens that cause infectious disease in humans is humans themselves. Human hosts are typically:

- people who are obviously ill with an infectious disease
- people who show no symptoms but are incubating an infectious disease
- people who are carriers of an infectious disease

Animals

Many people worry about animals spreading disease. In fact, animals aren't a common vehicle for diseases that affect humans. However, those that can be a source of pathogens include:

- dogs
- cats
- birds
- cattle
- rodents
- animals that live in the wild

Rabies and avian flu are examples of diseases that can be transmitted to humans by infected animals. Avian flu, or bird flu, is caused by a virus that birds can pass to one another. The virus usually doesn't affect humans, but when it does it can be deadly.

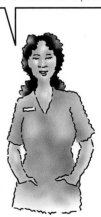

For every patient with a known infectious disease, there are probably five unknown carriers. You must practice infection control with all patients.

Insects

Insects are another source of disease. Flies and cockroaches carry many kinds of pathogens. Some insects feed on the blood of the reservoir host. When they bite another person, they can pass on the pathogens. For instance, ticks can cause Lyme disease, a bacterial disease that can affect the skin, joints, and nervous system. Some mosquitoes carry the West Nile virus, which can lead to swelling in the brain and spinal cord.

Common Infectious Diseases and How They Spread

Disease	How It Spreads
AIDS	direct contact or contact with contaminated needles
Chicken pox	direct contact or droplets
Hepatitis B	direct contact with infectious body fluid
Influenza	droplets in the air; direct contact with infected carriers or with contaminated articles such as used tissues
Measles	infected droplets in the air; direct contact with infected carrier
Mononucleosis	infected droplets in the air or contact with saliva
Pneumonia	infected droplets in the air or direct contact with infected mucus
Rabies	direct contact with saliva of infected animal, such as through an animal bite

Controlling Infections

An important part of your job as a medical assistant will be to help control and prevent infections in the medical office. One of the best ways to do this is to follow guidelines set by the Occupational Safety and Health Administration (OSHA) and the Centers for Disease Control (CDC).

MEDICAL ASEPSIS

Medical asepsis is a set of practices to keep an object or area free from microbes. These practices are sometimes called *clean techniques* because they prevent the spread of microorganisms within the medical office.

Clean Hands

Hand washing is the most important medical aseptic practice. You must follow a special technique, which is outlined for you in the Hands On procedure on page 32. Always wash your hands in these situations:

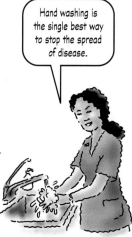

Hand washing is the single best way to stop the spread of disease.

- before and after patient contact
- after contact with any blood or body fluids

- after contact with contaminated material
- after handling specimens
- after coughing, sneezing, or blowing your nose
- after using the restroom
- before and after going to lunch and taking breaks
- before leaving for the day

Wear gloves when handling specimens or if you think you might come into contact with contaminated material. (You should always assume blood and body fluids are contaminated.) But even then, remember to wash your hands! To stop disease from spreading, you need to wash your hands before putting gloves on and after taking them off. The Hands On procedure on page 35 gives you step-by-step guidance on the proper way to remove contaminated gloves.

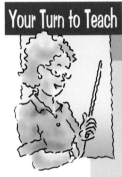

Your Turn to Teach   STOPPING THE SPREAD OF DISEASE AT HOME

As you work with patients, take time to teach them basic aseptic practices they can use at home.

- *Hand washing.* Remind patients that they can stop the spread of disease by washing their hands. Patients should wash their hands before and after meals; after sneezing, coughing, or blowing the nose; after using the bathroom; before and after changing a dressing; and after changing diapers.

- *Using tissues.* Encourage patients with respiratory symptoms (coughing and sneezing) to use tissues to cover their mouths and noses so they don't spread their illness through the air. Remind them to throw out used tissues right away and then wash their hands. Tissues are thin and it's easy for body fluids to soak through to a person's hands.

- *Changing bandages.* Explain procedures to patients and family members who will need to change bandages. Take care to demonstrate how to apply sterile dressings and clean bandages. To check their understanding, ask the patients or family members to repeat what you showed them.

- *Staying sanitary.* Talk to patients about how to dispose of waste from household members who have infectious diseases.

Clean Workplace

Medical asepsis also involves keeping the office clean. Areas to clean include examination and treatment rooms, waiting and reception areas, and clinical work areas.

- Take care to keep soiled linen, table paper, supplies, or instruments from touching your clothing. Always roll used table paper or linens inward so the unused side is facing out.
- Always think of the floor as contaminated! Anything dropped on the floor is no longer clean. It must be thrown away or cleaned to its former level of asepsis before being used.
- Clean tables, counters, and other surfaces often. If they become contaminated, they must be cleaned immediately. Microbes are less likely to live and grow on clean surfaces.
- Assume that body fluids and blood from any source are contaminated. Follow guidelines from OSHA and the CDC to stop the spread of disease. Protect yourself and your patients!

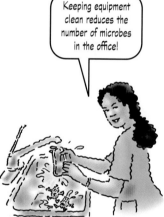

Keeping equipment clean reduces the number of microbes in the office!

LEVELS OF INFECTION CONTROL

Medical instruments, equipment, and supplies need to be kept clean to prevent the transmission of disease. There are different levels of infection control for the various kinds of tools—sterilization, **disinfection,** and **sanitization.** Each level has a different result and procedures.

Levels of Infection Control

Level of Control	Type of Control	Effect	Procedures
Low	Sanitization	removes contaminants	cleaning with soaps and detergents
Medium	Disinfection	destroys many pathogens	using different chemical solutions
High	Sterilization	destroys all microbes and spores	several different methods

Sanitization

The lowest level of infection control is sanitization—cleaning items using soap or detergent. Your goal is to reduce the number of microbes on objects or surfaces. Clean objects and surfaces thoroughly by rubbing and scrubbing using warm, soapy water. Any contaminants you can see should be removed. Sanitization must be done before disinfection or sterilization.

Disinfection

Disinfection offers an intermediate level of infection control. Using germicides or disinfectants, you can destroy many pathogens and other microbes. Disinfection doesn't destroy all microorganism or bacterial spores. But high levels of disinfection are almost as effective as sterilization.

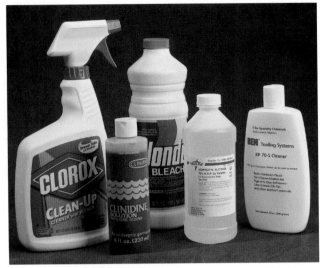

When used properly, bleach and other disinfectants can destroy many pathogens.

Types of Disinfectants. There are several procedures and many products for disinfecting. They provide three levels of infection control.

Improving Disinfection. Some disinfection methods work better than others. Here are some factors to consider:

- *Prior cleaning.* Disinfection is more effective if items are sanitized first.
- *Type of microorganism.* Some microbes are more resistant to certain methods and disinfectants than others.

Levels of Disinfection and Procedures

Level	Procedures	When to Use	Effect
Low	commercial products without tuberculocidal properties	routine cleaning; to clean objects or surfaces with no visible blood or body fluids	destroys many bacteria and some viruses; does NOT destroy *M. tuberculosis* or bacterial spores
Intermediate	commercial germicides that kill *M. tuberculosis*; solutions containing 1:10 dilution of household bleach (2 oz. of chlorine bleach per quart of tap water)	to clean instruments that have touched unbroken skin, such as blood pressure cuffs, stethoscopes, and splints	destroys many viruses, fungi, and some bacteria, including *M. tuberculosis*; does NOT destroy bacterial spores
High	immersion in approved disinfecting chemical for 45 minutes or according to guidelines on label; immersion in boiling water for 30 minutes (rarely used)	to clean reusable instruments that contact body cavities with mucous membranes, such as the vagina and rectum, that are not considered sterile	destroys most microorganisms except certain bacterial spores

- *Strength of the disinfecting solution.* Concentrated germicides are most effective. Disinfectants that are diluted with water may not kill as many pathogens.
- *Length of exposure.* Leave the object in germicide or disinfectant for the length of time recommended by the manufacturer.
- *Complexity of the object.* Objects with corners, edges, or rough spots may be more difficult to disinfect.
- *Temperature.* Many disinfectants work best at room temperature.

Sterilization

Sterilization offers the highest level of infection control. It destroys all forms of microorganisms, including bacterial spores. The four basic methods of sterilization are:

Disposable sterile supplies are for one-time use only.

- high pressure/ steam heat from an autoclave
- sterilization gases, such as ethylene oxide
- dry heat ovens
- immersion in approved chemical solutions

WHAT NEEDS TO BE STERILIZED?

Many of the instruments used in a medical office need to be sterilized. These types of equipment must be sterilized:

- instruments that break the skin
- instruments that contact areas of the body considered sterile, such as the bladder
- instruments that contact surgical incisions
- any instrument that becomes contaminated or soiled during a procedure

Some equipment comes in sterile, ready-to-use packages. Many medical offices use disposable sterile supplies. These supplies are used once and discarded immediately after use.

Guidelines for the Medical Office

The Occupational Safety and Health Administration is responsible for ensuring the safety of all workers. This federal agency makes and enforces safety rules for medical offices.

By law, a medical office must establish practices to keep employees healthy and safe. These practices must be written into a policy or procedure manual, or put in a separate infection control manual. They should be kept in a place where employees and OSHA inspectors can find them easily.

INSIDE AN INFECTION CONTROL MANUAL

The medical office must provide clear instructions to protect you from exposure to disease and **biohazardous** materials. Biohazardous means that the materials are capable of causing disease or infection. Biohazardous materials may be contaminated with pathogens. They present a risk to your health and the health of patients. It's important that the medical office where you work has written instructions for dealing with biohazards. Here are two key things the instructions should contain:

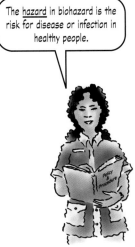

The <u>hazard</u> in biohazard is the risk for disease or infection in healthy people.

- *Exposure risk factor.* Written policy must include an **exposure risk factor** for each job description. This measures each employee's risk of being exposed to a communicable disease.

- *Exposure control plan.* Every medical office with more than 10 employees also must have a written **exposure control plan.** It explains what to do if employees or visitors are exposed to biohazardous material in spite of precautions.

WHAT'S YOUR RISK?

Not all medical assistants will have the same exposure risk factor. Administrative medical assistants have a low exposure risk, for instance. They require only minimal protection on the job. Clinical medical assistants have greater exposure to pathogens and therefore have a higher risk. They must have access to **personal protective equipment (PPE),** such as gloves, gowns, goggles, and/or face shields. The medical office also must provide immunization against hepatitis B at no charge.

Running Smoothly   EXPOSURE TO BIOHAZARDS

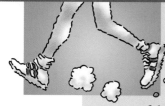

What should you do if you're exposed to a biohazard?

You're always careful, but one day your glove tears and a patient's blood gets on you. Now you must manage your exposure to this biohazard. Keep these safety procedures in mind.

- If the blood gets in your mucous membranes (eyes, nose, or mouth), you need to flush the area right away with water or saline.

- If you're stuck by a needle, you must let the site bleed. Then, clean the site with soap and water.

- Next, you must report the exposure to your employer right away. Your employer will need to follow OSHA guidelines to treat the exposure.

- You will need to be evaluated to determine if you may have come in contact hepatitis B, hepatitis C, or HIV.

- Your office must check the patient's medical records to check if they are infected with hepatitis B, hepatitis C, or HIV. If this information is not known, the patient should be asked to give consent to be tested. If the patient is infected with any of these bloodborne pathogens, you must be treated following OSHA standards to prevent illness.

- If the injury was caused by a needle, your employer must keep track of this in a sharps injury log.

THE EXPOSURE CONTROL PLAN

It's important to follow the guidelines in the exposure control plan for your medical office. If you think you or a patient has been exposed to a biohazard, apply first aid principles right away. Then, tell your supervisor, office manager, or office physician. Some kinds of exposures might require postexposure testing or procedures.

After exposure, you'll need to complete a report called an incident report or exposure report. In the report, you'll describe how the exposure occurred. The report can help your medical office change its policies to prevent this kind of exposure in the future. Your employer also must record the exposure on an OSHA log form.

> Take your personal protective equipment very seriously. It's your best protection against exposure to biohazardous materials.

OSHA's Form 300 (Rev. 01/2004)

Log of Work-Related Injuries and Illnesses

Attention: This form contains information relating to employee health and must be used in a manner that protects the confidentiality of employees to the extent possible while the information is being used for occupational safety and health purposes.

Year _____

U.S. Department of Labor
Occupational Safety and Health Administration

Form approved OMB no. 1218-0176

You must record information about every work-related injury or illness that involves loss of consciousness, restricted work activity or job transfer, days away from work, or medical treatment beyond first aid. You must also record significant work-related injuries and illnesses that are diagnosed by a physician or licensed health care professional. You must also record work-related injuries and illnesses that meet any of the specific recording criteria listed in 29 CFR 1904.8 through 1904.12. Feel free to use two lines for a single case if you need to. You must complete an injury and illness incident report (OSHA Form 301) or equivalent form for each injury or illness recorded on this form. If you're not sure whether a case is recordable, call your local OSHA office for help.

Establishment name _____

City _____ State _____

Identify the person				Describe the case		Classify the case										

Identify the person

(A) Case No.	(B) Employee's Name	(C) Job Title (e.g., Welder)	(D) Date of injury or onset of illness (mo./day)	(E) Where the event occurred (e.g. Loading dock north end)	(F) Describe injury or illness, parts of body affected, and object/substance that directly injured or made person ill (e.g. Second degree burns on right forearm from acetylene torch)

Classify the case

CHECK ONLY ONE box for each case based on the most serious outcome for that case:

Death (G)	Days away from work (H)	Remained at work		Enter the number of days the injured or ill worker was:		Check the "injury" column or choose one type of illness:					
		Job transfer or restriction (I)	Other recordable cases (J)	Away From Work (days) (K)	On job transfer or restriction (days) (L)	Injury (M)(1)	Skin Disorder (2)	Respiratory Condition (3)	Poisoning (4)	Hearing Loss (5)	All other illnesses (6)

Page totals | 0 | 0 | 0 | 0 | 0 | 0 | 0 | 0 | 0 | 0 | 0 | 0 |

Be sure to transfer these totals to the Summary page (Form 300A) before you post it.

	Injury (1)	Skin Disorder (2)	Respiratory Condition (3)	Poisoning (4)	Hearing Loss (5)	All other illnesses (6)

Public reporting burden for this collection of information is estimated to average 14 minutes per response, including time to review the instruction, search and gather the data needed, and complete and review the collection of information. Persons are not required to respond to the collection of information unless it displays a currently valid OMB control number. If you have any comments about these estimates or any aspects of this data collection, contact: US Department of Labor, OSHA Office of Statistics, Room N-3644, 200 Constitution Ave, NW, Washington, DC 20210. Do not send the completed forms to this office.

Page 1 of 1

REPORTING TO OSHA

If one or more of the following criteria are met, exposures to biohazardous material must be reported to OSHA. Your employer normally takes care of this task. Here's when an OSHA report must be made:

- The exposure was work-related and required medical treatment beyond first aid (such as medication or vaccination).

- The employee lost consciousness or had to be medically removed.

- The employee lost days at work or needed to transfer to another job.

- An accident involved an injury from a needle or a sharp object that was contaminated with another person's blood or another possibly infectious material.

- The exposure involved a known case of tuberculosis (TB) and resulted in a positive skin test for TB or a diagnosis of TB by a physician.

- A negative blood test for a contagious disease changed to a positive test after the exposure.

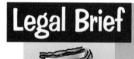

Legal Brief

STANDARD TRAINING ABOUT BLOOD-BORNE PATHOGENS

OSHA requires that newly hired medical office employees who will be exposed to blood have special training. The training must be repeated every year. It will include any new policies recommended by OSHA, the CDC, the Department of Health and Human Services, or the U.S. Public Health Service. The training should include these key points:

- descriptions of bloodborne diseases, how they are transmitted, and related symptoms

- the kinds of personal protective equipment available and its location in the medical office

- information about the risks of contracting hepatitis B and about the HBV vaccine

- the exposure control plan and postexposure procedures, along with follow-up care if an exposure occurs

PRACTICING STANDARD PRECAUTIONS

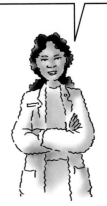

For safety reasons, remember to always treat blood and all other body fluids as contaminated.

Standard precautions are a set of procedures recognized by the CDC. The goal of the procedures is to reduce the transmission of microorganisms in any heath care setting, including medical offices.

You need to use standard precautions whenever you will be touching blood, body fluids, damaged skin, or mucous membranes. Here's a list of some important procedures.

- Wash your hands with soap and water after touching blood, body fluids, secretions, or other contaminated objects—whether you have worn gloves or not!

- You can use alcohol-based hand rub to decontaminate your hands if your hands are not visibly dirty or contaminated.

- Wear clean, nonsterile examination gloves if you think you might come into contact with blood, body fluids, secretions, mucous membranes, damaged skin, or contaminated objects.

- If you've touched infective material, change your gloves between procedures, even if the procedures involve the same patient.

- Wear equipment to protect your eyes, nose, and mouth. Keep your clothing clean by wearing a disposable gown, especially for procedures that might splash or spray blood, body fluids, or secretions.

- Dispose of single-use items appropriately. Don't disinfect them, sterilize them, or reuse them.

- Take care to avoid injuries before, after, and during procedures that involve scalpels, needles, or other sharp instruments.

- Don't recap used needles or bend or break them. When giving injections, make sure you have a sharps container within reach to throw away used needles.

- Place used disposable syringes, needles, and other sharps in the closest puncture-resistant container (sharps container).

- Use barrier devices such as mouthpieces or resuscitation bags as alternatives to mouth-to-mouth resuscitation.

PERSONAL PROTECTIVE EQUIPMENT

What kinds of personal protective equipment (PPE) are available to you? If you might be exposed to biohazardous materials in your work, you must have access to:

- disposable gowns, goggles, and face shields
- gloves—either latex or vinyl

You need to wear gowns, goggles, and face shields in any areas where splashing or splattering of airborne particles may occur. You must wear gloves whenever you perform a procedure that involves a risk of exposure to blood or body fluids. For example, you must wear gloves to:

- draw blood specimens
- dispose of biohazardous waste
- touch contaminated surfaces
- handle contaminated equipment
- give injections

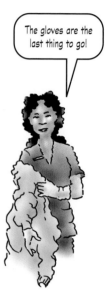

The gloves are the last thing to go!

Gloves should fit comfortably. Be sure to choose the right size for your hands. They should not be too loose or too tight. If you or patients are sensitive to the latex in regular examination gloves, an alternative must be made available.

Take care not to carry contaminants! After a procedure, remove face shields, gowns, and other protective barriers *before* you take off your gloves. Once you have removed the personal protective equipment, including your gloves, always wash your hands.

BIOHAZARD AND SAFETY EQUIPMENT IN THE MEDICAL OFFICE

The medical office where you work must offer the following protections from biohazardous and other dangerous materials.

- *MSDS binder.* Material safety data sheets (MSDS) are forms prepared by the manufacturers of all chemical substances used in a medical office. The binder in your office should contain sheets for all chemicals used in your workplace. Each sheet tells how to handle and dispose of the chemical and lists any protective gear you'll need. It also gives you information about the health hazards and other possible dangers of the chemical, the safety precautions you need to take when using it, and how to fight any fires involving it. These sheets also outline first aid in the event that you do have harmful exposure to the chemical.

- *Biohazard waste containers.* These are special containers used only for waste contaminated with blood, body fluids, or other potentially infectious material (OPIM). Sharps containers are one type of biohazard waste container. They are used to dispose of items that puncture or cut the skin.

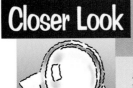

Closer Look

LATEX ALLERGY AND THE MEDICAL ASSISTANT

Many health care workers develop allergic reactions to latex. Latex is a product of the rubber tree. Proteins in latex can cause allergic reactions. Unfortunately, many products, including examination gloves, are made of latex.

Reactions to latex can range from mild to severe. Symptoms of a mild allergy are skin redness, rash, itching, or hives. A severe allergy can result in difficulty breathing, wheezing, or coughing.

You're most likely to see respiratory responses after gloves are removed. Powder inside the gloves goes into the air. It enters the respiratory system when you breathe. Protect yourself from latex allergy by following these guidelines.

- Use gloves that are not latex for tasks that don't involve contact or possible contact with blood or body fluids.

- Wear powder-free latex gloves if there's a chance you may contact blood or body fluids.

- Find out about other latex-free equipment, including blood pressure cuffs for taking a patient's blood pressure.

- Avoid using oil-based lotions or hand creams before putting on latex gloves. Oils can break down the latex and release the proteins that cause allergic reactions.

- Wash your hands thoroughly after removing latex gloves.

- Know the symptoms of latex allergy so you can recognize them in yourself, your coworkers, or patients.

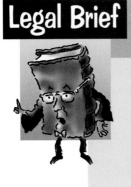

Legal Brief

WHO'S RESPONSIBLE FOR PERSONAL PROTECTIVE EQUIPMENT?

According to OSHA regulations, employers must make personal protective equipment available to their employees. If they do not, they can face significant fines.

Employees are responsible for using the personal protective equipment correctly and in the appropriate situations. Employees are also responsible for frequent hand washing.

- *Personal protective equipment.* Gloves and other PPE must be available for use in areas where there is a risk of exposure to blood or body fluids.

- *Eyewash station.* The eyewash basin can remove contaminants or chemicals that accidentally get in your eyes. For chemical exposure, the eyes should be washed for the amount of time recommended on the MSDS, or for at least 15 minutes. OSHA requires every laboratory to contain an eyewash station.

- *Immunization.* Employers are required by OSHA to provide immunization against bloodborne pathogens, such as hepatitis B, if vaccines are available. If the employee does not want the immunization, she must sign a waiver.

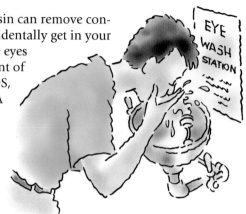

Pressing a lever starts a stream of water that forces open the caps of the eyewash station. Lower your face to the water stream to clean your eyes. You need to keep your face in the water stream until your eyes are clear of contaminants.

Handling Contamination in and Around the Office

Some of your duties as a medical assistant may involve keeping equipment and surfaces in the office clean. You'll need to follow proper procedures. To sanitize, clean off any soil you can see on surfaces and equipment using detergent or low-level disinfectant. Floors, examination tables, countertops, and cabinets all need to be cleaned routinely. They also must be cleaned when they've become soiled with blood or body fluids.

The Hands On procedures on pages 38 and 39 provide step-by-step guidelines for cleaning biohazardous contamination in examination or treatment rooms.

BIOHAZARD CLEANUP

Surfaces contaminated with biohazardous materials must be cleaned right away. You need to use an approved germicide or a diluted bleach solution to destroy microorganisms.

Some offices purchase commercial spill kits. These kits include all the materials you need to clean contaminated surfaces. Some kits may contain different materials depending on

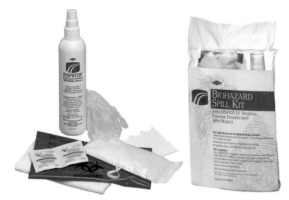

Most commercially prepared biohazard spill kits contain gloves, absorbent material, eye protection, and a biohazard bag for proper disposal.

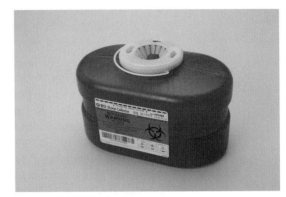

All sharps should be disposed of properly by placing them in a plastic puncture-resistant sharps container like the one shown here. Note the biohazard symbol on the sharps container.

the manufacturer. If your office doesn't purchase kits, you must gather the materials from the office yourself. It's a good idea to store them together in case a biohazardous spill occurs—you'll be ready for action! Here's what you'll need:

- clean examination gloves (both latex and vinyl should be available)
- gowns
- eye protection, such as goggles
- face shields and masks
- absorbent crystals, gel, or powder (such as sodium bicarbonate)
- a disposable scoop
- paper towels
- at least one biohazard waste bag (usually known as "red bags" in the office)
- a chemical disinfectant
- a sharps container or spill control barriers

If there's a large amount of contamination on the floor, you'll need disposable shoe covers. You don't want to spread microbes through the office on your shoes!

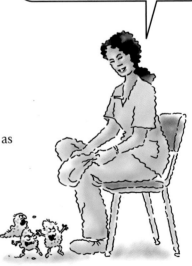

WHICH WASTE CONTAINER?

In the medical office, there are separate containers for disposing of different kinds of waste. You need to make sure you put waste in the right place.

Legal Brief   BIOHAZARD SPILL SUPPLIES

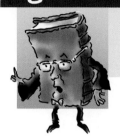

OSHA requires that spill kits or appropriate supplies for cleaning biohazardous waste be available in the medical office. Make sure you know where they're kept.

Regular Waste Container

The regular waste container is used only for waste that is not contaminated. Some examples include:

- paper
- plastic
- disposable tray wrappers
- packaging material

Liquids should be discarded in a sink or other washbasin, not in the plastic bag inside the regular waste container. This will keep you from having to clean up leaks and mess from the waste container.

When the plastic bag in the container is about two-thirds full, it should be removed from the waste can. Bring the top edges of the bag together and tie them, or use a twist tie. Follow your office policy and procedure for where to dispose of regular waste. Remember to put a fresh bag in the waste can!

Sharps Waste Container

The sharps waste container is used only for sharp objects that may puncture or injure someone. These include needles, microscope slides, used ampules, and razors. NEVER put any sharps in plastic bags. They need to go in an approved, puncture-resistant container for safety reasons.

Biohazard Waste Container

The biohazard waste container is used ONLY for waste contaminated with blood or body fluids. Some examples include:

- soiled dressings and bandages
- soiled examination gloves
- soiled examination table paper
- cotton balls and applicators that have been used on the body

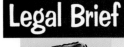

Legal Brief   DISPOSING OF INFECTIOUS WASTE

The Environmental Protection Agency (EPA) and OSHA set regulations and guidelines for disposing of hazardous materials. Individual states use these guidelines to determine their own policies.

Policies for disposing of infectious waste may be different in different states. You need to check your state and local regulations before making decisions about biohazardous waste.

YOUR MEDICAL OFFICE AND BIOHAZARD WASTE

Many medical offices are considered small generators of waste. This means they produce less than 50 pounds of waste each month. Hospitals and larger clinics that produce more than 50 pounds of waste each month are considered large generators. They must obtain a certificate of registration from the EPA. They also need to keep records of the quantity of waste and their disposal procedures.

Many facilities that are large generators use biohazard waste services. This ensures that they comply with state and federal laws and that biohazardous waste will be disposed of appropriately and safely.

Biohazard waste disposal services supply offices with appropriate waste containers. They pick up filled containers regularly. After they pick up filled containers, they dispose of waste according to EPA and OSHA guidelines.

The service keeps a tracking record. The record lists the type of waste, its weight in pounds, and its disposal destination. After the waste has been destroyed, the tracking record is sent to the medical office.

The tracking record must be kept in the office records for three years. It must be given to the EPA if an audit is performed to check whether the medical office is following regulations. States may have stiff penalties for violating disposal regulations, including fines and/or imprisonment.

Biohazard waste services determine their fees based on the type and amount of waste that is generated. Because of this, it's important to dispose of only biohazardous waste in these containers. You don't want your office to be charged for the removal of everyday trash. Follow the Hands On procedure on page 40 for disposing of hazardous waste.

Concerns About Hepatitis B and HIV

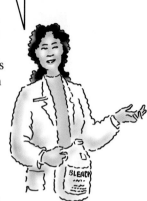

Luckily, HBV can be contained by proper use of standard precautions. It can be killed easily by cleaning with a diluted bleach solution.

As a medical assistant, you may worry about transmission of the hepatitis B virus (HBV) and the human immunodeficiency virus (HIV). You may already be familiar with public concerns about HIV. HBV also has been a hazard for health care professionals for many years.

There are good reasons to be concerned about HBV. It's more viable than HIV. HBV can survive in a dried state on counter surfaces and clinical equipment at room temperature for more than a week. That means there's a chance it can be spread through the medical office by direct contact, such as through contaminated hands or gloves.

PREVENTING EXPOSURE

HIV and HBV are both transmitted through exposure to blood and body fluids. If you have direct contact with surfaces that are contaminated, there is a possibility the virus can enter your body.

The virus can enter the body through accidental punctures with sharp objects contaminated with blood, such as used needles. It also might be able to enter through broken skin. Broken skin can result from a cut or wound. Several skin disorders also involve breaks in the skin:

- dry, cracked skin
- dermatitis
- eczema
- psoriasis

If you have one of these skin disorders, you need to be sure you wear PPE, especially if you think you might come into contact with blood or body fluids.

There's no vaccine to prevent infection by HIV, but you can protect yourself from HBV with the HBV vaccine. The HBV vaccine is given in a series of three injections. These injections normally produce immunity to the disease.

To test for immunity, it's recommended that you have a blood sample taken and tested six months after the last injection. The blood test checks for the presence, or titer, of antibodies against hepatitis B. If the test finds that you're not immune, the vaccine series can be repeated. Immunity to HBV can last as long as 15 years; however, this is a topic that is still being researched and debated in the medical world.

Legal Brief — YOUR RIGHT TO PROTECTION

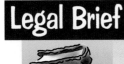

If your duties at work place you at risk for exposure to HBV, OSHA recommends that you be vaccinated to prevent infection. Your employer is required by law to provide the vaccine at no cost. Clinical medical assistants are at risk for HBV exposure and can receive the HBV vaccine.

If you choose not to receive the HBV vaccine, you must sign a waiver or release form. This form states that you are aware of the risks related to HBV. Individuals who contract hepatitis B may develop cirrhosis (damaged liver cells). They also may have a greater risk of developing liver cancer.

IF YOU'VE BEEN EXPOSED

If you've been exposed to blood or body fluids infected with HIV or HBV, the postexposure plan provides guidelines for what to do. The plan should include immediate blood testing. Your blood needs to be tested again at specific intervals, usually six weeks, three months, six months, nine months, and one year.

If you've already been immunized against HBV, further treatment is not normally needed. But if you haven't been immunized against HBV, you can receive hepatitis B immunoglobulin by injection to begin protecting your body right away. The series of immunizations for the HBV vaccine can be started to offer longer term protection.

Hands On — HAND WASHING FOR MEDICAL ASEPSIS   1-1

The hand-washing procedure should take two to three minutes.

1. Take off your rings and your wristwatch. It's not a good idea to wear rings when working with material that could be infectious. Rings can give microbes places to hide.
2. Stand close to the sink, but avoid touching it. The sink is considered contaminated. If you stand too close, you might contaminate your clothing.

Hands On

HAND WASHING FOR MEDICAL ASEPSIS (*continued*)

1-1

3. Using a paper towel, turn on the faucet. Adjust the temperature and then dispose of the paper towel. Warm water is best. Water that's too hot or too cold can crack or chap the skin on your hands and break one of your natural body barriers against pathogens.

4. Wet your hands and wrists under warm running water. Use a clean towel to push the soap dispenser. Then, apply soap and lather up! Rub your palms together and rub the soap between your fingers at least 10 times. The rubbing action will loosen microorganisms from between your fingers. You're removing transient flora and some resident flora, too.

5. Scrub the palm of one hand with the fingertips of the other using a circular motion. Then, switch hands to scrub the other palm. Friction helps remove microorganisms. You'll also need to scrub your wrists.

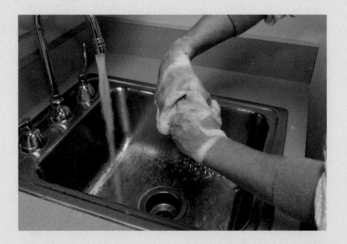

6. Rinse hands and wrists well under running warm water. Hold your hands below your elbows and wrists—that way microbes can flow from your hands and fingers, rather than back up your arms. Take care not to touch the inside of the sink—remember, it's considered contaminated.

(*continued*)

Hands On

HAND WASHING FOR MEDICAL ASEPSIS (*continued*)

1-1

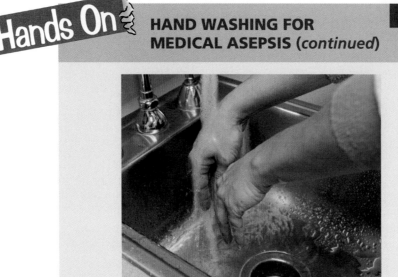

7. Next come the nails! Microbes can hide under your nails, too. Use an orangewood stick or nail brush to clean under each nail. Metal files or pointed tools might break the skin, creating an opening for microbes. You can clean your nails at the beginning of the day, before leaving for the day, or after touching potentially infectious material.

8. Use a clean paper towel to push the soap dispenser again. Use more liquid soap and warm, running water to wash your hands and wrists again. You need to wash away any microbes that might have been removed with the orange-wood stick.

9. Rinse your hands thoroughly again. Be sure to hold your hands lower than your elbows.

10. Dry your hands gently with a paper towel. They need to be completely dry to prevent your skin from drying and crack-ing. Discard the paper towel and used orangewood stick when you're finished.

11. Use a dry paper towel to turn off the faucets. Your clean hands shouldn't touch the faucet handles—they are also considered contaminated. Discard the paper towel.

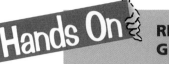 **REMOVING CONTAMINATED GLOVES**

1. To remove gloves, grasp the glove of your nondominant hand at the palm. (If you are right-handed, grasp the glove on your left hand.) Avoid grasping the glove at the wrist—you might transfer contaminants from your glove to your wrist. Make sure hands are pointed down and away from the body, preferably right over the biohazard container.

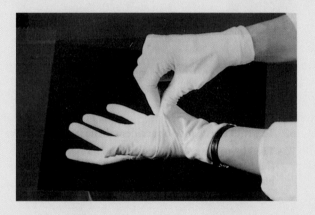

2. Tug the glove toward the fingertips of your nondominant hand.

3. Slide your nondominant hand out of the glove by rolling the glove against the palm of your dominant hand. You must be careful not to touch either glove with your bare hand.

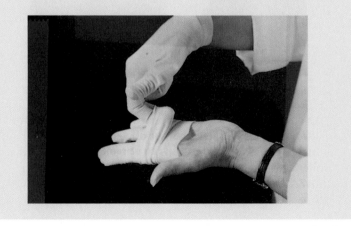

(continued)

Hands On   **REMOVING CONTAMINATED GLOVES** (*continued*)   **1-2**

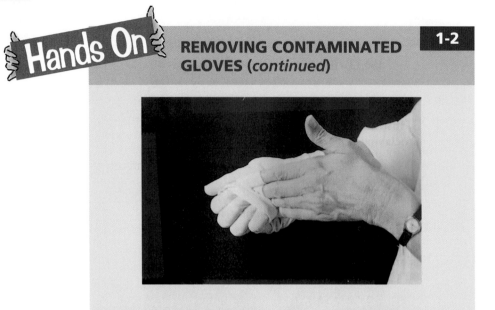

4. Keep holding the soiled glove in the palm of your dominant hand. Slip your bare fingers under the cuff of the glove you are still wearing. Be careful not to touch the outside of the glove! Skin can touch skin, but never the soiled part of the glove.

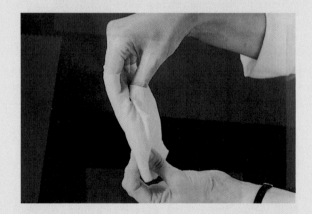

5. Stretch the glove of the dominant hand up and away from your hand. At the same time, turn the glove inside out. The glove you removed first should be balled up inside. All the soiled surfaces of the gloves should be inside. The first glove should be inside the second glove, and the second glove should be inside out.

Hands On

REMOVING CONTAMINATED GLOVES (continued)

1-2

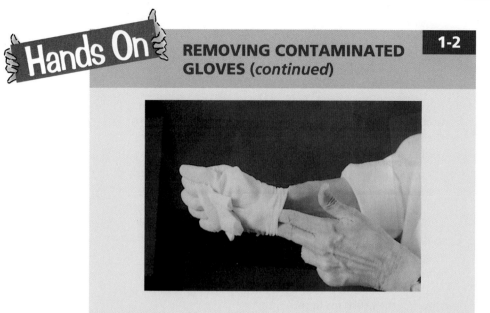

6. Discard the gloves as they are (without taking them apart) in a biohazard waste bin or bag.

7. Wash your hands. Wearing gloves doesn't replace the need for good hand washing.

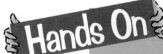

CLEANING EXAMINATION TABLES

1-3

1. Put on clean gloves. If there's a possibility of contact with used dressings, body fluids, or other contaminated items on the table, further protect yourself with a gown or apron, protective eyewear, and shoe coverings.

2. Even though you're wearing gloves, try to handle the soiled table paper or linen as little as possible. Fold it carefully so the most soiled surface is turned inward. This will help stop contaminants from getting into the air or touching your clothes.

3. Dispose of soiled table paper in a biohazard waste bag. If your office uses cloth linens, place them in a biohazard laundry bag in the examination room. Do not carry unbagged dirty linen through the office for laundering.

4. Spray the table with a commercial germicide or diluted bleach solution. Then, wipe with disposable paper towels. Discard the towels in the biohazard waste bag. Remove gloves and wash hands.

5. Apply new examination table paper or linens.

6. Dirty linens may be sent to an outside company for laundering. If they are laundered at the office, use normal laundry cycles and follow office policy and procedure. Follow the manufacturers' recommendations for the washer, detergent, and fabric.

Hands On

CLEANING BIOHAZARDOUS SPILLS

1-4

1. Put on your gloves first. If you think there will be any splashing, protect yourself! A gown or an apron will protect your clothing from contaminants. Wear protective eyewear and shoe coverings.

2. Follow your office policy for cleaning up spills. Use chemical gels, crystals, or powders to absorb the spill. Clean up the spill with disposable paper towels or a scoop. Be careful not to splash.

3. Dispose of paper towels and absorbent material in a biohazard waste bag. The bag will alert anyone handling the waste that it contains biohazardous material.

4. Spray the area with a commercial germicide or diluted bleach solution. Then, wipe with disposable paper towels. Be sure to discard towels in the biohazard waste bag.

5. Keeping your gloves ON, remove any protective eyewear. Discard the eyewear or disinfect it, depending on the policy in your office. Take off the gown or apron and shoe coverings. If they are disposable, put them in the biohazard waste bag. If they are reusable, put them in the biohazard laundry bag.

6. Place the biohazard waste bag in the biohazard waste bin for your office.

7. Take off your gloves and wash your hands thoroughly.

Hands On

GUIDELINES FOR WASTE DISPOSAL

1-5

1. Use separate containers for each type of waste. Sharps containers are only for sharps. Paper towels used for routine hand washing don't go in a biohazard waste bag.

2. Use only approved biohazard waste containers.

3. Fill sharps containers two-thirds full before disposing of them. Look for a fill line on the container to show you how much goes in.

4. If you need to move a filled biohazard waste container, make sure the bag is secure. A closure should be provided with the container.

5. Take extra care when the biohazard waste container is contaminated on the outside and wear gloves! Put the container inside another approved biohazard waste container. And be sure to wash your hands thoroughly afterward.

6. Place biohazard waste for pick up by the service in a secure, designated area.

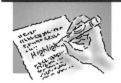

Chapter Highlights

- Medical assistants use specific procedures and practices to prevent the spread of microorganisms that carry disease.

- The human body has natural barriers to protect itself. These barriers can be overpowered by virulent pathogens, especially in a susceptible host.

- By understanding what microorganisms need to survive and how they are transmitted, the medical assistant can break the chain of infection.

- The medical assistant follows guidelines from OSHA and the CDC. These standard precautions will control and prevent infections in the medical office.

- Medical asepsis keeps office areas free of microorganisms. The medical assistant also teaches patients basic aseptic practices to prevent the spread of microorganisms in their homes. Hand washing is critical.

- Different tools require different levels of infection control. The highest level of infection control is sterilization. It destroys all microorganisms and spores.

- It's important for the medical assistant to know when and how to use different disinfection methods. There are three different levels of disinfection.

- Specific policies and regulations protect medical assistants from biohazardous materials and infectious disease. Written policies in the medical office outline the exposure risk factor for each employee. They also provide an exposure control plan.

- Medical assistants protect themselves and their patients by following strict procedures for cleaning biohazardous waste. Improper disposal of biohazardous waste can lead to fines or imprisonment.

- Many medical assistants worry about exposure to HIV and HBV. Knowing how these viruses are transmitted helps reduce the risks. Medical assistants have a legal right to a vaccine for HBV at no cost. Exposure to HIV or HBV requires follow-up testing.

Chapter 2

MEDICAL HISTORY AND PATIENT ASSESSMENT

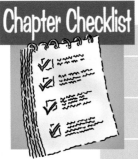

Chapter Checklist

- Obtain and record a patient medical history

- List the types of information included in each section of a medical history

- Describe the different techniques for collecting information in a patient interview

- Explain when to use open-ended and closed-ended questions during a patient interview

- Perform telephone and in-person screening

- Explain the difference between signs and symptoms

- Explain how a chief complaint and a present illness differ

- Summarize how to measure and record a patient's height and weight

- Obtain vital signs

- Explain the differences in taking a patient's temperature using the oral, rectal, axillary, and tympanic methods

- Explain how the body controls temperature and list the factors that influence it

- Describe how to assess and record a patient's respiration

- Identify body sites used for palpating a pulse

- Explain how to choose the correct blood pressure cuff size

- Describe the five phases of Korotkoff sounds

- Identify the factors that may affect blood pressure

Knowing a patient's past and current health information can help the physician diagnose the patient's present illness. A **diagnosis** is the process of identifying a disease or illness. As a medical assistant, you may play a large part in collecting the information the physician needs for a medical history and assessment.

- A patient's **medical history** is information about the patient's past and present health status. It also includes information about the health of family members and information about the patient's social habits, such as smoking.

- **Assessment** is the process of gathering information in order to determine the patient's problem. It begins with asking standard questions and recording the patient's answers. The methods you'll use to do this should be outlined in your office's policies and procedures manual.

The Medical History

As a medical assistant, you'll work with the physician and the patient to complete the medical history. Your role in this step will depend on the policies in your medical office. There are several ways that information for the medical history is obtained.

- Patients fill out a form during their first visit, before seeing the physician.

- Patients return a form that was mailed to them before their appointment.

- A medical assistant interviews the patient using a printed list of questions.

- The physician fills out the medical history form during her examination of the patient.

Even if the physician completes patients' medical histories, you should be familiar with the form. That way you'll be ready to assist the physician if you're asked.

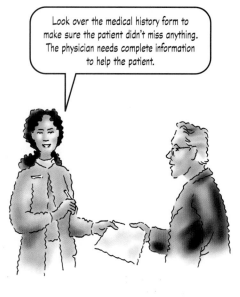

Look over the medical history form to make sure the patient didn't miss anything. The physician needs complete information to help the patient.

WHAT'S IN A MEDICAL HISTORY?

Medical history forms may be different for different medical specialties, but most forms have these main sections:

- demographic data
- past history (PH)
- review of systems (ROS)
- family history (FH)
- social history

Demographic Data

Demographic data is the patient's identifying information. Most of it is needed for the office's business operations. This information always includes the patient's name, address, and phone number. It also includes:

- the patient's emergency contact information
- the patient's gender, marital status, and race
- the patient's Social Security number
- the name, address, and phone number of the patient's employer
- the name, address, and phone number of the patient's insurance carrier
- the patient's health insurance policy number

Past History

The PH section collects information about the patient's past health status. This helps the physician plan the patient's current care. Here's the information this section usually gathers about the patient:

- allergies
- immunizations
- childhood diseases
- current and past medications, including over-the-counter medications and herbal supplements
- previous illnesses
- previous surgeries
- previous hospitalizations
- previous accidents

Review of Systems

The ROS section contains questions about each system of the patient's body. This helps reveal information a patient may have forgotten to note in the PH section, or thought was unimportant. The questions ask about overall health and specific symptoms or diseases that are related to each body system. The questions are usually in a sequence from head to toe.

Family History

This section of the medical history form asks for information about the health of the patient's close relatives. Some diseases or disorders have familial or hereditary links. A **familial disorder** is a problem that is unusually common within a family. **Hereditary disorders** are passed from parents to their offspring. In the FH section, health information is usually gathered about the patient's parents, brothers and sisters, and grandparents. If any immediate family member is deceased, the cause of death should be provided in the patient's medical history.

Social History

The social history section covers the patient's lifestyle. It includes information about marital status, occupation, education, and hobbies. It may also include information about:

- diet
- tobacco use
- alcohol use
- sexual history
- sleeping habits
- exercise

This information helps the physician understand how the patient's illness and any treatment may affect the patient's lifestyle. It also helps the physician see how the patient's lifestyle and illness may be related.

The social history also can be a guide to the need for patient education. The physician may want to address some patient behaviors in order to head off future problems. For example, high tobacco use or a diet high in fat may lead to later illnesses.

INTERVIEWING PATIENTS

To complete the medical history, you'll need to interview the patient. Your goal is to obtain accurate and relevant information. You'll find specific steps for obtaining a medical history in the Hands On procedure on page 86.

Professional Medical Associates – History Form

NAME: _____ DATE OF BIRTH: _____

What is the main reason for your visit to the doctor? _____

_____

Were you referred? _____ If so, by whom? _____

PAST MEDICAL HISTORY:

Are you allergic to any medication? _____

If so, list medications: _____

List current medications, dosage, and how many times a day you take them:

Medication   **Dose**   **Times A Day**

_____

_____

Alcohol Consumption: What type? _____ Amount _____ How Often? _____

                       History of Alcoholism? _____

When was your last TB or Tine test? _____

Have you ever had a positive test for tuberculosis? _____

When was your last Tetanus shot? _____

List all surgeries you have had in the past:

Date   **Type of Surgery**

_____

_____

List all past hospitalizations (not involving surgeries above):

Date   **Reason For Hospital Stay**

_____

_____

List all past problems with trauma (broken bones, lacerations, etc.):

_____

REVIEW OF SYSTEMS, PAST MEDICAL PROBLEMS:
If you have been told you have any of the problems listed below, or are having any of the problems listed below, please CIRCLE:

1. <u>GENERAL:</u> Weight loss, weight gain, fever, chills, night sweats, hot flashes, tire easily, problems with sleep, crying spells, history of cancer.

2. <u>SKIN:</u> Rash, sores that won't heal, moles that are new or changing, history of skin problems.

3. <u>HEENT:</u> Headache, eye problems, hearing problems, sinus problems, hay fever, dizziness, hoarseness, sores in your mouth that won't heal, dental problems.

   Do you chew tobacco or dip snuff? _____

4. <u>METABOLIC/ENDOCRINE:</u> Thyroid problems, diabetes or sugar problems, high cholesterol.

5. <u>RESPIRATORY:</u> Cough, wheezing, breathing problems, history of asthma, history of lung problems.

Do you smoke cigarettes or pipe? _____

How much? _____ For how long? _____

6. <u>BREAST (WOMEN):</u> Breast lumps, changes in nipples, nipple discharge, breast problems, family history of breast cancer. When was your last mammogram? _____

7. <u>CARDIOVASCULAR:</u> Heart murmur, rheumatic fever, high blood pressure, angina, heart problems, heart attack, abnormal heart rhythm, chest pain, palpitations, leg swelling, history of phlebitis or blood clots.

8. <u>GI:</u> Problems with appetite, swallowing, heartburn, nausea, vomiting, pain in the abdomen, constipation, diarrhea, blood in stool, history of ulcers, liver problems, hepatitis, jaundice, pancreas problems, gallbladder problems, or colon problems.

9. <u>REPRODUCTIVE (WOMEN):</u> Problems with irregular menstrual cycles, abnormal vaginal bleeding or discharge, history of sexually transmitted diseases, sexual problems.

AGE OF FIRST MENSES (PERIOD) _____ AGE OF MENOPAUSE _____

LAST PAP SMEAR _____ METHOD OF CONTRACEPTION _____

Obstetric History (Women)

NUMBER OF PREGNANCIES _____ PLEASE LIST AS FOLLOWS:

Delivery Date	Pregnancy Complications	Type Delivery	Baby's Weight

<u>MEN:</u> Problems with genital discharge, history of venereal diseases, sexual problems, prostate problems.

METHOD OF CONTRACEPTION _____

10. <u>UROLOGIC:</u> Problems with painful urination, urinary frequency, blood in urine, weak urinary stream, history of bladder or kidney infections, or kidney stones.

11. <u>MUSCULOSKELETAL:</u> Arthritis, back pain, cramps in legs.

12. <u>NEUROLOGIC:</u> Seizures, stroke, arm or leg weakness or numbness, black-out spells, memory or thinking problems, depression, anxiety, psychiatric problems.

13. <u>HEMATOLOGIC:</u> Anemia, bleeding problems, enlarged lymph nodes.

HAVE YOU EVER HAD A BLOOD TRANSFUSION? _____ DATE _____

FAMILY HISTORY:

List any medical problems that run in your family and which family members have these problems.

_____

_____

SOCIAL HISTORY:

MARITAL STATUS: _____

OCCUPATION: _____

EDUCATION: _____

HOBBIES: _____

WHAT DO YOU DO FOR ENJOYMENT? _____

Legal Brief HIPAA

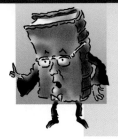

The Health Insurance Portability and Accountability Act (HIPAA) is a federal law that protects the privacy of health information. It requires that you treat the information in a patient's medical history as confidential. Patient records must be stored in a secure place. Only persons directly involved in the patient's care can access these records unless the patient gives specific permission.

Good Communication

It will be your responsibility to get accurate and useful information during the interview. A number of interviewing skills will help you do this.

Reflecting. *Reflecting* is repeating back what the patient said, using open-ended statements. For example, you might say, "So, you were saying your heart burn is bad when . . ."

Paraphrasing. *Paraphrasing* means rephrasing what the patient said in your own words. For example, you might say, "It sounds as if you're saying you have had heartburn and sour stomach for the past week."

Asking for Examples. Asking for examples allows you to clarify what the patient told you. For example, you might say, "Can you describe exactly the pain from the heartburn?"

Asking Questions. Asking questions can help you get more information or details about what the patient has said. For example, you might ask, "Does the heartburn seem to happen after eating certain meals or at a particular time of day?"

Summarizing. Summarizing, or recapping, the main points of what the patient said helps to make sure you understood the patient. For example, you might say, "Let me see if I have understood you correctly . . ." and then give a summary.

Allowing Silence. Allowing silence, or a pause, can be helpful during a conversation. It gives the patient a chance to think about what to say next.

DO YOU KNOW HOW TO LISTEN?

Listening involves more than using your ears! How you listen can be just as important as how you conduct the interview. By using active listening skills, you show that you're interested in what the patient is saying. Active listening can be shown through words (verbal) or body language (nonverbal). Here are two examples.

- *Verbal.* Show you're listening by occasionally using encouraging words or sounds such as "yes," "mm-hmm," or "ah."
- *Nonverbal.* Your body language shows you're listening when you nod, smile, or make frequent eye contact with the patient.

Before the Interview

Setting the right tone for the interview will encourage patients to relax. This will help you get more accurate information. Here are some pointers for setting the right tone.

- *Be prepared.* Make sure you're familiar with the medical history form and any previous medical history provided by the patient. New patients will have filled out a new patient questionnaire. Review the chart of a current patient for any updated information.

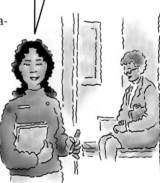

Be familiar with the forms before you talk to the patient. Shuffling papers can seem unprofessional!

- *Find the right location.* To keep patient information confidential, you need a private place to conduct the interview. Avoid public areas such as the reception area, where someone else might hear the patient's answers. You may be able to use a private office or examination room. Besides ensuring privacy, you'll also be cutting down on distractions. Interview the patient alone, unless he wishes family members to be present.

Getting Started

At the beginning of the interview, you need to put the patient at ease. Begin every patient interview by identifying yourself by name and title. Explain the purpose of the interview and how long it will take. Also tell the patient it will be kept confidential.

For example, you might say something like this: "Good morning, Ms. Johansen. My name is Jasmine, and I'm Dr. Martin's medical assistant. I'd like to ask you a few questions that will take about 15 minutes and help the doctor diagnose and treat you. Please be assured that all your responses will be kept in strict confidence."

Make sure to mention your credentials when talking to patients so they don't get the false impression that you're a nurse or physician.

First Impressions. You may be the first person the patient talks to in the office. The impression you make is critical! Your words and manner should communicate respect as well as concern for the patient. This professional but caring attitude will help you gain the patient's confidence. Some patients may not share information until that feeling of trust has been established.

Communication Barriers. Sometimes, patients may have difficulty expressing themselves. You also may have a hard time understanding a patient. As you speak to patients, assess whether there are any barriers to communication—things that will get in the way of each of you understanding the other. Here are some common communication barriers.

- The patient has difficulty with English.
- The patient has impaired vision or hearing.
- The patient has a mental or psychological limitation.

There are several ways to help patients understand what you're saying. You can help keep communication flowing by:

- avoiding highly technical or medical terminology
- paying attention to nonverbal behavior
- adjusting your questions to suit the situation
- maintaining good eye contact
- having a family member or caregiver there with the patient

Assessing the Patient

During the patient interview, listen carefully as the patient describes his medical problems. You need to identify **signs** and symptoms.

- *Signs* are objective information. That means they can be observed or seen by someone other than the patient. Some examples of signs are rash, bleeding, or coughing. Other signs may be found during the physician's examination.
- *Symptoms* are subjective information. They reflect changes in the body sensed by the patient. They're not usually

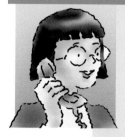

Ask the Professional — DEALING WITH AN ANXIOUS PATIENT

Q: *Yesterday, a patient who seemed anxious and upset came into the office. He looked upset the entire time he was there. I wasn't sure how to make him feel better. What could I have done?*

A: Some patients do feel anxious or worried when they visit a medical office. Sometimes people are anxious about being in a medical setting, or they may be worried about what they'll hear from the physician. It's important for you to show empathy and understanding. Here are some things to keep in mind.

- Acknowledge the patient's feelings using techniques such as reflecting or paraphrasing. Saying something like, "I understand that makes you feel worried," will reassure the patient that you're attentive to his concerns.

- Respond with facts, rather than reacting with emotions. You may feel impatient with a patient's questions or behavior, but the patient needs you to be both professional and calm.

- Protect the patient's privacy. Patients may feel anxious or vulnerable in a medical office. Discuss personal or medical information in the privacy of an examination room.

evident to anyone other than the patient. Examples include patient complaints such as headache, leg pain, nausea, or dizziness.

Sometimes, signs may indicate patient symptoms. A facial expression, such as wincing, may be a sign that a patient is in pain. If the patient is holding onto furniture or walls while walking, it could be a sign that the patient is feeling dizzy.

MAKING OBSERVATIONS

A good interview involves observation. This means noticing things about the patient's appearance or behavior. Some examples of observations you might make of physical status information are:

- pale or flushed skin
- visible bruises or injuries

You can also make observations about the patient's mental status. Some examples are:

- lethargy or tiredness
- crying
- confusion

When you write your observations in the patient's medical record, make sure you include only what you saw and heard. You should not record any judgments, opinions, or conclusions you might have made about what you observed. For example, you would not write that someone must have hit the patient because there were signs of bruising. Avoid making these assumptions.

CHIEF COMPLAINT AND PRESENT ILLNESS

After recording the patient's medical history, you need to find out why the patient has come to see the physician. To do this, you must determine the patient's chief complaint (CC) and present illness (PI).

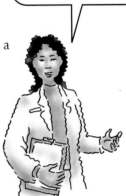

Not every patient who comes to the office is sick. The chief complaint can be the reason for the visit, like a yearly exam.

- *Chief complaint.* The **chief complaint** is the reason the patient is visiting the doctor. It's one statement describing the signs and symptoms that led the patient to seek medical care—for example, "I've had a headache for the past three days." The chief complaint is recorded for every visit, even if it's just a checkup.

- *Present Illness.* The **present illness** is a more specific account of the chief complaint. It includes an order of events, such as when the symptoms began, and any remedies the patient may have tried on his own.

Determining the Chief Complaint

Be sure to go over the patient's medical history form before you begin. Being as familiar as possible with the patient will help you get complete information.

Asking **open-ended questions** usually will lead the patient to reveal a chief complaint. Open-ended questions are those that encourage the patient to respond with more than one or two words. Some examples are, "What's the reason for your visit today?" or "Can you describe what's been going on?" Make sure you maintain eye contact so the patient knows you're listening actively.

Closed-ended questions most often require only a *yes* or *no* answer. They won't provide many details about the patient's condition. For example, "Do you have pain?" doesn't provide much information. However, you can use closed-ended questions to get specific information about the present illness, such as, "When did the pain first start?"

You should document the CC on the progress report form in the patient's record. Use the patient's own words in quotation marks whenever you can. Make sure the progress report includes the date, time of day, and your signature and credentials. The illustration below shows how to document a chief complaint.

Detailing the Present Illness

Once you've recorded the patient's chief complaint, you need to get more details about the patient's present illness, or PI. It's important to establish the chain of events associated with the illness.

For example, you must find out if the patient has tried any **over-the-counter medications.** These are medications available without prescriptions. They include aspirin, decongestants, antihistamines, and many others. They also include vitamins, natural drugs such as herbs, and some homeopathic medications.

Homeopathic medications are tiny doses of substances that would, in normal doses, produce the symptoms of the disease being treated. For example, Allium Cepa, which is made from onions, is a homeopathic remedy for a cold. It's used because

---

PROGRESS NOTES

Name: _____

Date: _____ SS#: _____

Address: _____

Occupation: _____ Phone (home)_____ (work)_____

DOB: _____ Age: _____

Drug allergies: _____

DATE	TIME	REMARKS
7/6/XX	08 00	CC: Pt. c/o "headache" and nasal congestion x2 days. Denies fever, earache, sore throat, or nasal drainage. S. Stine, CMA

This progress note shows the date and time of visit and the patient's CC.

onions make your nose run and eyes water when you cut them, just like a cold does.

Here's some questions you can ask to get information about the PI.

- *Chronology.* How and when did this first begin?

- *Location.* Can you explain or show me where the pain is?

- *Severity.* Can you describe the pain? Is the pain constant? When did the pain first begin? Are there times or movements that make the pain occur? (Some medical offices have patients rate the severity of the pain on a scale of one to ten, with ten being the worst pain they can imagine.)

- *Self-treatment.* What medications (both prescriptions and over-the-counter) and herbs have you taken? Have they helped?

- *Quality.* Does anything you do make the symptoms better? Worse?

- *Duration.* Have you had these symptoms before? If so, when and under what circumstances?

WHOSE IDEA WAS IT?

When you're trying to get accurate information, take care to keep your questions general. If you include details, patients may use your words instead of their own in their responses. Follow these tips for getting the information you need.

- Don't suggest answers by the way you ask questions. If you say, "Is the pain worse when you walk?" patients may say *yes* because they think that's what they're supposed to say.

- Don't coax patients by suggesting other symptoms. You may have an idea of what symptoms a patient is experiencing based on the chief complaint. But it's better to hear what the patient has to say than to make suggestions. Some patients will agree to the symptoms you describe, because they think they "should" be experiencing them.

- Use closed-ended questions to get specifics. Ask these questions only after patients have answered open-ended questions. For example, you might say, "How long have you had this pain?"

  See the Hands On procedure on page 87 for all the steps in documenting a chief complaint and present illness.

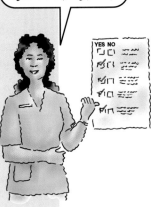

Try to avoid closed-ended questions, such as, "Is the pain sharp?" Some patients might agree to everything you say!

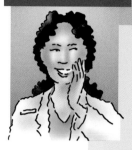

Secrets for Success

PRACTICE YOUR QUESTION-ASKING SKILLS

Asking good questions is critical for obtaining information. By becoming aware of the ways you use questions, you can improve your questioning skills. Here are some ways to practice using questions with friends and family.

- Think of three opportunities where you can use questions to probe for more information. Think about what kinds of questions you could ask.

- In a conversation, make it a point to ask a question to obtain more information or to get another person's opinion. Notice how the speaker responds to your question.

- Pay attention to your own tone of voice, body language, and behavior when you ask questions. Are you interested in learning more or provoking a response? Your attitude can have an effect on how your question comes across.

Anthropometric Measurements

In addition to collecting information about the patient's medical history and concerns, you may need to take physical measurements. Medical assistants take **anthropometric measurements,** or physical measurements of the patient's body. Typically, medical assistants measure the patient's height and weight. You need to document these measurements in the patient's medical record.

Measurements taken at the first visit are recorded as **baseline data.** Baseline data is used as a reference point to compare measurements at later visits. Usually, an adult's height is only recorded on the first visit and then once a year. The weight and vital signs are taken and recorded at each visit. You'll find an explanation of vital signs later in this chapter.

WEIGHT

You should take and record a patient's weight at each office visit. This is especially important for:

- infants
- children

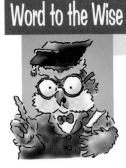

Word to the Wise

anthropometric (AN-thro-puh-MET-rik)

regarding measurements of the human body

- elderly patients
- pregnant patients

Other patients may need special monitoring if they're trying to lose or gain weight or if they're on medications that are calculated according to body weight. Certain diseases also require special monitoring.

Most medical offices have only one scale. It should be placed in a private location to keep patients from feeling uncomfortable. Several types of scales are used to measure weight:

- balance beam scales
- digital scales
- dial scales

Weight can be measured in pounds or kilograms, depending on the practices in your medical office.

Balance Beam Scale

Here are the steps to follow when weighing a patient using a balance beam scale:

1. Wash your hands.
2. Make sure the scale is properly balanced at zero.
3. Ask patients to remove shoes and any heavy outerwear or purses that could distort the reading. Have a place for the patient to sit while removing shoes.
4. Place a paper towel on the scale before the patient steps on. Because the patient will be standing in bare feet or stockings, the paper towel will prevent the spread of microorganisms.

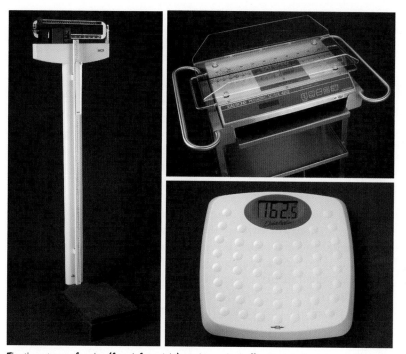

The three types of scales (from left to right) used in medical offices include the balance, dial, and digital scales.

5. Make sure the patient is facing forward on the scale without touching or holding onto anything if possible.

6. Slide the counterweights on the bottom and top bars from zero to the approximate weight of the patient. Always begin with the heavier weight bar (bottom). Each counterweight should rest securely in a notch with an indicator mark.

7. Adjust the counterweights by small amounts until the balance bar hangs freely at the exact midpoint.

8. To calculate the patient's weight, add the top reading to the bottom one. For example, if the heavier counterweight reads 100 and the lighter one reads 16 plus 3 small lines, the patient's weight is 116.75 pounds.

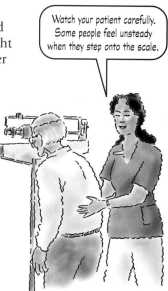

Watch your patient carefully. Some people feel unsteady when they step onto the scale.

9. Help the patient off the scale if necessary. You should stay close to the patient while he is on the scale. Anyone can lose his balance when getting on and off the scale, regardless of age.

10. Discard the paper towel. It also might be necessary to wipe the platform of the scale with a cleaning disinfectant.

11. Record the weight in the patient's medical record. Be sure to include the date, time, your signature, and your credentials. If you're measuring the patient's height at the same time, you can record them together.

Digital and Dial Scales

You will follow most of the same steps listed above when using a digital or dial scale. However, there are some differences.

On digital and dial scales, there aren't any counterweights to slide. When you weigh a patient on a digital scale, read and record the weight displayed on the digital screen. If you weigh a patient on a dial scale, an indicator arrow will rest at the patient's weight. Be sure to read the number from directly above the arrow. If you stand at an angle to read it, you won't see the correct measurement.

HEIGHT

Most balance beam scales have a moveable ruler at the back for measuring height. In some offices, a graph ruler is mounted on the wall. More accurate measures are obtained when a parallel bar is moved down against the top of a patient's head. Height is measured in inches or centimeters, depending on the physician's preferences.

Follow these steps to measure a patient's height using a scale with a ruler.

1. If this procedure isn't being done at the same time as the weight measurement, wash your hands first. Have the patient sit down and remove her shoes. Place a paper towel on the scale before the patient steps on.

2. Be sure the patient is standing straight with heels together and eyes straight ahead. The patient's posture must be erect for an accurate measurement. The best measurement of height is made with the patient's back to the ruler on the scale, but it's acceptable for the patient to face the ruler.

3. Hold the measuring bar perpendicular to the ruler.

4. Lower the measuring bar until it firmly touches the patient's head. Press lightly if the patient's hair is full or high. You don't want to include full hair in the height measurement!

5. Read the measurement at the point where the bar slides out of the scale. If measurements are in inches, convert them to feet and inches. For example, if the bar reads 65 plus two smaller lines, read it as 65.5. Since 12 inches equals one foot, the patient is 5 feet, 5.5 inches tall.

6. When you are finished measuring the patient's height, assist the patient in getting off the scale if necessary. Watch for signs that the patient is unsteady.

7. Have a place for the patient to sit to put on her shoes.

8. Record the patient's height in the medical record.

9. Discard the paper towel and wipe the platform of the scale with a cleaning disinfectant.

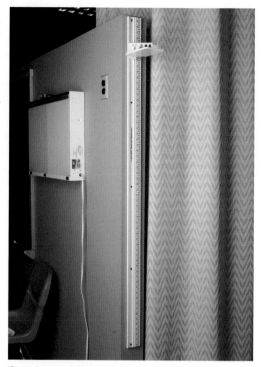

This wall-mounted ruler has a sliding bar like the moveable ruler on a balance beam scale.

PUTTING IT ON THE CHARTS

Here's an example of how to record a patient's height and weight on the medical chart:

02/10/2006 2:00 P.M. Ht. 5 feet, 5.5 inches; Wt. 116.75 lbs.
_____ Y. Torres, CMA

PHYSICAL MEASUREMENTS OF CHILDREN

An infant's height and weight is measured at every routine visit. You may also need to measure an infant's chest and head circumference. These measurements help the physician monitor the infant's growth and development.

Procedures for measuring an infant's weight and length (height) are somewhat different from those for older children and adults. Pediatric weights and heights are often recorded on a growth chart as well as in the patient's medical record. The growth chart provides a graph of the child's growth patterns.

Measuring Infant Length

To measure infant length, you need an examining table with clean table paper and a tape measure. Always wash your hands first. Explain the procedure to the parent. Ask the parent to remove the infant's clothing, except for the diaper. Follow these steps for measuring infant length.

1. Wash your hands.
2. Place the infant on a firm examination table covered with clean table paper. You need a firm surface for accurate measurements! If you're using a measuring board, it should be covered with clean paper.
3. Hold the infant's head at the midline. Fully extend the infant's body by grasping the knees and pressing them flat onto the table. Most infants stay in a flexed position, so you need to extend the legs to get an accurate measurement. Be gentle, but firm. If you need help, ask the parent or a coworker to help you. A footboard against the soles of the infant's feet will give the most accurate measurement.
4. Mark the table paper with your pen at the top of the infant's head. Make a second mark on the paper at the infant's heel.
5. Using the measuring tape, measure between the marks on the paper.
6. Record the length in the infant's medical record and on the growth chart.
7. Clean the area and wash your hands.

Measuring Infant Weight

Infant weight is measured using a scale designed for infants. Follow these steps to find an infant's weight.

1. Wash your hands.
2. Either carry the infant or have the parent carry the infant to the scales.
3. Place protective paper on the scale and balance the scale. The balance beam must be centered before each use.
4. Remove the infant's diaper just before placing the infant on the scale. For the most accurate weight, infants should be weighed without any clothing. Cool air against the infant's skin may cause voiding so be sure to cover the private area of infant boys. In some offices, the infant is weighed in a diaper, as long as it is dry and clean. If so, you need to note that the infant wore a dry clean diaper.
5. Place the infant on the scale. Keep one of your hands over or near the infant on the scale at all times. Larger infants who can sit may be weighed while sitting. Sitting can help

to make the experience less frightening.

6. Quickly move the counter-weights to balance the apparatus exactly.

7. Pick up the infant. Ask the parent to replace the infant's diaper if it's been removed.

8. Record the weight in the infant's medical record and on the growth chart.

9. Clean the area and wash your hands.

Other Pediatric Measurements

You also may need to measure and record the head and chest circumference of an infant. Head circumference refers to the measure around the largest part of the infant's head. Chest circumference is the measurement around the chest. You'll use a flexible cloth or paper measuring tape. Follow these steps to obtain the head and chest circumference of an infant.

1. Wash your hands.

2. First, place the infant supine (lying on the back with face upward) on an examination table, or ask the parent to hold the infant.

3. Measure around the head above the eyebrow and posteriorly at the largest part of the occiput, the bone forming the back of the skull.

4. Record the infant's head circumference on the growth chart and in the infant's medical record.

5. Now measure around the chest (with clothing removed) at the nipple line. Be sure to keep the tape measure at the

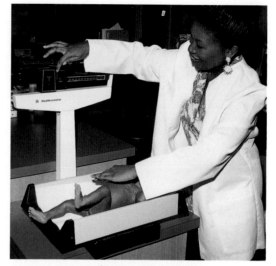

Most infants are weighed lying down.

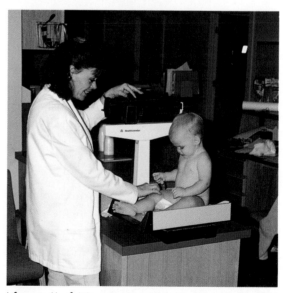

Infants capable of sitting up may be weighed while sitting, especially if this makes the procedure less upsetting for them.

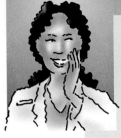

Secrets for Success

USING THE CORRECT WORDS FOR ORIENTATION

In medical terminology, specific terms are used to refer to directions and positions. Learning these terms will help you improve your understanding of medical instructions or notes.

- *Anterior* means toward the front.
- *Posterior* means toward the back.
- *Lateral* means to the left or right side of the body.
- *Medial* means toward the middle or inside of the body.
- *Superior* means toward the head, or above.
- *Inferior* means farther from the head, or below.
- *Proximal* means near the origin or point of attachment.
- *Distal* means away from the origin or point of attachment.
- *Midline* means in the middle or center of something.

same level anterior and posterior (front and back). This ensures the most accurate reading.

6. Record the infant's chest circumference on the growth chart and in the infant's medical record.

7. When you're finished with both measurements, wash your hands and clean the equipment.

ON THE CHARTS

All the infant's measurements are recorded in his medical record. Here's an example of how you would chart all of these measurements:

10/15/2006 9:45 A.M. Wt. 14 lb. Length 24 in. Head 15 in. Chest 17 in. _____ B. Brady, CMA

Vital Signs

In addition to anthropometric measurements, medical assistants may be required to measure patient **vital signs.** (In some offices these are called **cardinal signs.**) Vital signs are physical measurements of basic body functions. Measuring vital signs provides information about the basic body systems that keep a person alive. Medical assistants often measure and record four different vital signs.

- *Temperature* (T) is the internal heat produced by the body.
- *Pulse rate* (P) is the beating of the heart, felt in an artery and heard with a stethoscope.
- *Respiratory rate* (R) is the speed at which a patient breathes, heard with a stethoscope or seen.
- *Blood pressure* (BP) is the force of blood pressing on arteries as it circulates in the body.

The table below is a summary of normal ranges for vital signs for newborns to elderly adults.

Normal Ranges for Vital Signs

Age	Pulse (beats per minute)	Respirations (breaths per minute)	Blood Pressure— Systolic (mmHg)*	Blood Pressure— Diastolic (mmHg)*	Temperature (°F)**
Newborn (0–4 weeks)	120–160	40–60	greater than 60		
Infant (1–12 months)	100–120	25–30	70–95		97.5–100.4
Children (1–8 years)	80–100	15–30	80–110		97.0–99.7
Adolescents	60–100	12–20	118–132	70–82	97.8–99.1
Adults	60–100	12–20	80–130	60–90	
Elderly adults	55–70	12–20	80–130	70–90	96.4–99.5

*According to American Heart Association guidelines, patients with blood pressure readings above 115/75 have an increased risk of cardiovascular complications. Also, a systolic pressure from 120 to 139 or a diastolic pressure from 80 to 89 is considered the warning range for possible high blood pressure.

**Oral temperatures are not taken on infants and very young children as they are unable to safely keep the thermometer in their mouths for the necessary length of time.

VITAL SIGNS—TEMPERATURE

The body temperature reflects a balance between the heat produced by the body and the heat lost by the body. The body produces heat in two ways:

- the body's **metabolism,** or the normal physical and chemical processes that occur inside the body
- muscle movement

The body loses heat through normal processes, such as:

- **respiration,** or breathing
- elimination of waste products
- conduction, or transmission through the skin

Vital signs give the physician vital information. Make sure you write them down in the medical record accurately.

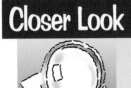

Closer Look — THE TRANSFER OF HEAT

Body heat is always changing. Heat transfer occurs when there is a difference in heat content between two areas. Measuring temperature is actually measuring heat transferred from one space to another. The following table lists the main ways heat is transferred to and from the body. The illustration shows a common example of each mechanism of heat transfer.

Mechanisms of Heat Transfer

Mechanism	Definition	Example
Radiation	Diffusion or spreading out of heat by electromagnetic waves.	The body gives off waves of heat from uncovered surfaces.
Convection	Heat is produced by motion between areas of unequal density.	An oscillating fan blows cool air across the surface of a warm body.
Evaporation	Liquid is converted to vapor.	Body fluid (perspiration) radiates from the skin.
Conduction	Heat is transferred during contact between two objects.	The body transfers heat to an ice pack, melting the ice.

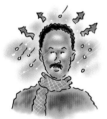 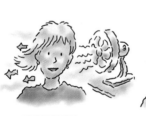 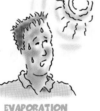

RADIATION   **CONVECTION**   **EVAPORATION**   **CONDUCTION**

Each mechanism of heat transfer described in the table is illustrated here.

The average body temperature is around 98.6° Fahrenheit (F) or 37.0° Celsius (C). A patient with a temperature within the average range (shown in the table on page 63) is **afebrile**. A patient with a temperature above normal is considered **febrile,** or has a fever.

Hot Places

You need to be familiar with the different methods and sites for measuring body temperature.

- *Oral.* An oral thermometer is placed in the mouth under the tongue. This is the most commonly used thermometer.

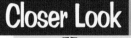

FAHRENHEIT OR CELSIUS?

Clinical thermometers may use either the Fahrenheit or the Celsius scale. As a medical assistant, you should know how to convert temperatures from one scale to the other. You also need to be aware of how temperature readings differ depending on how the temperature is taken. This table shows normal temperatures in both the Fahrenheit and Celsius scales, as well as the variations in temperature among body sites.

Temperature Comparisons

	Fahrenheit	Celsius
Oral	98.6	37.0
Rectal	99.6	37.6
Axillary	97.6	36.4
Tympanic	98.6	37.0

- *Rectal.* A rectal thermometer is gently inserted in the rectum. This method is often used for infants.
- *Axillary.* To measure temperature, a thermometer is placed under the armpit.
- *Tympanic.* A tympanic thermometer is one that is inserted into the ear canal.
- *Temporal scanner.* The thermometer is placed lightly on the forehead, used for infants over three months.

There are also disposable thermometers that can be used once and then thrown away. These can typically be placed in the mouth, or under the armpit. Some disposable thermometers can be attached to the forehead.

Glass Thermometers

Glass thermometers are used to measure oral, rectal, and axillary temperatures. They consist of a glass tube and a silver bulb, which is filled with non-hazardous mineral spirits or an alcohol-based substance.

Glass thermometers are shaped differently for oral and rectal use.

- Rectal thermometers have a rounded or stubbed bulb. The end opposite the bulb is usually color-coded red.

- Thermometers with a long, slender bulb are used for axillary or oral temperatures. They are often color-coded blue.

It's important that these different types of thermometers are cleaned and stored separately.

You'll find information on how to take an oral temperature with a glass thermometer in the Hands On procedure on page 88. Steps for taking a rectal temperature are in the Hands On procedure on page 90. Taking axillary temperatures is detailed in the Hands On procedure on page 93.

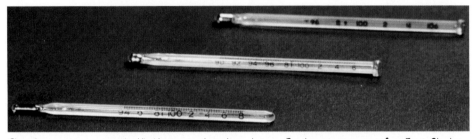

Glass thermometers once contained liquid mercury, a hazardous substance. But they are now mercury free. Front: Slender bulb, oral. Center: Rounded bulb, red tip, rectal. Back: Blue tip, oral.

READING A GLASS THERMOMETER

When a glass thermometer is placed in position for a certain length of time, the patient's body heat expands the liquid in the tube. The liquid rises in the glass tube and stays there until you shake it back down into the bulb.

There are two main scales for glass thermometers.

- *Fahrenheit thermometer.* The glass stem of the Fahrenheit thermometer is calibrated with lines and numbers showing temperature readings in even degrees (94°, 96°, 98°, and so on). Uneven numbers (95°, 97°, 99°, and so on) are marked only with a longer line. Between both even and uneven numbers, four smaller lines show 0.2-degree increments of temperature. Looking at the level of the liquid in the thermometer will give you the temperature reading.

- *Celsius thermometer.* The glass stem of the Celsius thermometer has markings to show each degree. Between each degree, there are ten smaller markings to show 0.1-degree increments. For example, if the liquid rises to the third small line past the line marked 37, the temperature reading to record is 37.3°C.

Electronic Thermometers

Electronic thermometers consist of a base unit and an attached temperature probe. The base unit is battery-operated, so it can be carried to where you need to use it. Electronic thermometers have inter-changeable temperature probes for different uses. The probes are color-coded red for rectal read-ings and blue for oral or axillary readings.

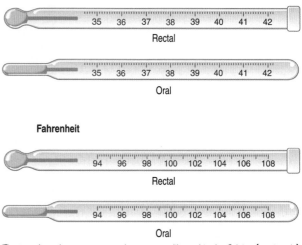

The two glass thermometers on the top are calibrated in the Celsius (centigrade) scale, and the two on the bottom use the Fahrenheit scale. Note the blunt bulb on the rectal thermometers and the long thin bulb on the oral thermometers.

When the probe is positioned properly, it senses the body tempera-ture. A digital readout shows in the window of the handheld base.

Before using an electronic thermometer, place a disposable probe cover over the probe. Be careful to not contaminate the probe cover by touching it or placing it on a surface. When you're done taking the patient's temperature, discard the probe cover in a biohazard waste container. Sanitize and disinfect the thermometer according to your office's policy. For other guide-lines on how to take a temperature with an elec-tronic thermometer, see the Hands On procedure on page 95.

Tympanic Thermometers

These battery-powered thermometers are sometimes called aural thermometers, because they are inserted into the ear. The end of the thermometer is covered with a disposable cover. When it's in place, pressing a button emits infrared light inside the ear. The light bounces off the tympanic membrane, or eardrum.

A sensor in the thermometer measures the tem-perature of the blood in the tympanic membrane. The temperature reading is displayed on a digital screen on the unit within two seconds. If used correctly, this is a highly reliable method for measuring temperature. How-ever, you should not use a tympanic thermometer when the

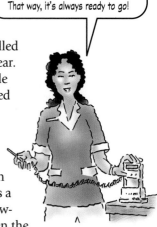

Keep the electronic thermometer in a charging unit when it's not being used. That way, it's always ready to go!

patient has a buildup of ear wax or an ear infection. The steps for using the tympanic thermometer can be found in the Hands On procedure on page 96.

Disposable Thermometers

Disposable thermometers are designed for one use only. They're fairly accurate, but not as accurate as glass, electronic, or tympanic thermometers. They register temperature quickly by showing color changes on a strip. This makes them useful for simple screenings in settings such as schools or day-care centers.

Other disposable thermometers for young children take the form of sucking devices or pacifiers. However, these are not used in the medical office setting.

HOW THE BODY CONTROLS TEMPERATURE

A patient's temperature is influenced by heat produced or lost by the body. However, temperature is controlled by the hypothalamus, an area at the base of the brain.

When the body is too warm, the hypothalamus sets off **vasodilation**—a

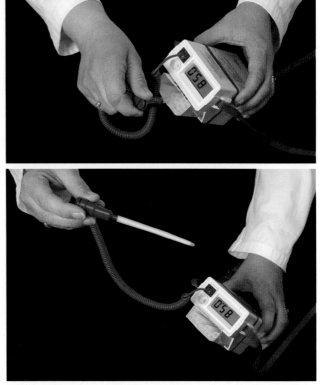

Even though an electronic thermometer is placed in a disposable sheath before use, it still must be sanitized after each use. Check the manufacturer's instructions for cleaning methods.

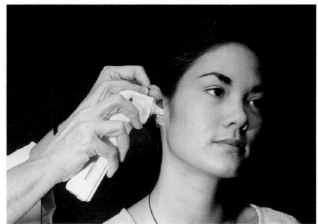

If used properly, the tympanic thermometer will give a reading comparable to the oral thermometer.

process where blood vessels widen or dilate. The result is that excess heat is carried to the surface of the body in the blood. The hypothalamus also signals an increase in perspiration, or sweating. Perspiration cools the body as moisture evaporates from the skin.

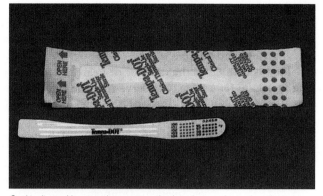

On this disposable paper thermometer, the dots change color to show the body temperature.

If the body is too cool, the hypothalamus begins **vasoconstriction,** or the narrowing of blood vessels. Less blood reaches the surface of the body, reducing heat loss. The person may also begin shivering, a process that generates more heat.

Factors Influencing Temperature Control

Temperature changes may be a sign of disease, but there are several other factors that cause temperatures to vary.

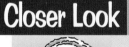

Closer Look   RECORDING PATIENTS' TEMPERATURES

Temperature readings from different parts of the body shouldn't be taken as equal. A reading of 98.6°F is considered average for oral thermometers, but readings from other sites may be slightly different.

- Rectal temperatures are generally 1°F *higher* than oral temperatures. This is because of the blood supply and tightly closed environment of the rectum. A rectal temperature of 101°F is the equivalent to an oral temperature of 100°F.

- Axillary temperatures are usually 1°F *lower* than oral temperatures. It's difficult for patients to keep the axilla, or armpit, tightly closed. An axillary temperature of 101°F is the equivalent of an oral temperature of 102°F.

- Tympanic thermometers give similar readings to oral thermometers as long as they are used properly.

When you record a temperature in a patient's chart, you'll need to write where you took the measurement as well as the temperature itself—for example, *101°F, axillary.*

- *Age.* Children usually have higher temperatures than adults because of their higher metabolisms. On the other hand, elderly people have lower metabolisms and lower temperatures. The temperatures of infants and the elderly are easily affected by the environment.
- *Gender.* Women have slightly higher temperatures than men, especially at time of ovulation.
- *Exercise.* When you exercise, you burn more calories for energy. That raises the body temperature.
- *Time of day.* Body temperature is usually lowest in the early morning, before you become physically active.
- *Emotions.* Temperature typically rises when you're under stress and falls when you're experiencing depression.
- *Illness.* Disease can cause high or low body temperatures.
- *Heat or cold.* Hot or cold beverages as well as a hot or cold environment can affect temperature.

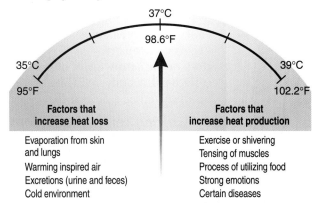

Various factors, including some you might not normally think of, can affect the body's balance between heat loss and heat production.

Fever!

Fever is a rise of body temperature. It often results from a disease process such as a bacterial or viral infection.

A fever of 102°F or higher (rectally) or 101°F or higher (orally) is referred to as **pyrexia.** An extremely high temperature, 105°F to 106°F, is called **hyperpyrexia.** Hyperpyrexia is considered dangerous because the intense body heat may destroy cells in the brain or other vital organs.

A rise in body temperature also can result from exercise, anxiety, or **dehydration**—a loss of fluids from the body. However, these causes are unrelated to disease and are not considered fevers.

STAGES IN THE FEVER PROCESS

The fever process has several well-defined stages.

1. *Onset.* The onset, or beginning of the fever, may be abrupt or gradual.

2. *Course.* The course is how long the fever lasts. It can range from a day or so to several weeks. There are several ways to describe a fever's course. If a fever is constant over its entire course, it's called a **sustained** fever. If it occurs off and on over its course, it's known as a **remittent** fever. An **intermittent** fever is one that occurs at intervals. If after a period of normal readings, the fever returns, it's called a **relapsing** fever.

3. *Resolution.* The return to normal is the resolution. If the resolution occurs abruptly, it's called a crisis. If the resolution is more gradual, it's referred to as lysis.

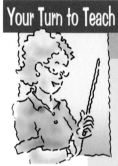

Your Turn to Teach

WHAT PATIENTS NEED TO KNOW ABOUT FEVER

Understandably, patients are often concerned about fevers. When talking to a patient about a fever, explain that a rise in temperature is usually a natural response to disease. Therefore, a patient's attempts to "bring down a fever" may slow the disease recovery process. However, if the patient is uncomfortable or the fever is abnormally high, it should be brought down to about 101°F. The body's natural defenses may still be able to destroy the pathogen without extreme discomfort to the patient.

After consulting with the physician, you can instruct patients about several different comfort measures.

- Drink clear fluids, as tolerated, to rehydrate body tissues. (Patients should use caution when drinking clear fluids if nausea and vomiting are present.)

- Keep clothing and bedding clean and dry, especially after **diaphoresis** (sweating).

- Avoid becoming chilled. Chills cause shivering, which raises the body temperature.

- Rest and eat a light diet, as tolerated.

- Use antipyretics, or fever-reducing agents, to stay comfortable.

- Don't give aspirin products to children under 18. Aspirin has been associated with Reye's syndrome, a potentially fatal disorder, following cases of viral illnesses and varicella zoster (chicken pox).

VITAL SIGNS—PULSE

The rate and power of the heartbeat is measured using a pulse. As the heart beats, blood is forced through the arteries. This causes the arteries to expand. When the heart relaxes, the arteries relax as well. The expansion and relaxation of the arteries can be felt at different parts of the body. These locations are called pulse points. The most commonly used pulse points are the:

- carotid
- apical
- brachial
- radial
- femoral
- popliteal
- posterior tibial
- dorsal pedis

Taking a Pulse

For many pulse points, you can determine the pulse rate through **palpation.** Palpation is using your sense of touch to examine the patient. To palpate a pulse, you place two or three fingers over one of the pulse points. You can use any of the following combinations of fingers:

- index and middle finger
- middle and ring finger
- index, middle, and ring finger

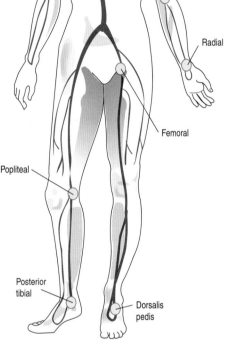

This drawing shows the location of the arteries most commonly used as pulse points.

You don't want to use your thumb to palpate a pulse. This is because your thumb has its own pulse. If you used your thumb, you could be counting your own pulse and not the patient's pulse.

When you press on a pulse point with your fingers, each expansion of the artery counts as one heartbeat. You should be able to find a pulse in arteries supplying blood to the **extremities,** or the patient's arms and legs. A pulse in arteries supplying blood to one of the extremities tells you that oxygenated blood is flowing to that limb. Steps for measuring the radial pulse are detailed in the Hands On procedure on page 97.

Sometimes, you may use a stethoscope to help you listen for the heartbeat. For example, you'll need a stethoscope to measure the apical pulse. You place the bell on the patient's body over the apex of the heart and listen for the pulse.

Only fingers are used to palpate a pulse.

Pulse Characteristics

When you palpate the pulse, there are three different characteristics you should notice: rate, rhythm, and volume.

Rate. The number of heartbeats per minute is the pulse rate. You can assess the rate by palpating the pulse and counting each heartbeat while watching the second hand of your watch. To get an accurate reading, you count the number of beats for a full minute. Another method is to count the number of beats for 30 seconds and multiply the number of beats by 2; however, this cannot be used when taking an apical pulse. When taking an apical pulse, you must count the beats for a full minute.

Rhythm. The interval between each heartbeat or the pattern of the beats is referred to as the rhythm. Normally, there's a regular pattern. Each heartbeat occurs at a regular, consistent rate. You need to document any irregular rhythm in the patient's chart and inform the doctor.

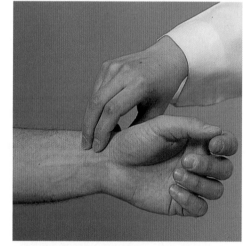

This picture shows the correct finger position for finding a radial pulse.

Volume. The volume refers to the strength or force of the heartbeat. It's described in words such as *soft, bounding, weak, thready, strong,* or *full.* You should record a description of the pulse volume in the patient's chart. Be sure to tell the doctor about any abnormal volume.

Factors Affecting Pulse Rates

Many different factors can affect the rate, rhythm, and volume of the heartbeat. Some of them include:

- *Time of day.* The pulse is usually lower early in the morning than later in the day.

- *Gender.* Women have a slightly higher pulse rate than men.
- *Body type and size.* Tall, thin people usually have a lower pulse rate than shorter, stockier people.
- *Exercise.* Heart rate increases with exercise because blood needs to circulate faster in the body.
- *Stress or emotions.* Anger, fear, excitement, and stress will raise the pulse; depression will lower it.
- *Fever.* Fever increases the pulse rate. Cell metabolism increases in the presence of fever. The heart rate increases as the body works to supply oxygen and nutrients to cells. The pulse may rise as much as ten beats per minute for each degree of fever.
- *Medications.* Many medications may raise or lower pulse rates, either as a desired effect or as an undesired side effect.

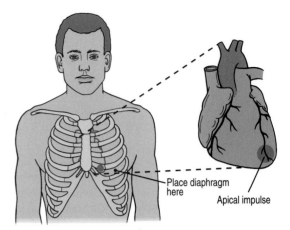

Place diaphragm here

Apical impulse

This diagram shows the location of the apical pulse in relation to the clavicle and ribs.

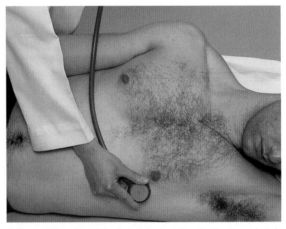

Unlike the other pulse points, the apical pulse is heard rather than palpated.

- *Blood volume.* Loss of blood volume due to **hemorrhage** (a dramatic loss of blood) or dehydration can increase pulse rate. Cell metabolism increases, so the heart rate increases to supply more nutrients to cells.

TYPICAL PULSE RATES

The average pulse rate for an adult ranges between 60 and 80 beats per minute. However, pulse rates change with age. The table on the next page shows how pulse rates differ at different stages of life.

Variations in Pulse Rate by Age

Age	Beats per Minute
Birth to 1 year	110–170
1–10 years	90–110
10–16 years	80–95
16 years to midlife	60–100
Elderly adult	55–70

When the Pulse Is Hard to Find

Medical assistants usually measure pulse rate from the radial artery in the arm. It's convenient for both the medical assistant and the patient. Sometimes, the radial pulse may be irregular or hard to palpate. The next best choice is to listen to the apical pulse.

Peripheral pulses, or pulses found in the arms or legs, are sometimes hard to detect. Another way to measure peripheral pulses that are hard to palpate is to use a Doppler unit.

The Doppler unit is a small electric device that's used to listen to the pulse. It has three parts:

- a main box with control switches

- a probe

- an earpiece unit that plugs into the main box

The probe contains a transducer—a device which allows you to hear the pulse. The earpiece resembles the earpiece of a stethoscope. It can be detached so that everyone in the room can hear the sounds, if desired.

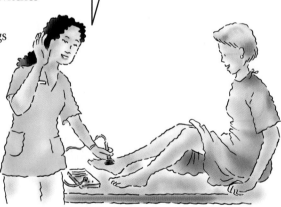

Ah...now I hear it. A Doppler unit amplifies the sound of a pulse that is difficult to palpate.

USING A DOPPLER UNIT

Here are the steps to follow in using a Doppler unit.

1. *Apply gel.* A coupling or transmission gel should be applied to the pulse point before you place the end of

the probe on the area. The gel creates an airtight seal between the probe and the skin. The seal helps transmit the sound.

2. *Find the pulse.* With the machine on, hold the probe at a 90-degree angle to the patient's skin. Press lightly to make sure the probe makes contact. Move the probe in small circles in the gel until you hear the pulse. The Doppler unit will emit a loud pumping sound with each heartbeat. Adjust the volume control if necessary.

3. *Clean up.* After you assess the rate and rhythm of the heartbeat, clean the patient's skin with a tissue or soft cloth. You'll also need to use a tissue or cloth to clean off the probe. Don't use alcohol or water to clean the probe. It can damage the transducer.

VITAL SIGNS—RESPIRATION

You may think of respiration as just breathing. But the term also refers to the exchange of gases between the air you breathe and the blood in your body. During respiration, the body takes in oxygen and pushes out carbon dioxide. Respiration has two parts.

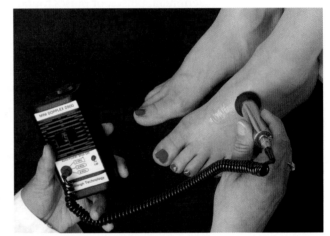

A Doppler device is used to take a dorsalis pedis pulse.

- *External respiration* involves exhalation, or breathing out, and inhalation, or breathing in. It's the process of moving air through the respiratory system. Air travels to the alveoli, tiny air sacs in the lungs. In the alveoli, oxygen is absorbed into the bloodstream.

- *Internal respiration* is the exchange of gases between the blood and the cells that make up body tissues.

The Respiration Process

Respiration is controlled by the respiratory center in the brain stem. Chemosensors in the carotid arteries monitor the level of carbon dioxide in the blood. They provide feedback to the respiratory center.

The diaphragm is a muscle between the chest and abdomen that the body uses for breathing. As a patient breathes in, the diaphragm contracts and flattens out. The rib cage lifts and expands. Air flows into the lungs. The medical term for this inhalation process is **inspiration.**

During **expiration,** or exhalation (breathing out), the diaphragm relaxes, moving upward into a dome-like shape. This allows the rib cage to contract. Air in the lungs flows out of the chest cavity.

Normal Respiration Rates

Like heart rates, respiratory rates change with age.

- Infants can have 25 to 60 respirations per minute, depending on their age.
- In children, 15 to 30 respirations per minute are normal.
- Adults normally range from 12 to 20 respirations per minute.

Respiration rates also are affected by temperature. Patients with an elevated body temperature usually also have increased pulse and respiratory rates.

Measuring Respirations

You can measure respirations by observing the rise and fall of the patient's chest. This is usually done as part of the pulse measurement. Here are some things to keep in mind:

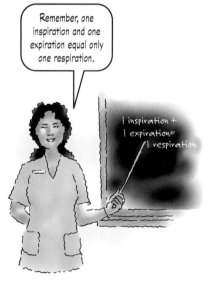

Remember, one inspiration and one expiration equal only one respiration.

1 inspiration + 1 expiration= 1 respiration

- Try not to make patients aware that you're counting respirations. Patients often change their breathing action if they know they are being watched.
- Count the number of respirations in a full minute, or for 30 seconds and multiply by 2.
- You also can use a stethoscope to listen to respirations if necessary.

More guidance on measuring respirations can be found in the Hands On procedure on page 98.

Respiration Characteristics

There are three main characteristics of respirations: rate, rhythm, and depth.

Closer Look   THE APGAR SCORE

Vital sign measurements are part of the Apgar score. The Apgar score is a method for describing the general health of newborns at one minute and five minutes after delivery. Obstetricians, pediatricians, and delivery room personnel use it to assess newborns who may need to be watched more closely. Five signs are assessed:

- heart rate
- respiratory effort
- muscle tone
- response to a suction catheter in the nostril
- color

A perfect score for each sign is two. A total absence of any sign is zero. A perfect Apgar score of ten indicates all of the following things about a newborn.

- Heart rate is greater than 100 beats/minute.
- Respirations are eupneic (the infant is breathing normally) or the baby is crying.
- Muscle tone is good and the baby is active.
- Baby coughs or sneezes in response to the suction catheter.
- Skin is pink, with no acrocyanosis (blue color in the extremities).

Most babies have one-minute scores of seven to nine. Many may have a bit of acrocyanosis until their respiration is fully established. Babies with one-minute scores of less than four usually require medical assistance. They often need oxygen to help them with their breathing.

Rate. The number of respirations occurring in one minute is the respiration rate.

Rhythm. The time or spacing between each respiration is referred to as the rhythm. Normally, respirations are equal and regular. If the rhythm is abnormal, you need to document it in the patient's chart. You would write *irregular* after the respiration rate and notify the doctor.

Depth. The depth refers to the volume of air being inhaled and exhaled. When a person is at rest, the depth should be regular and consistent. There are normally no noticeable sounds other than those involved in the regular exchange of air.

> Abnormal sounds during inspiration or expiration can be a sign of disease.

Respirations that are abnormally deep or shallow must be documented in the patient's record. You also need to document any abnormal sounds, such as crackles (wet or dry sounds), popping sounds, or wheezes (high-pitched sounds). You must also inform the doctor of these abnormalities.

VITAL SIGNS—BLOOD PRESSURE

Blood pressure is the measurement of the pressure of blood in an artery as it's forced against the artery walls. It's measured in two phases of the **cardiac cycle,** or heartbeat. The cardiac cycle lasts from the beginning of one heartbeat to the beginning of the next. There are two pressure phases in each cycle:

- *Systolic pressure.* The phase of the cardiac cycle when the heart muscle contracts is known as **systole.** As the heart contracts, it forces blood to move through chambers of the heart known as the atria and ventricles. The highest pressure level during contraction is recorded as the systolic pressure.

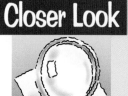

Closer Look   DESCRIBING ABNORMAL BREATHING

Medical professionals use specific terms to describe respiration when they document abnormal breathing.

- Tachypnea—a respiratory rate that is much faster than normal
- Bradypnea—a respiratory rate that is much slower than normal
- Dyspnea—difficult or labored breathing
- Apnea—no respiration
- Hyperpnea—abnormally deep, gasping breaths
- Hyperventilation—a respiratory rate that greatly exceeds the body's oxygen demand
- Hypopnea—shallow respirations
- Orthopnea—inability to breathe lying down; the patient usually has to sit upright to breathe

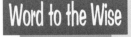

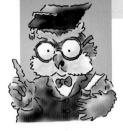

Word to the Wise

sphygmomanometer (SFIG-mo-muh-NOM-ih-ter)
an instrument used to measure blood pressure

- *Diastolic pressure.* A second phase in the cardiac cycle occurs as the heart pauses to rest and refill. During **diastole,** the pressure in the arteries drops. The pressure level recorded during this phase is called the diastolic pressure.

Measuring Blood Pressure

To measure blood pressure, you need to use a stethoscope and a **sphygmomanometer,** or blood pressure cuff. You need to record both the systolic pressure and the diastolic pressure. These two numbers are written as a fraction, with the systolic pressure over the diastolic pressure—for example, 120/80.

Three types of sphygmomanometers are commonly used in medical offices. They differ in terms of how readings are displayed.

- Aneroid sphyg-momanometers display blood pressure readings on a circular dial.
- Column sphygmo-manometers display blood pressure readings using mercury-free liquid in a glass tube.
- Automated blood pressure monitors inflate the cuff when a button is pushed and show the results as numbers on a digital readout

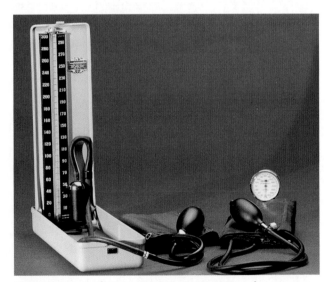

The two basic types of sphygmomanometers are the mercury-free column sphygmomanometer (left) and the aneroid sphygmomanometer (right).

These blood pressure monitors are calibrated to measure blood pressure in millimeters of mercury (mmHg). That means a blood pressure reading of 120/80 indicates the amount of force needed to raise a column of mercury to the 120 mm calibration mark on the tube during systole and to 80 mm during diastole.

CHOOSE THE RIGHT SIZE

Before taking a patient's blood pressure, assess the size of the patient's arm and then choose the correct cuff size. Different cuff widths are available for infants to obese adults. The width of the cuff should be 40 to 50 percent of the circumference of the arm.

To determine the correct size, hold the narrow edge of the cuff at the midpoint of the upper arm. Wrap the width, not the length, of the cuff around the arm. The cuff width should reach not quite halfway around the arm.

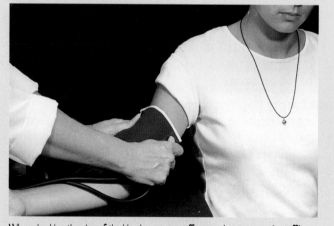

When checking the size of the blood pressure cuff, remember to wrap the cuff's width, not its length, around the patient's arm. The cuff's width should reach not quite halfway around the arm.

Getting a Reading

The sphygmomanometer is attached to a cuff by a rubber tube. A second rubber tube is attached to a hand pump with a screw valve. After the cuff is wrapped around the patient's upper arm, you use the hand pump to inflate an air bladder inside the cuff. The screw valve turned clockwise keeps the air from escaping.

As the cuff inflates, it presses against the brachial artery. This pressure stops blood from flowing through the artery. When you slowly turn the screw valve counterclockwise, the pressure decreases. Blood begins to flow through the artery again. With a stethoscope, you listen to the sounds the blood makes as it begins flowing again. Different sounds indicate the systolic and diastolic pressures. You can find specific steps for taking blood pressure in the Hands On procedure on page 99.

Korotkoff Sounds. These sounds are named for a Russian physician, Nicolai Korotkoff, who first described them. A different sound marks each phase as the cuff deflates. Only the sounds of phase 1 and phase 5 are recorded as blood pressure.

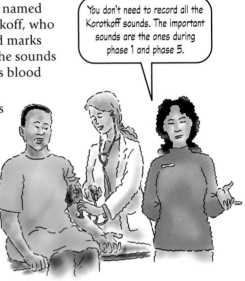

You don't need to record all the Korotkoff sounds. The important sounds are the ones during phase 1 and phase 5.

- phase 1—faint tapping sound; this marks the systolic blood pressure.
- phase 2—soft swishing sound
- phase 3—rhythmic, sharp, distinct tapping
- phase 4—soft tapping sound that becomes faint
- phase 5—the last sound heard; this is the patient's diastolic blood pressure.

Auscultatory Gap. In patients with a history of **hypertension,** or high blood pressure, you may experience an auscultatory gap during phase 2 of the Korotkoff sounds. An auscultatory gap is the loss of any sounds for a drop of up to 30 mmHg after the first sound is heard.

You need to be aware of the possibility of this gap. It can lead to errors in blood pressure readings. The last sound heard at the beginning of the gap may be inaccurately recorded as the diastolic pressure. It's important to watch the dial or column liquid carefully until you're sure you've heard the last sound before noting the diastolic pressure.

Normal Blood Pressure

The average adult blood pressure is 120/80. Athletes may have a lower normal blood pressure because their cardiovascular systems are highly conditioned.

Sometimes, blood pressure drops suddenly when the patient moves from a sitting or lying position to a standing position. This drop is called **postural hypotension** or *orthostatic hypotension.* It can cause symptoms such as vertigo, or dizziness. It also may cause fainting. Be careful when asking patients to change

Running Smoothly

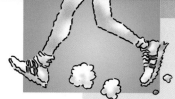

SHUNTS, MASTECTOMIES, AND BLOOD PRESSURE

Some patients require special attention when taking blood pressure.

- A dialysis shunt is a surgically made access port that allows a patient with little or no kidney function to be connected to a dialysis machine. Taking blood pressure in the arm with the shunt could permanently damage the shunt. Don't do it! If the shunt is damaged, the patient cannot receive dialysis until a surgeon puts in a new shunt.

- Patients who have had a mastectomy (surgery to remove a breast) should also not have blood pressure taken in the arm on the affected side. That side of the body may have impaired circulation because of the surgery.

Medical records of patients who have had a mastectomy or who have a dialysis shunt should clearly show that no blood pressure measurements or blood draws are to be performed on the designated arm. You should be able to use the other arm to measure blood pressure.

Most patients are aware of the importance of not taking blood pressure or specimens from the affected arm. Although they will probably alert you before you make a mistake, it's always best to check the medical record first!

from lying down to sitting or standing, and remind patients to move slowly.

Pulse Pressure. The difference between systolic and diastolic readings is called the pulse pressure. For the average adult blood pressure of 120/80, the pulse pressure is 40 (120 − 80 = 40).

The normal range for pulse pressure is 30 to 50 mmHg. As a general rule, the pulse pressure should be no more than one-third of the systolic reading. If the pulse pressure is much larger or smaller, you need to notify the physician.

Diseases Affecting Blood Pressure. Blood pressure readings depend on the elasticity of the artery walls, the strength of the heart muscle, and the quantity and thickness of the blood. Any diseases that affect these body structures will affect blood pressure readings. Some diseases affect the size and elasticity of the arteries.

- *Arteriosclerosis* refers to a number of diseases that cause narrowing and hardening of the artery lumen, the space inside the arteries. Arteriosclerosis causes artery walls to thicken and lose elasticity.
- *Atherosclerosis* is a specific type of arteriosclerosis in which **plaque** builds up in the linings of arteries. Plaque is deposits of fatty substances and cholesterol. These deposits cause arteries to narrow and harden, reducing blood flow.

How Health Affects Blood Pressure

Sometimes a patient's family history can be a factor in a patient's blood pressure. But good general health practices can help keep the arteries and the heart healthy. Some general health practices and patient history that may affect blood pressure include:

- dietary habits
- alcohol use
- tobacco use
- exercise habits (amount and type of exercise)
- previous heart conditions

Along with the patient's general health, there are many other factors than can affect blood pressure readings.

- *Age.* As the body ages, blood vessels begin to lose elasticity. More force is needed to expand artery walls. The buildup of plaque from the process of atherosclerosis also increases the force needed for blood flow.
- *Activity.* Exercise temporarily raises blood pressure. Inactivity or rest usually lowers the pressure.
- *Weight.* People who are obese, or even just overweight, are at increased risk for developing high blood pressure.
- *Stress.* During stress, the body releases a hormone called epinephrine (also known as adrenaline). This hormone increases the heart rate and raises the blood pressure.
- *Body position.* Blood pressure normally lowers when a person is supine, or lying down on her back.
- *Medications.* Some medications lower blood pressure and others may raise it.

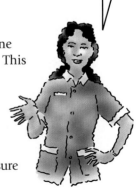

So many factors can affect blood pressure. Physicians usually diagnose high blood pressure when there have been three or four elevated readings over a period of time.

What Can Go Wrong

As a medical assistant, you need to be concerned about getting accurate assessments of vital signs. There are many possible sources of errors in taking blood pressure readings. It's important to be aware of them—and to try to avoid them. Sources of errors include:

- wrapping the cuff improperly
- failing to keep the patient's arm at the level of the heart while taking blood pressure readings
- failing to support the patient's arm on a stable surface while taking a blood pressure reading
- recording the auscultatory gap as the diastolic pressure
- failing to keep the pressure gauge at eye level
- applying the cuff over the patient's clothing and attempting to listen through clothing
- allowing the cuff to deflate too rapidly or too slowly
- failing to wait one to two minutes before rechecking the same arm
- using the wrong size cuff

If you do get a reading that is not within normal limits, recheck the blood pressure before reporting it. You might have made an error!

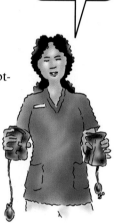

Size is important! A blood pressure measurement can be wrong by as much as 30 mmHg if the cuff size is incorrect.

Hands On   INTERVIEWING THE PATIENT   2-1
TO OBTAIN A MEDICAL HISTORY

This procedure should take about 10 to 15 minutes.

1. Gather the supplies you need—a medical history form or questionnaire and a black ink pen.

2. Review the medical history form before you speak to the patient so that you're familiar with the order of the questions and the type of information needed.

3. Take the patient to a private and comfortable area of the office. You want to ensure confidentiality and prevent distractions!

4. Sit facing the patient so you're both at the same eye level. Standing above the patient may make the patient feel threatened or uncomfortable.

5. Introduce yourself and explain the purpose of the interview.

6. Ask the appropriate questions and document the patient's responses. Make sure you determine the CC and PI.
   - Be sure to use language the patient can understand.
   - No matter what the patient tells you, be professional.
   - Take care that your words and actions don't show judgmental attitudes. You want your patient to trust you!

7. Maintain frequent eye contact to show that you're listening. This reassures the patient you're interested in what she is saying.

8. If appropriate, explain to the patient what to expect during the medical examination or procedures. Keeping the patient informed may help decrease anxiety.

9. When the interview is finished, thank the patient for cooperating. Offer to answer any questions the patient may have.

Charting Example:
07/10/06 11:00 A.M. CC: New patient checkup. Medical history form complete and in chart. Patient indicates no physical or health problems at this time. Family history of colon cancer and hypertension noted. _____ E. Parker, CMA

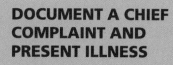

DOCUMENT A CHIEF COMPLAINT AND PRESENT ILLNESS

2-2

This procedure should take 10 minutes or less.

1. Gather supplies, including the patient's medical record containing a cumulative problem list or progress note form.

2. Review the new or established patient's medical history form. Being as familiar as possible with the patient will help you get complete information about the CC and PI.

3. Greet the patient by name and escort him to the examination room. Using the patient's name helps develop rapport and may ease any patient anxiety. Correctly identifying the patient also can help prevent mistakes!

4. Use open-ended questions to find out why the patient is seeking medical care. Be sure to maintain eye contact so the patient is aware that you're actively listening.

5. Determine the PI using open-ended and closed-ended questions. Use several open-ended questions first. Then use closed-ended questions to get more specific information.

6. Document the CC and PI on the cumulative problem list or progress report form. Include the date, time, CC, PI, and your signature (first initial, last name, and title). Use only correct medical terminology and approved abbreviations.

7. When you've finished asking questions, thank the patient for cooperating. Explain that the physician will be in soon for the examination. If you give a time frame about when the physician will arrive, be honest.

Charting Example:
06/06/2006 9:45 A.M. CC: Pt. c/o headache and nausea 3 × days. Has taken ibuprofen for the pain with "some relief." The pain is a "dull ache" in the frontal area of the head and face. No emesis. Face flushed, skin warm and dry. T 98.8°F, P 88, R 24, BP 190/110 (L) sitting. _____ S. Vincer, CMA

Hands On

MEASURING ORAL TEMPERATURE USING A MERCURY-FREE GLASS THERMOMETER

2-3

This procedure should take 10 minutes.

1. Gather the following supplies: a glass mercury-free oral thermometer with a blue top, a disposable plastic sheath, tissues or cotton balls, gloves, a biohazard waste container, and disinfectant solution. Then, wash your hands and put on gloves.

2. Dry the thermometer if it has been stored in a disinfectant solution. To dry the thermometer, use tissues or cotton balls to wipe the thermometer from the bulb up the stem. A dry thermometer will slip easily into the sheath.

3. Carefully check the thermometer for chips or cracks. A damaged thermometer could injure the patient!

4. Check the thermometer reading. Hold the stem at eye level and turn it slowly to see the liquid in the column.

5. If the reading is above 94°F, shake down the thermometer. The liquid inside must be below 94°F to provide an accurate temperature reading.
   - Grasp the thermometer carefully at the end of the stem using your thumb and forefinger.
   - Snap your wrist several times.
   - Be careful not to hit the thermometer against anything when snapping your wrist.

6. Insert the thermometer into the plastic sheath.

7. Greet the patient by name. Explain the procedure and ask about any eating, drinking of hot or cold fluids, gum chewing, or smoking within the last 15 minutes.
   - Any of these could alter the oral reading.
   - Wait 15 minutes before taking the reading or choose another method.

8. Place the thermometer under the patient's tongue to one side of the frenulum, a small strip of tissue that connects the tongue to the floor of the mouth. This area has the highest blood flow and will give the most accurate reading.

9. Ask the patient to keep the mouth and lips closed. This prevents air from entering the mouth and causing an

Hands On

MEASURING ORAL TEMPERATURE USING A MERCURY-FREE GLASS THERMOMETER (*continued*)

2-3

inaccurate reading. Remind the patient not to bite down on the thermometer.

10. Leave the thermometer in place for three to five minutes.
    • Three minutes is long enough if the patient has no evidence of fever.
    • If the patient is noncompliant and frequently talks or opens her mouth, the thermometer should be left in place for five minutes.
    • It also should be left in place for five minutes if the patient is febrile.
    • While you're waiting for a temperature reading, you can take the patient's pulse, respirations, and blood pressure.

11. When the time is up, remove the thermometer from the patient's mouth. Be sure to wear gloves!

12. Then, remove the sheath by holding the edge of the sheath with the thumb and forefinger of one hand and pulling down from the open edge over the length of the thermometer to the bulb. The soiled area should now be inside the sheath. Discard the sheath in a biohazard waste container.

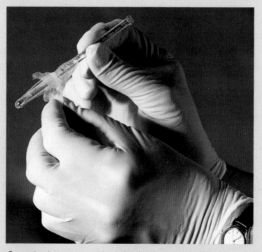

Grasp the thermometer with one hand and remove the sheath inverting the plastic toward the bulb. This way, the soiled area is inside the sheath.

(*continued*)

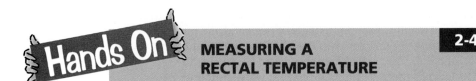

MEASURING ORAL TEMPERATURE USING A MERCURY-FREE GLASS THERMOMETER (*continued*)

2-3

13. Hold the thermometer horizontal at eye level. Note the level of liquid that has risen into the column.

14. Sanitize and disinfect the thermometer according to office policy. Remove your gloves and then wash your hands.

15. Record the temperature reading in the patient's medical record. Remember, procedures are not considered done if they are not recorded. The vital signs are usually recorded together.

Charting Example:
08/23/2006 8:30 A.M. T 100.2° (O) _____ J. Barth, CMA

MEASURING A RECTAL TEMPERATURE

2-4

This procedure should take ten minutes.

1. Gather the following supplies: a glass mercury-free rectal thermometer with a red top, a disposable plastic sheath, tissues or cotton balls, gloves, a biohazard waste container, lubricant, and disinfectant solution. Then, wash your hands and put on gloves.

2. Dry the thermometer if it has been stored in a disinfectant solution. To dry the thermometer, use tissues or cotton balls to wipe the thermometer from the bulb up the stem. A dry thermometer will slip easily into the sheath.

3. Carefully check the thermometer for chips or cracks. A damaged thermometer could injure the patient!

4. Check the thermometer reading. Hold the stem at eye level and turn it slowly to see the liquid in the column.

Hands On

MEASURING A RECTAL TEMPERATURE (*continued*)

5. If the reading is above 94°F, shake down the thermometer. The liquid inside must be below 94°F to provide an accurate temperature reading.
   - Grasp the thermometer carefully at the end of the stem using your thumb and forefinger.
   - Snap your wrist several times.
   - Be careful not to hit the thermometer against anything when snapping your wrist.

6. Insert the thermometer into the plastic sheath.

7. Spread lubricant onto a tissue and then from the tissue onto the sheath of the thermometer. Don't apply lubricant directly onto the thermometer. Lubricant should always be used for rectal insertion to prevent patient discomfort.

8. Greet the patient by name and explain the procedure.

9. Ensure the patient's privacy by placing the patient in a side-lying position facing the examination room door, if possible. If the door is opened, a patient facing the door is less likely to be exposed. Drape the patient appropriately. The side-lying position facilitates exposure to the anus.

10. Visualize the anus by lifting the top buttock with your non-dominant hand. Never insert the thermometer without first having a clear view of the anus.

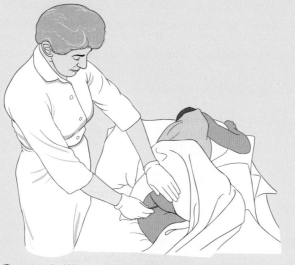

The patient should be in a side-lying position and draped appropriately to ensure patient privacy and comfort.

(*continued*)

Hands On

MEASURING A RECTAL TEMPERATURE (continued)

2-4

11. Gently insert the thermometer past the sphincter muscle. The thermometer should be inserted about 1.5 inches for an adult, 1 inch for a child, and 0.5 inch for an infant.

12. Release the upper buttock and hold the thermometer in place with your dominant hand for three minutes. The thermometer will not stay in place if you don't hold it. Replace the drape to ensure the patient's privacy, but don't move your dominant hand.

13. After three minutes, remove the thermometer and sheath. Discard the sheath in a biohazard waste container. You need to remove the sheath before reading the thermometer to get an accurate reading.

14. Hold the thermometer horizontal at eye level and note the temperature reading.

15. Give the patient a tissue to wipe away excess lubricant.

16. Sanitize and disinfect the thermometer according to office policy. Then, remove your gloves and wash your hands.

17. Record the temperature reading in the patient's medical record. Be sure to mark the letter *R* next to the reading, to show the temperature was taken rectally. Temperatures are presumed to have been taken orally unless otherwise noted.

Note: Infants and very small children may be held in your lap or over your knees for this procedure. Hold the thermometer and the buttocks with your dominant hand while securing the child with your nondominant hand. If the child moves, the thermometer and your hand will move together, avoiding injury to the anal canal.

Charting Example:
04/18/2006 10:30 A.M. T 101.4° (R) _____ Y. James, CMA

Hands On

MEASURING AN AXILLARY TEMPERATURE

This procedure should take 15 minutes.

1. Gather the following supplies: a glass mercury-free oral thermometer with a blue top, a disposable probe cover, tissues or cotton balls, gloves, a biohazard waste container, and disinfectant solution. Then, wash your hands and put on gloves.

2. Dry the thermometer if it has been stored in a disinfectant solution. To dry the thermometer, use tissues or cotton balls to wipe the thermometer from the bulb up the stem. A dry thermometer will slip easily into the sheath.

3. Carefully check the thermometer for chips or cracks. A damaged thermometer could injure the patient!

4. Check the thermometer reading. Hold the stem at eye level and turn it slowly to see the liquid in the column.

5. If the reading is above 94°F, shake down the thermometer. The liquid inside must be below 94°F to provide an accurate temperature reading.
   - Grasp the thermometer carefully at the end of the stem using your thumb and forefinger.
   - Snap your wrist several times.
   - Be careful not to hit the thermometer against anything when snapping your wrist.

6. Insert the thermometer into the probe cover. Be careful not to contaminate the sheath by touching it or placing it down on any surface.

7. Explain the procedure to the patient. Expose the patient's axilla. Don't expose more of the patient's chest or upper body than is necessary. It's important to protect the patient's privacy at all times.

8. Place the bulb of the thermometer deep in the axilla. Bring the patient's arm down, crossing the forearm over the chest. This position provides the best skin contact with the thermometer. It also provides a closed environment. Drape the patient appropriately for privacy.

(continued)

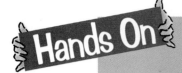 **MEASURING AN AXILLARY**
TEMPERATURE (*continued*)

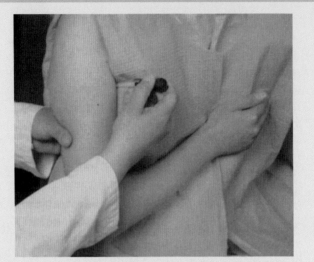

With the thermometer in the axilla, the arm should be down, and the forearm should be crossed across the chest.

9. Leave the thermometer in place for ten minutes. Axillary temperatures take longer than oral or rectal ones. You shouldn't need to hold the thermometer in place unless the patient doesn't understand that the arm must stay down.

10. At the appropriate time, remove the thermometer.
    - Remove the probe cover by holding the edge of the cover with the thumb and forefinger of one hand and pulling down from the open edge over the length of the thermometer to the bulb. The soiled area should now be inside the cover.
    - Discard the probe cover in a biohazard waste container.

11. Hold the thermometer horizontal at eye level and note the temperature reading.

12. Sanitize and disinfect the thermometer according to office policy. Then, remove your gloves and wash your hands.

13. Record the temperature reading in the patient's medical record. Be sure to mark an *A* beside it. This indicates the reading was axillary. Temperatures are presumed to have been taken orally unless otherwise noted.

Charting Example:
02/01/2006 3:45 P.M. T 97.8° (A) _____ B. DeMarcus, CMA

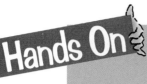

MEASURING TEMPERATURE USING AN ELECTRONIC THERMOMETER

2-6

This procedure should take five minutes.

1. Gather the following supplies: an electronic thermometer with an oral or a rectal probe, a disposable probe cover, lubricant, tissues, gloves (for rectal temperature), and a biohazard waste container. Wash your hands and put on gloves.

2. Greet the patient by name and explain the procedure.

3. Choose the most appropriate method (oral, axillary, or rectal). Attach the appropriate probe to the battery-powered temperature unit.

4. Insert the probe into the probe cover. All probes fit into one size probe cover.
   - Covers usually are carried with the unit in a specially fitted box attached to the back of the unit.
   - If you use the last probe cover, be sure to attach a new box of covers to the unit to be ready for future patients.

5. Position the thermometer appropriately, depending on the method you are using. If measuring the temperature rectally, take care to apply lubricant to the probe cover and hold the probe in place.

6. Wait for the electronic unit to beep when it senses that the temperature is no longer rising. This usually occurs within ten seconds.

7. After the beep, remove the probe. Note the temperature reading on the digital display screen on the unit.

8. Discard the probe cover in a biohazard container by depressing a button, usually on the end of the probe. Replace the probe in the slot on the unit, but make sure you've noted the temperature reading first! Most units automatically shut off when the probe is put back into the unit.

9. Remove your gloves if you are wearing them and wash your hands. Then, record the temperature in the patient's medical record. Record the reading in the same way as if you were using a glass thermometer. Indicate a rectal reading with an *R*, an oral reading with an *O*, and an axillary reading with an *A*.

Charting Example:

11/28/2006 10:15 A.M. T 101° (O) _____ D. Snap, CMA

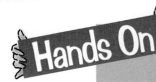

MEASURING TEMPERATURE USING A TYMPANIC THERMOMETER 2-7

This procedure should take five minutes.

1. Gather the following supplies: a tympanic thermometer, disposable probe covers, and a biohazard waste container. Wash your hands.

2. Greet the patient by name and explain the procedure.

3. Insert the ear probe into the probe cover. Always put a clean probe cover on the ear probe before taking a temperature.

4. With your nondominant hand, straighten the patient's ear canal. Place the end of the ear probe in the patient's ear with your dominant hand.
   - For most patients, you straighten the ear canal by pulling the top posterior part of the outer ear up and back.
   - For children under three, pull the outer ear down and back.

5. With the ear probe properly placed in the ear canal, press the button on the thermometer. The reading will be shown on the digital display in about two seconds.

6. Remove the probe and note the reading. Discard the probe cover in a biohazard waste container. Probe covers are for one use only. Then, wash your hands.

7. Record the temperature on the patient's record in the same way that you record temperatures for a glass thermometer. Be sure to indicate that the tympanic temperature was taken.

Charting Example:
04/15/2006 2:25 P.M. T 99.4°tympanic _____ M. Smythe, CMA

Hands On

MEASURING THE RADIAL PULSE

2-8

This procedure should take three to five minutes.

1. Wash your hands first.

2. Greet the patient by name if you haven't already done so and explain the procedure. In most cases, the pulse is taken at the same time as other vital signs.

3. Position the patient so the arm is relaxed. The arm should be supported either on the patient's lap or on a table. If the arm is not supported, or the patient is uncomfortable, it may be hard to find the pulse.

4. Use the index, middle, and ring fingers of your dominant hand to find the pulse.
   - Don't use your thumb—it has a pulse of its own that can be confused with the patient's pulse.
   - You may place your thumb on the opposite side of the patient's wrist to steady your hand.

5. Press your fingers on the pulse point. Press firmly enough to feel the pulse. Pressing too firmly can cause the pulse to disappear.
   - If the pulse is regular, count it for 30 seconds, watching the second hand of your watch. Multiply the number of pulsations by 2 since the pulse is always recorded as the number of beats per minute.
   - If the pulse is irregular, count it for a full 60 seconds. Otherwise, the measurement may be inaccurate.

6. Record the pulse rate in the patient's medical record with the other vital signs. Make a note and notify the doctor if the rhythm is irregular and the volume is thready or bounding.

Charting Example:
06/16/2006 11:30 A.M. Pulse 78; irregular and thready. Doctor notified. _____ E. Kramer, CMA

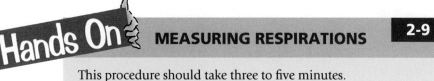

Hands On   **MEASURING RESPIRATIONS**   2-9

This procedure should take three to five minutes.

1. Wash your hands.

2. Greet the patient by name if you haven't already.

3. Observe carefully for the easiest area to assess respirations. Some patients have abdominal movement instead of chest movement during respirations.

4. In most cases, respirations are measured at the same time as the pulse. After counting the radial pulse, continue to watch the second hand of your watch. Begin counting respirations. Count a complete rise and fall of the patient's chest as one respiration.
   - It's best not to inform the patient that you are counting respirations. A patient who is aware that you are counting respirations may alter his breathing pattern.

5. If the breathing pattern is regular, count the respiratory rate for 30 seconds. Then multiply by 2. If the pattern is irregular, count for a full 60 seconds. Otherwise, the measurement may be inaccurate.

6. Record the respiratory rate in the patient's medical record along with the other vital signs. Also, note the rhythm if irregular. Mark down any unusual sounds, such as wheezing.

Charting Example:
08/17/2006 8:45 A.M. Respirations 30. Rapid, shallow, and labored. Doctor notified. _____ J. Thompson, CMA

Hands On   MEASURING BLOOD PRESSURE   2-10

This procedure should take five minutes.

1. Wash your hands and gather a sphygmomanometer and a stethoscope.

2. Greet the patient by name and explain the procedure.

3. Position the patient with the arm to be used supported with the forearm on the lap or a table. The patient's right arm is commonly used, unless there is a medical reason not to, such as a recent surgery. This will be noted in the patient's medical record. Note the optimal positioning of the arm.
   - The arm should be slightly flexed, with the palm upward. This makes it easier to find and palpate the brachial artery.
   - The upper arm should be level with the patient's heart. If the upper arm is higher or lower than the heart, the reading may be inaccurate.

4. Expose the patient's arm. Clothing over the area can block out the sounds you'll need to hear. If the sleeve is pulled up, ensure it isn't tight. A too-tight sleeve can act as a tourniquet, decreasing the flow of blood and causing an inaccurate blood pressure reading. Make sure the patient's legs are not crossed and ask the patient to not talk during the procedure.

5. Palpate the brachial pulse in the antecubital area—the region of the arm in front of the elbow.
   - Center the deflated cuff directly over the brachial artery.
   - The lower edge of the cuff should be one to two inches above the antecubital area.
   - If the cuff is too low, it may interfere with placement of the stethoscope and cause noises that obscure the Korotkoff sounds.

6. Wrap the cuff smoothly and snugly around the arm. Secure the cuff with the Velcro edges.

7. Hold the air pump in your dominant hand, with the valve between your thumb and forefinger. Turn the valve screw clockwise to tighten it. The cuff will not inflate with the valve open.
   - Be careful not to make the valve screw so tight that it's hard to release. You need to be able to loosen it with one hand after the cuff is inflated.

(continued)

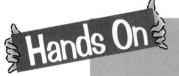

MEASURING BLOOD PRESSURE (*continued*)

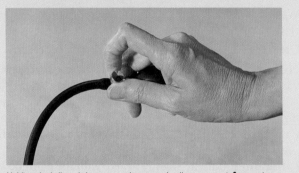

Holding the bulb and the screw valve properly allows you to inflate and deflate the cuff easily.

8. First, determine a reference point for how far you need to inflate the cuff.
   - While palpating the brachial pulse with your nondominant hand, inflate the cuff.
   - Note the point or number on the dial or glass tube column at which you no longer feel the brachial pulse.
   - This will give you a reference point for reinflating the cuff when taking the blood pressure.

9. Deflate the cuff by turning the valve counterclockwise. Wait at least 30 seconds before reinflating the cuff. The waiting time allows blood circulation to return to the extremity.

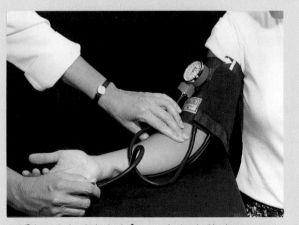

Palpate the brachial pulse before auscultating the blood pressure.

Hands On

MEASURING BLOOD PRESSURE (*continued*)

2-10

10. Clean the earpieces of the stethoscope with an alcohol wipe. Place the stethoscope earpieces in your ears with the openings pointed slightly forward. Stand about 18 inches from the manometer with the gauge at eye level to reduce the chances of making an error while taking the reading.

11. Place the diaphragm of the stethoscope against the brachial artery and hold it in place with your nondominant hand. Don't press too hard or you may obliterate the pulse. On the other hand, if you don't press firmly enough, you may not hear the sounds.
    * The stethoscope tubing should hang freely without touching or rubbing any part of the cuff. If the stethoscope rubs or touches any other objects, environmental sounds may make the Korotkoff sounds impossible to hear.

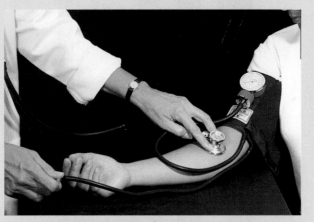

Hold the stethoscope diaphragm firmly against the brachial artery.

12. With your dominant hand, turn the screw near the bulb just enough to close the valve. Inflate the cuff.
    * Pump the valve bulb to about 30 mmHg above the number you noted during step 8.
    * Inflating more than 30 mmHg above the baseline is uncomfortable for the patient and unnecessary. But if you don't inflate the cuff enough, the systolic reading may be inaccurate.

(*continued*)

Hands On

MEASURING BLOOD PRESSURE (*continued*)

2-10

13. Once the cuff is inflated appropriately, turn the valve counterclockwise. You want to release the air at about 2 to 4 mmHg per second.
    - Releasing the air too fast will cause missed beats.
    - Releasing it too slowly will interfere with circulation.

14. Listen carefully while watching the gauge. Aneroid and mercury-free measurements are always made as even numbers, because of the way the manometer is calibrated.
    - Note the point on the gauge at which you hear the first clear tapping sound. This is the systolic sound or Korotkoff phase 1.

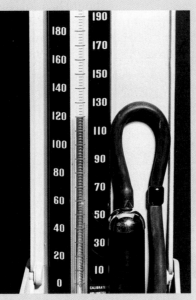

Step 14A. The meniscus on the mercury-free column in this example reads 120 mmHg.

15. Continue to listen and deflate the cuff. When you hear the last sound, note the reading, and quickly deflate the cuff.
    - The last sound heard is the Korotkoff phase 5 sound. It is recorded as the diastolic pressure or the bottom number.
    - If you are unsure of the reading, wait 1 to 2 minutes before repeating the procedure. Never immediately reinflate the cuff.

Hands On

MEASURING BLOOD PRESSURE (continued)

2-10

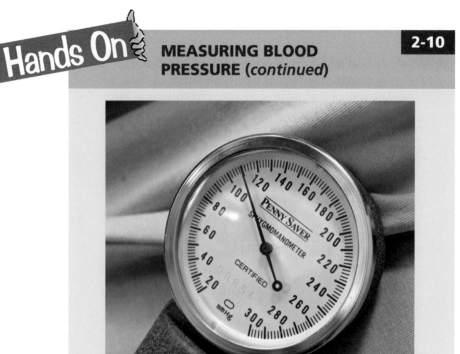

Step 14B. The gauge on the aneroid manometer reads 110 mmHg.

16. Remove the stethoscope earpieces from your ears. Remove the cuff and press any remaining air from the bladder of the cuff.
    - If this is the first reading or a new patient, the physician may also want a reading in the other arm or in another position.
    - In some patients, blood pressure varies between the arms or in different positions such as lying or standing.

17. When all readings are finished, put the equipment away and wash your hands.

18. Record the reading. The systolic pressure is always written as a fraction over the diastolic pressure (for example, 120/80). Note which arm was used—RA for right arm, or LA for left arm. Record the patient's position if other than sitting.

Charting Example:
11/28/2006 3:30 P.M. T 98.6°(O), P 78, R 16, BP 130/90 (LA) sitting, 128/88 (LA) standing _____ Y. Torres, CMA

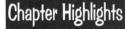

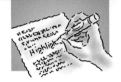

- Medical assistants may need to collect information for the patient's medical history and medical assessment. The role of the medical assistant in collecting information depends on the policies of the medical office.

- The medical history provides the physician with a basis for asking questions during an examination. It also helps the physician understand how the patient's illness and lifestyle interact.

- During an assessment, patients are interviewed to establish signs and symptoms of illness. For each visit, a chief complaint and present illness are documented in the patient's record.

- Physical measurements also provide information about a patient's health. Medical assistants may collect anthropometric measurements and measure vital signs.

- Anthropometric measurements for adults typically include height and weight. Pediatric measurements may also include head and chest circumference.

- Body temperature reflects the balance between heat produced and heat lost by the body. The type of thermometer used for measuring temperature depends on the practices of the medical office.

- Four different methods for taking temperature are oral, rectal, axillary, and tympanic. The method must be documented in the patient's medical record, along with the reading.

- Pulse and respiration rates are often measured at the same time. Three important characteristics of the pulse are the rate, rhythm, and volume. Important characteristics of respirations are the rate, rhythm, and depth.

- Blood pressure is measured during two phases of the cardiac cycle called systole and diastole. Five phases of Korotkoff sounds can be identified with a stethoscope. The systolic pressure reading is measured during phase 1. The diastolic pressure reading occurs during phase 5.

- Measuring blood pressure can be tricky. By being aware of possible sources of errors, medical assistants can make sure their readings are accurate.

Chapter 3

ASSISTING WITH THE PHYSICAL EXAMINATION

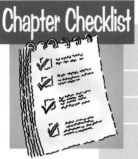

Chapter Checklist

- Identify the medical assistant's responsibilities before, during, and after the physical examination

- List the supplies typically needed in an examination room

- Prepare and maintain examination and treatment areas

- Explain the use of the common and specialized instruments used in a physical examination

- Describe the six basic techniques for examining patients

- Prepare patients for and assist with routine and specialty examinations

- Describe the basic examination positions and their uses

- Explain the typical procedures for examining different body structures

- List the basic sequence of the physical examination

- Explain how the physician tests posture, gait, and reflexes

- Teach patients how to recognize cancer warning signs

- List the guidelines for general physical examinations, immunizations, and cancer screening

Some patients will come to the medical office only for a physical examination. A complete physical exam allows the physician to assess the patient's general state of health. It helps the physician to detect signs and symptoms of disease.

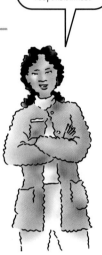

You can play an important role in each part of patient assessment. Be sure you know your responsibilities.

Physical Examinations

New patients usually get a complete physical exam to give the physician baseline information about their health. Then the physician can use this information as a reference for future comparisons. It also can help the physician in diagnosis—identifying a disease or condition.

Other patients come to the office for routine examinations. These are performed at regular intervals. They help maintain a patient's health and prevent disease.

The physical examination is part of the process of patient assessment. Assessing a patient has three phases:

- the medical history
- the physical examination
- any laboratory and diagnostic tests

YOUR RESPONSIBILITIES FOR PHYSICAL EXAMINATIONS

Your duties will depend on your office's policies and practices. But here are some of the things you may be responsible for:

- assisting with or taking the medical history
- preparing the patient for examination
- assisting the physician during the examination
- collecting specimens for diagnostic testing

INSTRUMENTS AND SUPPLIES

Many different instruments are used during the physical exam. They help the examiner see, hear, or feel the areas of the patient's body that are being assessed. In most cases, the physician is the one who uses the instruments. However, you should be familiar with the instruments and supplies so you're prepared to assist.

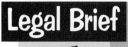
WHY YOUR PRESENCE MAY BE REQUIRED

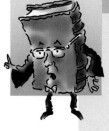

Depending on the policies in your medical office, you may be required to remain in the room during the physical examination. The American Medical Association (AMA) recommends that a third party—someone other than the physician and patient—be present during a physical examination. Your presence provides legal protection for the physician if there are any misunderstandings or accusations by the patient.

Even if the medical assistants in your office do not routinely remain in the room during a physical exam, you may be asked to do so if the patient requests your presence.

Instruments should be kept in a special tray or drawer in each examination room. The exact instruments and supplies you'll find there depend on the preferences of the physician. But some basic supplies always should be available during the physical examination. These include the following:

- *Tape measure.* A standard flexible tape measure is used to take measurements of parts of the patient's body. The units on the tape measure may be in inches or centimeters, depending on the physician's preference.
- *Gloves.* Latex and latex-free gloves must be in the examining room for use whenever there may be contact with body fluids or broken skin.

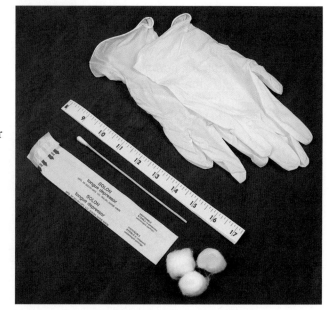

Common supplies used in the adult physical examination include gloves, a tape measure, cotton-tipped applicators, and tongue depressors.

- *Tongue depressors.* This thin disposable tool is used to press down the tongue during examination of the mouth and throat.
- *Cotton-tipped* **applicators.** These cotton-tipped swabs can have many uses during the exam, including testing sensory reactions and collecting samples.

Percussion Hammer

This instrument is sometimes called a reflex hammer. It is used to test **neurological reflexes.** These are responses by the body's nervous system to specific stimuli. The percussion hammer has a stainless steel handle and a hard rubber head. It's used to test reflexes by striking **tendons.** These are tough cords of tissue that connect muscle to bone.

The tip of the handle also may be used on the sole of the foot to assess the **Babinski reflex**—an abnormal reflex where stroking the sole of the foot causes the big toe to move upward. The Babinski reflex is a sign of brain or spinal cord injury (except in children under two where it is the normal response). Normally, stroking the sole of the foot results in the toes curling downward in the plantar reflex.

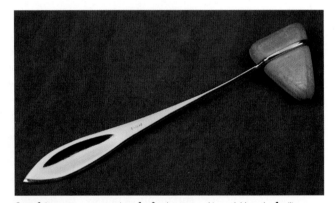

One of the most common styles of reflex hammers, this model has the familiar triangular rubber tip.

Tuning Fork

The tuning fork is used to test hearing. It's a stainless steel instrument with two prongs at one end and a handle at the other. The examiner strikes the instrument against her hand, causing the

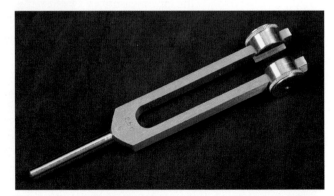

The tuning fork helps the physician determine whether the patient needs additional auditory tests.

prongs to vibrate. The vibrating prongs produce a humming sound. While it's vibrating, the examiner places its handle against a bony area of the patient's skull, near one of the ears. The patient is asked to describe what, if anything, he is hearing in that ear. The results of this test may lead the physician to order additional auditory tests.

Nasal Speculum

This stainless steel instrument is inserted into the nostril to help the examiner see inside. The nasal **speculum** also may be available in a disposable form. A speculum is a tool designed to allow examiners to investigate body cavities. Using the nasal speculum, the physician inspects:

- the lining of the nose
- the nasal membranes
- the septum, a thin wall between the nostrils that divides the two nasal cavities

A nasal speculum can help physicians see some nasal abnormalities.

Otoscope

The otoscope allows the examiner to see inside the ear canal and inspect the **tympanic membrane.** Also known as the ear drum, the tympanic membrane is a thin, oval membrane between the outer ear and middle ear. It transmits sound vibrations to the inner ear.

The otoscope has a stainless steel handle at one end. At the other end is a head that consists of three parts:

- a light
- a magnifying lens
- a cone-shaped hollow speculum

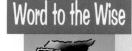

Word to the Wise

speculum (SPEK-yuh-luhm)

a medical tool that enlarges and separates the opening of a body cavity so the examiner can see the interior

The speculum is covered with a disposable cover before it's placed in the ear canal.

Some otoscopes are portable. Batteries in the handle provide power for the light. Other otoscopes are part of a unit attached to a wall. The unit is plugged into an electrical outlet to provide power.

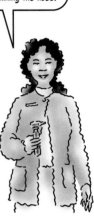

Some otoscopes may have a specialized nasal speculum tip for examining the nose.

Ophthalmoscope

The ophthalmoscope allows the examiner to inspect the interior structures of the eyes. Like the otoscope, the ophthalmoscope has a handle at one end and a head with several parts:

- a light
- a magnifying lens
- an opening to view the eye

Some units are portable, with batteries in the handles. A portable unit also may have a common handle with otoscope or ophthalmoscope tips that can be attached for different examinations.

Stethoscope

You're probably familiar with the stethoscope, an instrument used for listening to body sounds. It has a bell with a diaphragm at one end. Flexible rubber tubing connects the bell to two earpieces. The earpieces have plastic or rubber tips that must be adjusted and directed inward before they are placed in the examiner's ears.

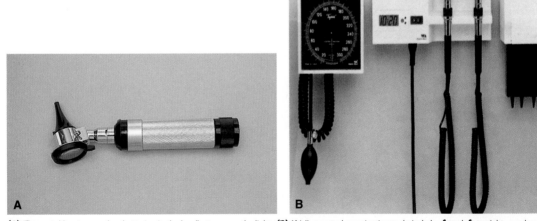

A

B

(A) The portable otoscope has batteries in the handle to power the light. (B) Wall-mounted examination tools include, from left to right, a sphygmomanometer with a cuff, an ophthalmoscope, an otoscope, and a dispenser for disposable otoscope speculum covers.

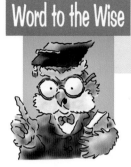

ophthalmoscope (off-THAL-muh-skope)

a medical tool used to inspect the interior structures of the eyes

The diaphragm is placed on the patient's body, and the examiner listens to sounds through the earpieces. The stethoscope is typically used to listen to sounds of the:

- heart
- lungs
- intestines
- carotid arteries

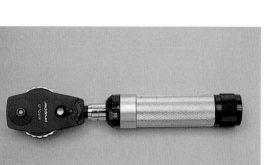

This portable ophthalmoscope is used to examine the retina and other parts of the eye's interior.

INSTRUMENTS AND SUPPLIES FOR SPECIALIZED EXAMINATIONS

Some medical specialties may require extra equipment and supplies. Along with the basic instruments already described, you may need to be familiar with some specialized equipment.

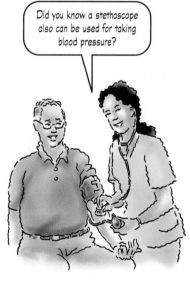

Did you know a stethoscope also can be used for taking blood pressure?

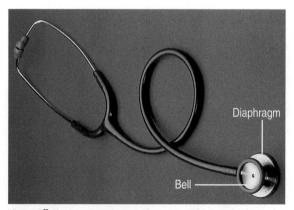

Diaphragm

Bell

It's not difficult to use a stethoscope, but you must be trained to know what to listen for.

Closer Look

GETTING THE LIGHTS RIGHT

Special lights help the physician see more clearly during physical exams. It's your responsibility to make sure all these lights are in working order.

- *Overhead examination light.* Some offices have an adjustable overhead examination light.
- *Gooseneck lamp.* This is a floor lamp with a movable stand that bends at the neck. The physician may use this lamp when overhead lighting is not good enough.
- *Penlight.* This small light is the size and shape of a ballpoint pen. It can be carried conveniently in a pocket. If no penlight is available, a small flashlight is a good substitute. These small lights provide extra light to a specific area, such as the eye, nose, or throat.

While assisting the physician, you may be asked to direct the examination light or the gooseneck lamp toward a specific area of the body. The physician usually holds the penlight.

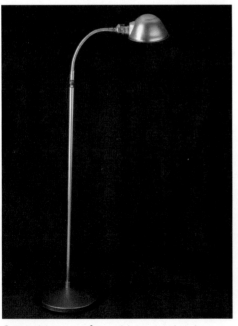

Gooseneck lamps are often used during gynecological examinations.

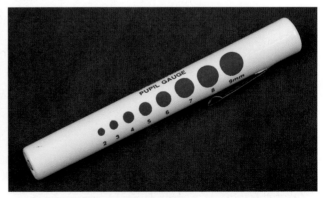

The penlight offers a directed beam of light for more precise illumination.

Ear, Nose, and Throat

An otorhinolaryngologist (ear, nose, and throat specialist) may wear a head light or head mirror during examinations. The instrument consists of a light or mirror attached to a headband. A head light provides direct light to the area being examined. A mirror reflects light from the examination light into the area.

Other special instruments help the physician look at the throat and the **larynx**—the part of the throat that contains the vocal cords.

- The laryngeal mirror is a stainless steel instrument with a long slender handle and a small round mirror. It's used to examine areas of the patient's throat and larynx that may not be directly visible.

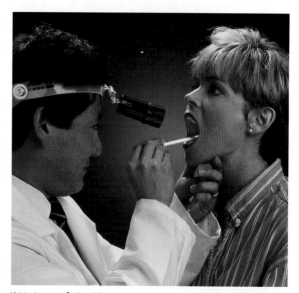

- The laryngoscope consists of a handle and a head. The handle is similar to the battery handle of an otoscope or ophthalmoscope. The head has a small light. Different blades can be attached to the head to help the examiner see the larynx or vocal cords. The blades may be curved or straight.

With the use of a head light, the physician can have both hands free to examine the patient.

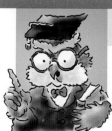

Word to the Wise   **Otorhinolaryngologist** (O-to-RI-no-LAR-in-GOL-uh-jist)

a physician who specializes in treating disorders and diseases of the ears, nose, and throat

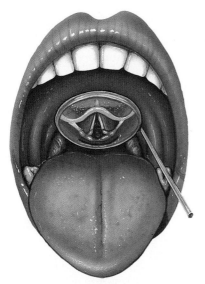

The laryngeal mirror gives the examiner a good view of a patient's throat and larynx.

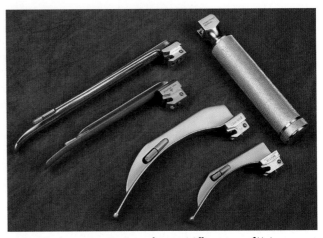

One laryngoscope handle can fit several different types of blades.

For Women Only

A general physical examination of female patients may include a pelvic examination and a **Papanicolaou (Pap) smear.** A Pap smear is a sample of secretions and cells of the vagina or

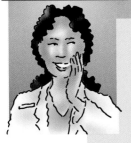

Secrets for Success

SPECIAL ROLES FOR CLINICAL MEDICAL ASSISTANTS

Clinical medical assistants who work in specialized medical offices may need to be familiar with other supplies and instruments. Some examples of specialized medical assistants include:

- *Ophthalmic medical assistants* help with eye care and assist ophthalmologists. Some of their duties may include testing eye muscle function or teaching patients how to use and care for contact lenses. They also maintain optical instruments related to eye examinations and eye care.

- *Podiatric medical assistants* help podiatrists—physicians who are trained to care for feet and treat foot disease. These medical assistants may need to make castings of feet, develop x-rays, or assist with foot surgery.

cervix—the lower part of the uterus where vagina and uterus join. The smear is examined with a microscope to detect any abnormal cells, including cancer cells.

Vaginal Speculum. The vaginal speculum is an instrument made of stainless steel or disposable plastic. It's inserted into the vagina to expand the opening. The physician can then examine internal reproductive structures or obtain the cells needed for a Pap smear.

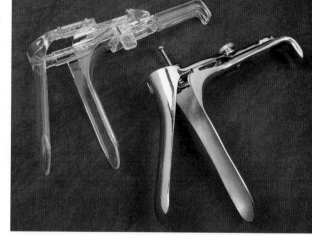

A vaginal speculum may be either plastic or metal. Metal specula are often warmed before use.

Cell Collection. The physician has special instruments to collect vaginal or cervical cells.

- *Cotton-tipped applicator.* This applicator is larger than the small cotton-tipped swabs with which you may be familiar. Often, it is used to remove excess vaginal secretions or to apply medications during gynecological examinations.

- *Ayre spatula* or *cervical scraper.* This scraper is about six inches long and is made of plastic or wood. At each end, there is a different tip. One end has a tip with an irregular shape. It is placed in the cervical opening and rotated to collect a specimen. The other end of the scraper has a rounded tip. This end may be used to collect a specimen from the vagina.

- *Histobrush.* This brush is made of nylon or plastic with soft bristles at one end. It may be used to obtain cells for a Pap smear.

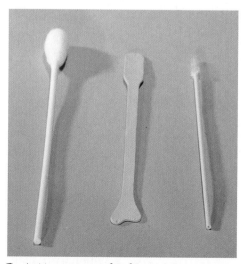

The physician may use any of the following during a pelvic exam to obtain samples for laboratory testing: cotton-tipped applicator (<u>left</u>), Ayre spatula (<u>center</u>), and histobrush (<u>right</u>).

In a traditional Pap smear, cells collected with the scraper, spatula or brush are transferred to a glass slide. In a newer, more accurate test called a Thin Prep Pap Smear, the cells are removed from the brush or plastic spatula by swirling it in a special liquid preservative. The glass slide or solution is then sent to a laboratory for processing and analysis.

Lubricant

Lubricant is a water-soluble gel used to reduce friction. It can be used for both male and female physical exams. In females, lubricant allows a vaginal speculum to be inserted easily during the pelvic examination. After cells are obtained for a Pap smear, lubricant may be used for a **bimanual examination.** In a bimanual examination, two fingers from a gloved, lubricated hand are inserted into the vagina. The other hand is placed on the abdomen. This allows the physician to palpate internal structures in the pelvic cavity. Lubricant also may be used for rectal examinations in both male and female patients and during prostate exams for males.

> Even though you won't perform some of these exams, you'll want to be familiar with what the physician is doing so you can help and document information.

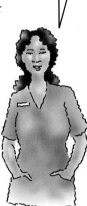

EXAMINATION TECHNIQUES

The physician uses several different techniques during an examination. These techniques help the physician gather information about the patient's health. There are six basic techniques:

- inspection
- palpation
- manipulation
- percussion
- auscultation
- mensuration

> Breath odors aren't just unpleasant—they can indicate disease! A fruity smell may be a sign of diabetes.

Inspection

Inspection is looking at areas of the body to observe physical features. The physician inspects the patient both with the naked eye and with instruments. Inspection may be done using room lighting or using a special light source. The physician reviews the patient's general appearance, including:

- movements
- color of skin and membranes
- contours or shapes
- **symmetry** (equality of size and shape) or **asymmetry** (inequality of size and shape)
- odors

Palpation

As you learned in Chapter 2, palpation is touching or moving body areas with the fingers or hands. The physician palpates areas of the body for several reasons:

- to determine pulse characteristics
- to detect the presence of growths, swelling, tenderness, or pain
- to assess the size, shape, and location of organs
- to assess skin temperature, moisture, texture, and elasticity

Palpation performed with both hands is called bimanual palpation. Palpation performed with the fingers only is a **digital examination.**

Manipulation

When the physician moves the patient's joints or body parts, it is called **manipulation.** She moves the patient's limbs to check **extension** and **flexion.** Extension is a movement of the joint that increases the angle between the bones at the joint. Flexion refers to bending a limb at the joint to decrease the angle between the bones. Extending and flexing the joints helps the examiner determine the **range of motion (ROM)**—the ability of the joint to go through normal motions.

Percussion

The **percussion** technique involves tapping or striking parts of the body with the hand or an instrument to produce sounds. Percussion allows the physician to determine the position, size, and density of the air or fluid that is inside a body organ or cavity. Two types of percussion are performed with the hand.

- *Direct percussion* refers to striking the body with a finger.
- *Indirect percussion* is placing a finger on an area of the body and then striking the finger with a finger of the other hand.

For both kinds of percussion, the physician listens for sounds and feels the vibrations.

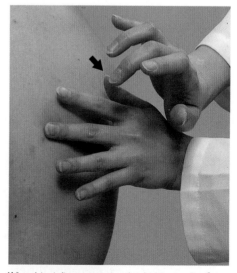

When doing indirect percussion, the physician taps her finger instead of the patient directly.

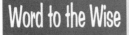

Word to the Wise

Auscultation (AW-skuhl-TAY-shun)

the act of listening to sounds within the body to evaluate the heart, lungs, intestines, or fetal heart tones

Auscultation

In **auscultation,** the examiner listens to body sounds. She places a stethoscope or her ear directly on areas of the patient's body. Areas of the body that can be auscultated include:

- the heart
- the lungs
- the abdomen
- blood vessels

Mensuration

Mensuration is the process of measuring. It includes measurement of:

- the patient's height
- the patient's weight
- the pressure of the patient's grip
- the flexion and extension in an extremity
- the size and depth of a wound

In some cases, head, chest, or waist circumference is measured. The length and circumference of a patient's limb may also be measured. If the patient is pregnant, her uterus may be measured as well.

The Medical Assistant's Role

As a clinical medical assistant, you can have five areas of responsibility in assisting with physical examinations:

- preparing the examination room
- preparing the patient

- assisting the physician
- assisting with follow-up procedures
- cleaning the examination room

PREPARING THE EXAMINATION ROOM

Medical assistants are usually asked to prepare examination rooms. The room should be clean, well-lighted, well-ventilated, odor free, and at a comfortable temperature for the patient. You must check several things in getting the room ready.

> Be prepared! Check the batteries in otoscopes, ophthalmoscopes, and laryngoscopes every day and replace them if necessary.

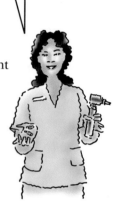

- *Examination table.* The table should be cleaned between patients with an approved disinfectant. You must remove used table paper and replace it with clean paper.
- *Equipment.* Part of your job is to make sure the equipment is in working order at the beginning of each day. It should all be clean and ready to use.
- *Supplies.* Make sure the room has a supply of gloves, cotton-tipped applicators, and other supplies needed during an examination.

You'll find specific steps for preparing and cleaning the examination room in the Hands On procedure on page 142.

PREPARING THE PATIENT

After the room is ready, you can call the patient to the treatment area. Call for the patient by name and escort her to the examination room. You'll find details about preparing the patient for the physical examination in the Hands On procedure on page 144.

Your good interpersonal skills are essential when dealing with each patient. You want to put the patient at ease and increase her confidence in you and the physician. Treat each patient as an individual. Speak clearly with a confident tone of voice as you explain any procedures.

> Remember, your goal is to create a positive, supportive, caring, and friendly atmosphere.

Gathering Information

Before the physician sees the patient, you may be responsible for recording the patient's medical history, chief complaint, and vital signs (as explained in Chapter 2). If a urine specimen is needed, follow the appropriate steps.

- explain how to obtain the specimen
- direct the patient to the washroom
- explain what to do with the specimen once it has been collected

Ask the Professional   BRIDGING CULTURAL DIFFERENCES

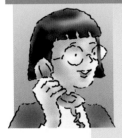

Q: *Some of the patients who come to our office have different cultural backgrounds. How do I help them understand what I need them to do?*

A: Patients from different cultures may have expectations and reactions to treatment that are based on their experiences in other countries. To help patients who may not be familiar with medical procedures in the United States, you need to provide careful explanations and lots of reassurance. You also must be sensitive to the fact that people from another culture may have practices and values that are different from your own.

- Listen carefully to the patient's concerns. If you don't understand something, ask the patient to repeat it. Be aware that in some cultures, the husband speaks for his wife and she will not speak to you directly.

- Explain the examination procedures clearly. Details that are obvious to you may not be clear to your patient. Be aware that in some cultures, direct eye contact, touching or getting too close to the patient, or pointing with your finger are considered rude or disrespectful.

- You may need to explain why the patient needs to disrobe during the procedure. Tell the patient that you will help to keep him or her covered as much as possible. Explain that the physician only looks at one part of the body at a time during the examination. Be aware that in some cultures, a female's clothing may not be removed unless a female family member is present.

- Make sure the patient knows that you and the physician will both protect his privacy. Offer extra drapes if you think it will help the patient feel more at ease. Be aware that in some cultures, a female health care worker cannot touch a male patient.

- Talk to the physician if the patient doesn't want to follow your instructions. Maybe the physician and the patient can reach a compromise that will allow the examination to be performed.

Getting Ready for the Examination

In the examination room, give the patient instructions for disrobing. You'll need to explain which clothes to remove and how to put on an examination gown. Depending on the type of exam to be performed, patients may wear the gown with the opening at the front or at the back. For example, a patient who's having a breast exam needs to wear the gown so it opens at the front.

Medical assistants normally leave the room while the patient undresses. This protects the patient's privacy.

Patients with Special Needs

Some patients may need extra assistance to get ready for the examination.

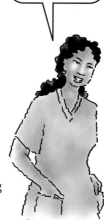

> Part of your job is to keep patients safe. If a patient is unsteady or seems confused, wait with him or her until the physician arrives.

- Elderly patients or patients with physical disabilities may use wheelchairs, walkers, or canes to move from place to place. In the examination room, they may need your help to disrobe, to move onto the examination table, and/or to move into different positions during the examination.
- Pregnant patients may need help to move onto the examination table or to assume different positions during the examination. Some examination positions may not be suitable for women in the later stages of pregnancy. (You'll read about examination positions shortly.)

The Hands On procedure on page 145 provides steps for assisting a patient in a wheelchair. To learn more about helping pregnant women during the physical examination, read the Hands On procedure on page 147.

WAITING FOR THE PHYSICIAN

After the patient is dressed appropriately, there are some things you can do to be sure the patient is ready for the physician.

- Ask the patient to sit on the exam table. Some patients may need your help to get onto the table.
- Cover the patient's legs with a drape.
- Place the chart outside the examining room door.

When the patient is ready, you can notify the physician that the patient is ready.

Running Smoothly   PROTECTING PATIENTS' PRIVACY

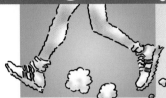

You may encounter patients who aren't able to undress themselves. Patients who might require help disrobing include elderly patients, patients who are very weak or ill, and young children. You should provide assistance when necessary. Remove the patient's clothing and cover exposed areas quickly with a gown or a sheet. Here are some more tips for protecting patient privacy:

- Make sure the door is closed or that the patient is in a screened area when changing.

- Don't ask a patient who is wearing a gown to walk through public areas, such as the waiting room, to get to other rooms.

- Expose only the body parts that are needed for the examination. Use drapes to cover exposed body areas.

ASSISTING THE PHYSICIAN

As a medical assistant, your responsibilities involve assisting the physician as well as the patient.

- *Helping the physician.* You may need to hand the physician instruments or supplies or direct an examination light. For legal reasons, you also may be required to remain in the room when a male physician examines a female patient or when a female physician examines a male patient.

- *Helping the patient.* You may need to help the patient get into the proper position. You'll also need to adjust the drape to expose only the parts of the body being examined.

The steps to follow in assisting with a physical examination are described in the Hands On procedure on page 148.

Moving the Patient

During a physical examination, the physician needs to check many different body parts. The patient may need to take a certain position so the physician can see or palpate the area. You may need to help by guiding the patient into the position.

Move the patient's body slowly. Watch for signs that the patient feels uncomfortable. You may be able to provide a small pillow or slightly adjust a position to help the patient feel more at ease.

Patient Examination Positions

As the patient changes positions, be sure to adjust the drapes to protect patient privacy. Here are the different patient examination positions. You also can review the table on page 126 to see the typical uses for each examination position and the instruments the physician will need.

Erect or Standing Position. In the erect or standing position, the patient stands erect and faces forward with the arms at the sides.

Sitting Position. In the sitting position, the patient sits erect at the end of the examination table. The feet are supported on a footrest or stool. Because the back is not supported, this position may be difficult for weak or elderly patients. Another option is the supine position.

Supine Position. In the supine position, the patient lies on his back with arms at the sides. A pillow may be placed under the head for comfort. Most patients are comfortable in this position.

Dorsal Recumbent Position. In the dorsal recumbent position, the patient is supine. The legs are separated, and the knees are bent with the feet flat on the table. Because the knees are bent, this position places less stress on the back. Some elderly patients or patients with back pain may find this position more comfortable than the supine position.

Lithotomy Position. The lithotomy position is similar to the dorsal recumbent position. However, the patient's feet are in stirrups instead of flat on the table. The stirrups should be level with each other, about 12 inches out from the edge of the table. You may help patients move their feet in and out of the stirrups. Moving both feet at the same time prevents back strain. For patients who have difficulty getting into this position, the dorsal recumbent position is an alternative.

Sims' Position. In Sims' position, the patient lies on the left side, with the left arm and left shoulder behind the body. The right leg and arm are sharply flexed on the table. The left knee is slightly flexed. Patients who are uncomfortable lying on their sides, such as those with hip joint problems, may find this position difficult.

Prone Position. In the prone position, the patient lies on the abdomen with the head supported and turned to one side. The arms may be under the head or by the sides, depending on which is more comfortable for the patient. Patients who are obese or in their later stages of pregnancy should not be asked to take this position. It may also be too uncomfortable for elderly patients or patients with breathing difficulties.

Knee-Chest Position. In the knee-chest position, the patient kneels on the table with the arms and chest on the table, hips in the air, and back straight. The patient's head is turned to one side. You may need to help guide the patient into the correct position. Elderly patients, pregnant patients, or obese patients may find this position difficult.

Fowler's Position. In the Fowler's position, the head of the examination table is elevated 80 to 90 degrees. The patient's torso is upright, and the legs are extended on the examination table (sitting with legs out in front).

Semi-Fowler's Position. In the semi-Fowler's position, the examination table head is elevated 30 to 45 degrees. The patient is in a half-sitting position with the knees slightly bent.

Trendelenburg Position. In the Trendelenburg position, the patient lies supine on the table. The lower end of the table is raised about 30 degrees so the head is lower than the feet and legs. This position is not used commonly in a medical office setting.

Reverse Trendelenburg Position. In the reverse Trendelenburg position, the patient lies supine on the table with the head higher than the feet and legs. The head of the table is elevated about 30 degrees to reach this position.

Ask the Professional   PROVIDING REASSURANCE

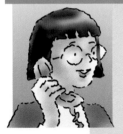

Q: *While I was assisting the physician during an examination, I noticed that the patient seemed to be grimacing and wincing as if in pain. What should I do in that situation?*

A: While you're assisting the physician, watch the patient for signs of anxiety or discomfort. Sometimes patients may verbally express discomfort during the examination. Other times, their body language or facial expressions may indicate their feelings. Being supportive and reassuring will help patients feel more comfortable and less anxious. Sometimes an alternative body position may need to be tried in order to make the patient more comfortable.

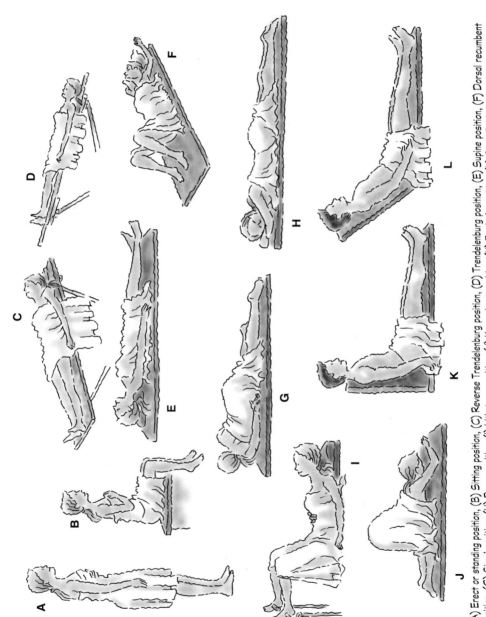

(A) Erect or standing position, (B) Sitting position, (C) Reverse Trendelenburg position, (D) Trendelenburg position, (E) Supine position, (F) Dorsal recumbent position, (G) Sims' position, (H) Prone position, (I) Lithotomy position, (J) Knee-chest position, (K) Fowler's position, (L) Semi-Fowler's position.

Examination Positions and Their Uses

Position	Body Parts Examined	Equipment, Instruments, and Supplies Needed
Sitting	General appearance	
	Head, neck	Stethoscope
	Eyes	Ophthalmoscope, penlight
	Ears	Otoscope, tuning fork
	Nose	Nasal speculum, penlight, substances to smell
	Sinuses	Penlight
	Mouth	Glove, tongue blade, penlight
	Throat	Glove, tongue blade, penlight, laryngeal mirror, laryngoscope
	Axilla, arms	
	Chest	Stethoscope
	Breasts	
	Upper back	Stethoscope
	Reflexes	Percussion hammer
Supine	Chest	Stethoscope
	Abdomen	Stethoscope
	Breasts	
Lithotomy, dorsal recumbent, Sims'	Female genitalia and internal organs	Gloves, vaginal speculum, Ayre spatula, histobrush, lubricant, microscopic slide or liquid preparation
	Female rectum	Glove, lubricant, fecal occult blood test
Standing	Male genitalia and hernia	Gloves
	Spine, posture, gait, coordination, balance, strength, flexibility	
Dorsal recumbent, Sims'	Male rectum	Gloves, lubricant, fecal occult blood test
	Prostate	Glove, lubricant
Prone	Back, spine, legs	
Knee-chest	Rectum	Glove; lubricant; anoscope, proctoscope, or sigmoidoscope; fecal occult blood test
	Female genitalia	Glove, lubricant, vaginal speculum, Ayre spatula, histobrush
	Prostate	Glove, lubricant
Fowler's	Head, neck, chest	Stethoscope
Trendelenburg	Chest, abdomen, pelvis, legs, feet	Stethoscope
Reverse Trendelenburg	Head, chest, abdomen, legs, feet	Stethoscope

FOLLOW-UP PROCEDURES

The physician may have left the room, but your responsibilities are not over. Here's what you should do after the examination.

- Offer to help the patient return to a sitting position.
- Ask the patient to dress—and leave the room unless the patient needs your help.
- Give the patient instructions about what to do after dressing.

> Check the medical record to make sure everything has been accurately documented before releasing it to the billing department. This helps the patient and the medical office.

In many offices, the patient dresses and stays in the examination room. Then the medical assistant comes back to the room and gives the patient further instructions. In other offices, patients are told to go to the front desk to:

- schedule future appointments
- receive further instructions
- receive prescriptions
- address billing issues

During the examination, the physician may order follow-up treatment or procedures that need to be performed afterward. You may need to provide assistance by performing those procedures or giving instructions to the patient. Examples of some common follow-up tests the physician may order are listed in the table below. You'll learn more about follow-up procedures in Chapter 6.

Follow-Up Tests and the Medical Assistant

Test	Purpose	Medical Assistant's Role
Blood work: complete blood count (CBC), blood chemistry	Blood tests are the most commonly performed medical tests. They provide information about the patient's general health status and can be used to detect various diseases, such as anemia and heart disease.	With special training, the medical assistant might draw specimens for blood tests ordered by the physician.
Urinalysis	A series of tests may be performed to examine the urine's appearance and acidity and the presence of proteins and sugars. These tests are used to detect infection and/or disease.	Medical assistants need to instruct the patient on proper collection techniques for the urine sample.
Chest x-ray	Chest x-rays can be used to detect abnormalities of the lungs, heart, large blood vessels, ribs, and thoracic spine.	Only qualified x-ray technicians will obtain a chest x-ray. Medical assistants may need to provide directions to the office where the x-ray will be taken.

CLEANING THE EXAMINATION ROOM

Before you call the next patient, you'll need to clean the examination room. This includes cleaning all reusable equipment with appropriate disinfectants. You also must make sure any used disposable supplies or equipment have been discarded properly. (You read about how to do this in Chapter 1.) After you clean the examination table, cover it with clean paper to prepare the room for the next patient.

The Physical Examination

To help you know what might be expected of you in assisting the physician, it's a good idea to be familiar with what occurs during a physical exam. It usually follows an orderly sequence:

- examination of specific areas of the body—head and neck; eyes, ears, nose, and sinuses; mouth and throat; chest, breasts, abdomen, groin, genitalia, and rectum; legs

- test of reflexes

- observation of posture, gait, and coordination; tests of balance and strength

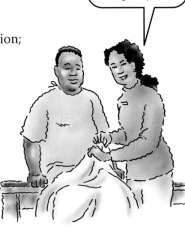

The examination begins with the patient seated on the examining table. The patient should have a drape over the lap and legs for privacy.

EXAMINING THE BODY

Throughout the examination, the physician observes the patient's general appearance, behavior, speech, posture (the position of the body and its limbs), nutritional status, hair distribution, and skin. Now let's take a detailed look at the specific parts of the body the physician examines.

Head and Neck

The physician inspects the patient's skull, face, scalp, and hair. These structures also are palpated for size, shape, and symmetry. This includes looking for nodules, masses, and local trauma or injury. The patient may be asked to roll his head in all directions to assess the range of motion. This allows the physician to check for any limitations of movement. She also may palpate several structures in his neck.

- *Trachea.* This main airway for the passage of air to the lungs is sometimes referred to as the "windpipe."

- *Lymph nodes* or *lymph glands.* These small bean-shaped structures help fight infections. There are some lymph nodes located on the anterior neck.

- *Thyroid.* This gland is located in front of the neck below the larynx. It produces substances that regulate metabolism and growth. The thyroid is palpated for size and symmetry. The patient may be asked to swallow to facilitate palpation.

- *Carotid arteries.* These are large blood vessels located on both sides of the neck. They supply oxygen-carrying blood to the brain. The carotid arteries may be palpated and auscultated for abnormal sounds.

Eyes

The medical assistant often performs a visual acuity test with the patient before the physician's examination. You can learn the steps for performing this test in the Hands On procedure on page 151. For some patients, a color vision test may be performed. The Hands On procedure on page 153 provides details for performing this test.

Along with looking at the results of vision tests, the physician also examines several structures of the eye.

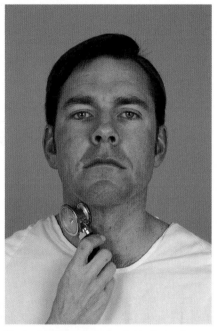

Blood makes abnormal sounds called bruit when it moves through diseased blood vessels. Bruit often results from narrowing or blockages in arteries.

- *Sclera.* Sclera is the fibrous tissue that covers the eye. It is the white part of the eye. It's checked to be sure the color is normal.

- *Pupil.* The pupil is a round opening in the eye that allows light to pass through. It is the black center part of the eye. The physician uses a penlight to check that the pupils of the patient's eyes are equal in size. She also checks to make sure the patient's pupils are round in shape and react normally to light. Normal pupil reaction is recorded as **PERRLA,** which means that the pupils are equal, round, and reactive to light and **accommodation.** Accommodation refers to the ability of the pupils to adjust when focusing on objects at different distances.

- *Eye movement.* The physician may ask the patient to watch movements of her fingers to assess eye movements.

Normal eye movement is documented as EOM intact, or **extraocular** eye movement intact. Extraocular refers to outside the eye. This notation means that the eyes move appropriately to track moving objects.

- *Peripheral vision.* The ability to see things off to the side while looking straight ahead is known as **peripheral** vision.

- *Retina.* The retina is the light-sensitive area at the back of the eye. It may be assessed using the ophthalmoscope. The ophthalmoscope allows the physician to look inside the eye and examine the condition of the retina. The physician also looks at the blood vessels in the eye to check for any signs of disease there.

Ears

The outer ear is palpated for size, shape, and symmetry. The physician inspects the ear canal and any **cerumen,** or ear wax, using an otoscope. The physician also examines the tympanic membrane, or ear drum. The tympanic membrane is checked for color and whether it is intact. Normally, it's pearly gray and concave. Infection can cause discoloration of the tympanic membrane. Fluids behind the ear drum can cause it to bulge outward.

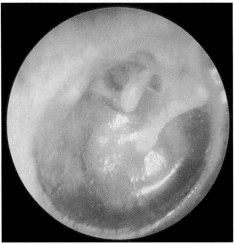

A normal tympanic membrane looks like this when viewed though an otoscope.

Nose and Sinuses

The physician may examine both the exterior and the interior of the patient's nose. The exterior is palpated for any abnormalities. The interior is inspected using a nasal speculum and light.

- *Nasal septum.* The physician checks the position of the **nasal septum** for deviation. The nasal septum is a thin wall that separates the nasal cavities. Sometimes, it can be displaced to the left or right as a result of injury. A damaged nasal septum can block the nasal passage.

- *Nostrils.* The physician also inspects the nostrils to check the color of the **mucosa,** or the membrane lining the cavity. She looks for discharge, lesions, obstructions, swelling, tenderness, or **polyps.** Polyps are soft growths on membrane linings. They may be **benign** (harmless) or **malignant** (cancerous).

The physician might test the patient's sense of smell. The patient closes his eyes and tries to identify a common substance such as alcohol, peppermint, lemon, or strawberry by smell alone.

After inspecting the nose, the physician also may inspect or palpate the paranasal **sinuses.** Sinuses are air-filled cavities in the bones of the skull and face. The paranasal sinuses are located near and are connected to the nose. A special technique called **transillumination** may be used to look at the sinuses. In transillumination, the room is darkened, and a penlight or flashlight is placed against the patient's upper cheek or periorbital ridge (the body ridge around the eyes).

Mouth and Throat

The physician inspects the mucous membranes of mouth, gums, teeth, tongue, tonsils, and throat. Supplies and instruments used to examine these structures include:

- clean gloves
- a light source
- a tongue blade
- a laryngeal mirror, if necessary

The examiner also assesses general dental hygiene and the functioning of salivary glands. The goal is to look for abnormalities in the oral cavity, such as color, ulcerations, or nodules.

Chest

The patient's gown is removed to the waist so the physician can examine the anterior chest. She observes the general appearance and symmetry of the chest and breast area. The respiratory rate and pattern are noted, as well as any obvious masses or swelling.

Palpation of the chest includes the axillary lymph nodes and the area over the heart. The physician may use percussion to assess underlying structures. Using a stethoscope, she auscultates the lungs for abnormal breath sounds. The patient may be asked to take several deep breaths. The physician also assesses heart sounds and the apical pulse.

The posterior chest is also inspected and palpated. The physician examines the muscles of the back and spine. Percussion of the back helps her assess the lungs. With a stethoscope, the physician listens to posterior lung sounds. Again, the patient may be asked to take deep breaths to facilitate the examination.

BREAST EXAMINATION

Breasts may be palpated in both male and female patients. The supine position is preferred for palpation. In this position, the breast tissue flattens out, making abnormalities easier to feel.

The tissue examined includes the:

- breast
- nipple
- tissue extending up to the clavicle, or collarbone (a bone that makes up part of the shoulder)
- tissue under the axilla
- tissue down to the bottom of the rib cage

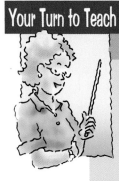

Your Turn to Teach

BREAST SELF-EXAMINATION FOR FEMALE PATIENTS

Your goal is to help your patient learn how to properly perform her own breast examinations. Use a breast model if one is available, or an instruction sheet containing illustrations like the ones shown on the following pages. Wash your hands for infection control before handling any teaching aids.

1. Explain why the breasts should be examined regularly. Tell the patient that she needs to check for lumps, dimples, and thickened areas, as these could be signs of malignancy. She should be encouraged to examine her breasts at the same time each month, about a week after her menstrual period. Note that early detection leads to early diagnosis and treatment.

2. Tell your patient that her breast tissue needs to be examined in three different positions for the most thorough examination.
   - *In front of a mirror.* Explain that she should disrobe and inspect her breasts in front of a mirror. She needs to first place her hands on her hips and then raise her arms above her head. Tell the patient that she needs to look for any changes in the breast contour, or any swelling, dimpling of the skin, or changes in the nipple. Regular inspection will show her what is normal for her.

Your Turn to Teach

BREAST SELF-EXAMINATION FOR FEMALE PATIENTS (*continued*)

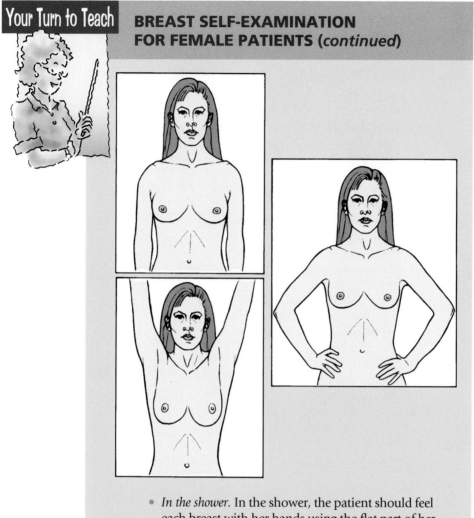

- *In the shower.* In the shower, the patient should feel each breast with her hands using the flat part of her first three fingers. Tell her to use her right hand to lightly press over all areas of her left breast. She should use her left hand to examine her right breast in the same way. Explain that she needs to check for any lumps, hard knots, or thickenings. Tell the patient that doing this in the shower will be easier because her hands will glide more smoothly over wet skin.
- *Lying down.* After showering, the patient should lie down and place a pillow or folded towel under her right shoulder. This helps distribute the breast tissue more evenly on the chest. Her right hand is placed

(continued)

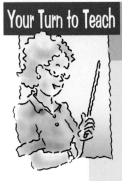

Your Turn to Teach

BREAST SELF-EXAMINATION FOR FEMALE PATIENTS (*continued*)

behind her head. She should examine her right breast using the flat part of the fingers of her left hand. Describe how to use small, circular motions, beginning at the outermost top of the breast and moving clockwise around it. Remind the patient to palpate every part of the breast tissue, moving her fingers in toward the nipple. When she is finished, she will place the towel or pillow under the left shoulder and repeat the procedure, using her right hand to examine her left breast.

3. Tell the patient also to check for any abnormal discharge from her nipples. To do this, she should gently squeeze each nipple using her thumb and index finger. Tell her that she should report any abnormal knots, lumps, thickening, or discharge to the physician.

4. Provide the patient with a patient education instruction sheet or pamphlet, if available.

5. Document your teaching in the patient's chart.

Charting Example:
03/02/2007 2:15 P.M. Pt. given written and verbal instructions on performing monthly breast self-examination. She verbalized understanding. Advised to contact office for any problems or abnormalities. _____E. Smith, CMA

Abdomen and Groin

After examining the breasts, the drape is lowered to expose the body from the abdomen to the pubic area. The patient's chest is draped or gowned to just below the breasts.

The abdomen is inspected for contour, symmetry, and pulsations from the aorta—the main artery that carries blood from the heart to the body. The aorta extends from the heart down the center of the thoracic and abdominal cavities.

The physician also uses the stethoscope to listen to bowel sounds. Percussion may be used to determine the outlines of the abdominal organs. Palpation is used to assess organ enlargement, masses, pain, or tenderness.

The lower abdomen and groin are palpated to assess enlargement of the **inguinal lymph nodes.** Inguinal means related to the groin region. Palpation also is used to look for a **hernia.** This is a structure or organ protruding through the muscle or tissue that normally surrounds it. Hernias often result from a weak area or tear in the muscle. The physician also may palpate the femoral arteries, large arteries of the thigh which pass through each side of the groin.

Genitalia and Rectum—Male Patients

The physician follows a routine series of steps in examining the male genitalia and rectum.

1. The physician puts on clean gloves to examine the external male genitalia and the rectum. The genitalia are inspected to check for symmetry, lesions, swelling, masses, and hair distribution. The scrotal contents may be visualized using the transillumination technique in a darkened room. The scrotum is palpated for testicular size, contour, and consistency.

2. The patient is then asked to bear down as if having a bowel movement. The physician places a gloved index finger upward along the side of the scrotum in the inguinal ring to check for a hernia.

3. To check the patient's anus for lesions or hemorrhoids, the physician has him bend over the exam table or placed in Sims' position. The physician inserts a lubricated gloved finger into the anus and palpates the rectal sphincter muscle and prostate gland for size, consistency, and any masses. The prostate gland is a gland in men that produces the fluid part of semen.

After the rectal exam, an **occult** blood test, or test for hidden blood, may be performed on any stool obtained from the

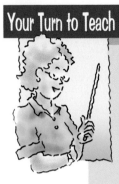

TESTICULAR SELF-EXAMINATION

It will take about ten minutes to teach a male patient how to perform a testicular self-examination. Using a testicular model or pictures, explain to the patient how to examine each testicle. (Wash your hands for infection control before touching these aids.)

1. Tell the patient to gently roll each testicle between his fingers and thumb to check for lumps and thickenings. Tell him to roll each testicle in a horizontal motion and then in a vertical one. Both hands should be used to check each testicle to make sure all areas are palpated.

2. Explain that at the top of each testicle is a cord-like structure called the epididymis, which stores and transports sperm. The patient should be able to identify this structure to avoid mistaking it for an abnormal growth or lump.

3. Instruct the patient to report any abnormal lumps or thickenings to the physician.

4. Provide the patient with an instruction sheet, if one is available.

5. Document your teaching in the patient's chart.

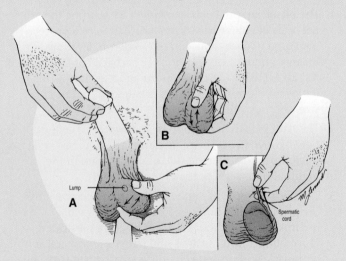

Lump

A

B

C

Spermatic cord

1. Use both hands to palpate the testis. The normal testicle is smooth and uniform in consistency.
2. With the index and middle fingers under the testis and the thumb on top, roll the testis gently in a horizontal plane between the thumb and fingers (A).
3. Feel for any evidence of a small lump or abnormality. Follow the same procedure and palpate upward along the testis (B).
4. Locate and palpate the epididymis (C), a cord-like structure on the top and back of the testicle that stores and transports sperm. Also locate and palpate the spermatic cord.
5. Repeat the examination for the other testis, epididymis, and spermatic cord. It is normal to find that one testis is larger than the other.
6. If you find any evidence of a small, pea-like lump or if the testis is swollen (possibly from an infection or tumor), consult your physician.

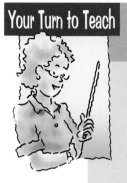

Your Turn to Teach

TESTICULAR SELF-EXAMINATION
(*continued*)

During the procedure, make sure you encourage the patient to ask questions. You need to ensure that the patient understands the procedure.

Charting Example:

12/13/2007 3:45 P.M. Pt. given verbal and written instructions on testicular self-examination. He verbalized understanding. Advised to contact office for any problems or abnormalities. _____ C. Brook, RMA

gloved finger. After the examination of these areas, hand the patient tissues to wipe off any excess lubricant.

Genitalia and Rectum—Female Patients

The female genitalia and rectum usually are examined with the patient in the lithotomy position. One corner of the drape extends over the genitalia, and the other corner covers her chest. A gooseneck lamp is used to direct light on the vaginal area. There are several steps involved in this exam.

1. Wearing clean gloves, the physician inspects the external genitalia for lesions, edema or swelling, cysts, discharge, and hair distribution.

2. The physician inserts the vaginal speculum. This allows the physician to easily inspect the vaginal mucosa and cervix. A Pap smear from the cervix is obtained, and the speculum is removed.

3. The physician performs a bimanual examination to palpate internal reproductive organs. During this examination, the physician checks the organs for size, contour, consistency, and any masses.

Specific information for assisting with the pelvic examination is provided in the Hands On procedure on page 155.

Sometimes, a **rectovaginal** examination is performed to examine the posterior uterus and vaginal wall. The physician places a gloved index finger in vagina and a gloved and lubricated middle finger in rectum at same time.

The rectum is usually inspected and palpated for lesions, hemorrhoids, and sphincter tone. A stool specimen may be obtained from the gloved finger and tested for occult blood.

Legs

The legs are visually inspected and checked for **varicose veins.** These are abnormally large, twisted blood vessels just below the skin that can cause pain, swelling, or itching. Peripheral pulse sites are palpated with the patient in the supine position. These sites may be palpated again with the patient in a standing position.

POSTURE, GAIT, AND REFLEXES

With the patient in the standing position, the physician also may check the patient's general posture. The patient may be asked to walk or perform other movements so the physician can assess **gait** and **coordination.**

- *Gait* refers to the style or way in which a person walks.
- *Coordination* is the way the muscles and groups of muscles work together during movement.

The physician may ask the patient to do a balance test. In this test, the patient stands with feet together and eyes closed. Other aspects of body movements that may be tested are the range of motion and the strength of the arms and legs.

REFLEXES

To test body reflexes, the patient needs to be in a sitting position. The physician strikes several tendons with a percussion hammer. Here's a list of the tendons that are typically tested.

- The *biceps tendon*—a tendon of the large muscle on the front of the upper arm.
- The *triceps tendon*—the tendon of the muscle on the back of the upper arm that extends the elbow.
- The *patellar tendons*—sometimes known as the patellar **ligaments.** Ligaments are similar to tendons. They are tough bands of tissue that connect bones or cartilage. The patellar tendons connect the patella, or kneecap, to the leg bone known as the tibia.
- The *Achilles tendon*—a large band of tissue connecting the muscle on the back of the leg (the gastrocnemius muscle) to the bone in the heel. This is the largest tendon in the human body.
- The *plantar tendons*—several tendons on the sole of the foot.

General Guidelines for Physical Exams

How often should patients have a complete physical examination? Physicians may vary in their recommendations, but here are some general guidelines.

- For patients ages 20 to 40, physical examinations may be performed every one to three years.
- For patients over 40, a physical examination every year is recommended.

If a patient has a medical condition, it may be necessary to have physical examinations more often. At age 40, all patients should have a baseline **electrocardiogram (ECG or EKG)**—a test that records the electrical activity of the heart. Follow-up ECGs may be performed as necessary.

> The patient can move to a supine position when the physician checks the plantar reflexes.

SCREENING FOR COLON AND RECTAL CANCER

Beginning at age 50, patients should be tested for colon and rectal cancer. There are several different approaches recommended for colon and rectal cancer screening.

- *Annual rectal examinations and fecal occult blood tests.* Patients with increased risk for developing colon or rectal cancer may begin screening earlier or have screening more often.
- *Flexible sigmoidoscopy.* In this procedure, the physician examines the lining of the rectum and lower part of the colon with a flexible, lighted tube. This test is recommended every five years. It also may be used in conjunction with annual fecal occult blood tests.
- *Colonoscopy.* Another method of examining the colon is the colonoscopy—a test in which a long, flexible instrument with a light and lens on the end is inserted into the rectum and colon. It allows physicians to examine the lining of the colon and rectum for abnormalities. Some physicians recommend a colonoscopy at age 50. If the results are normal, this test is recommended every 10 years.

IMMUNIZATIONS FOR ADULTS

Immunizations are not just for children. Some immunizations are recommended for adults.

- A tetanus booster should be given every ten years, or sooner if the patient has an open wound.

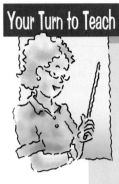

Your Turn to Teach

TEACHING WARNING SIGNS

You should take every opportunity to teach patients about signs that might signal health problems. You can teach patients to recognize the early warning signs of cancer. One way to help patients remember the signs is the acronym CAUTION:

C <u>C</u>hange in bowel or bladder habits

A <u>A</u> sore that doesn't heal

U <u>U</u>nusual bleeding or discharge

T <u>T</u>hickening, lumps, or changes in the shape of breasts or testicles

I <u>I</u>ndigestion or difficulty swallowing

O <u>O</u>bvious change in a wart or mole

N <u>N</u>agging cough or hoarseness of the voice

Other important signals that should not be ignored are frequent, severe headaches and persistent abdominal pain.

You also need to tell patients what signs to watch for in their children.

- continual crying for no obvious reason
- unexplained nausea and vomiting
- general failure to thrive
- spontaneous bleeding or bleeding that does not stop
- bumps, lumps, masses, or swelling anywhere on the body
- frequent stumbling for no apparent reason

- One injection of pneumonia vaccine is recommended for all adults over age 65 years, and one or two injections for younger adults with certain health problems.
- Adults born after 1957 should be vaccinated for mumps, measles, and rubella unless they are already immune to these diseases.
- Influenza vaccine for influenza A and B should be given annually after age 50, and after age 19 for persons with certain health problems.
- A series of three hepatitis B injections is recommended for adults who work in certain high-risk occupations or engage in certain high-risk activities.

- A series of two hepatitis A injections is recommended for adults who work in certain high-risk occupations, who engage in certain high-risk activities, or who have certain blood disorders or liver disease.

GUIDELINES FOR WOMEN

There are several general guidelines for women, regarding gynecological and breast examinations.

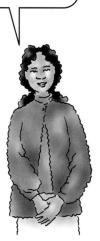

As with most cancers, early detection of breast cancer can save lives.

- *Pap smear.* The first Pap smear is recommended at ages 18 to 20. After the first Pap smear, it's recommended that women have a Pap smear every year.

- *Breast examination.* A physician should examine the breasts every one to three years for women ages 20 to 39 to detect lumps and thickenings that could be malignancies. For women age 40 and older, an annual breast examination is recommended. Patients also should perform regular breast self-examinations. They may detect abnormalities that should be reported to their physicians.

- *Mammogram.* These x-rays of the breast are used to detect abnormalities or disease. Annual mammograms are recommended from the age of 40. If a patient is at risk for developing breast cancer, a physician may recommend mammograms earlier and more often.

Hands On

CLEANING AND PREPARING THE EXAMINATION ROOM

3-1

1. Wash your hands and put on clean gloves. If there's a chance of contact with soiled dressings, body fluids, or other contaminated items, put on personal protective equipment such as a gown or apron, protective eyewear, and shoe coverings.

2. Discard all disposable waste in the appropriate biohazard, sharps, or regular waste container.
   - Any broken glass requires special care. Use a dustpan and brush, or forceps if necessary, to pick up glass fragments and dispose of them properly. They may be contaminated!
   - Remove soiled examination table paper and linens (follow the steps listed in the Hands On procedure *Cleaning Examination Tables* in Chapter 1).
   - Remove all soiled reusable instruments for disinfection or sterilization. (See Chapters 1 and 4 for information on disinfection and sterilization techniques.)

3. Remove your gloves and wash your hands. Then put on new gloves to continue your task. Using disposable paper towels, remove any visible soil from countertops, cabinets, or other surfaces in the room.

4. Wipe all surfaces with an approved disinfectant. Take care to clean every surface to prevent the spread of microorganisms.

5. Check the protective coverings on equipment in the office. If they are soiled, clean or replace them. Disinfect office equipment and allow it to air dry before replacing any protective coverings.

6. Dispose of your paper towels in the biohazard waste container. Remove your gloves. They also must go into the biohazard waste container. Then wash your hands.

7. Check all supplies normally kept in the room, such as cotton, patient gowns, and instruments. Restock any supplies as necessary, following your office's policy.

8. Set up equipment and supplies needed for the next examination, including clean examination paper (refer to the

Hands On

CLEANING AND PREPARING THE EXAMINATION ROOM (*continued*)

3-1

Hands On procedure *Cleaning Examination Tables* in Chapter 1). Be sure to check that equipment such as otoscopes or ophthalmoscopes are working properly.

9. Select the proper gown for the patient and place it on the clean examination table. Set out any clean drapes needed for the examination.

10. Return any unused supplies and items to their proper places.

Hands On

PREPARING THE ADULT PATIENT FOR THE PHYSICAL EXAMINATION

3-2

1. Wash your hands.
2. Greet the patient by name and escort him to the prepared examining room. Identifying the patient by name helps to prevent errors.
3. Explain the procedure. This may help the patient feel less anxious.
4. Obtain and record the patient's medical history and chief complaint.
5. Measure and record the patient's vital signs, height, weight, and visual acuity. These measurements help give the physician an overall picture of the patient's health.
6. If the physician requires it, instruct the patient to obtain a urine specimen. Even if a urine specimen is not part of the physical examination, an empty bladder makes abdominal and/or pelvic examinations more comfortable. Direct the patient to the bathroom.
7. Once the patient has returned, provide instructions for disrobing and explain how to put on the gown (open in the front or the back).
   - The gown must open in the direction that provides the best accessibility for the examination.
   - Leave the room unless the patient needs help. (Elderly and disabled persons may need help disrobing and/or putting on the gown.)
8. Help the patient sit on the edge of the examining table. The sitting position is often the first position used by the physician. Cover the patient's legs with a drape.
9. Place the chart outside the examination room and notify the physician that the patient is ready. Alerting the physician helps prevent delays.

Hands On

ASSISTING WITH PATIENTS IN WHEELCHAIRS

3-3

1. Wash your hands and greet the patient by name. If you think you'll need help moving the patient, ask another staff member to assist you. Don't risk hurting yourself by trying to move the patient alone.

2. Bring the wheelchair as close as possible to the end of the examination table. Locate the wheelchair at a 90-degree angle to the table to minimize the distance for moving the patient. Lock the wheels to stop the wheelchair from moving.

3. Check to make sure the patient is wearing shoes or slippers with nonskid soles. Then place the patient's feet on the floor by lifting the patient's feet and adjusting the wheelchair's foot and leg supports.
   - Keep your own feet in front of the patient's feet to prevent the patient from slipping.
   - For some patients, you may need to place a footstool in front of the table to support their feet.

4. If you're moving the patient yourself, face the patient and ask the patient to hold onto your shoulders. Your knees should be in line with the patient's knees.
   - Bending your knees slightly will lower your body and make it easier for the patient reach you. It also helps to avoid injury to your back when you lift the patient.

5. Place your arms under the patient's arms and around the patient's body. Prepare the patient by explaining that you will count to three and then lift. If possible, the patient can help by supporting some of her body weight.

6. Count to three and lift the patient. Turn toward the examination table. The back of the patient's knees should touch the table.

7. Lower the patient onto the examination table. If the patient can't sit without support, help the patient into a supine position. Otherwise, keep the patient in a sitting position.

8. If you're moving the patient with someone else, decide which one of you will turn the patient toward the examination table during the transfer. Usually, the stronger person turns the patient.

(continued)

Hands On

ASSISTING WITH PATIENTS IN WHEELCHAIRS (*continued*)

3-3

9. You and your helper should both face the patient with your knees slightly bent. Each of you should have one knee in line with the patient's knees. The patient will put one hand on each person's shoulder.

10. Place one of your arms around the patient. Your helper should do the same. Lock your wrists together to provide extra support. On the count of three, lift the patient together.

11. One person turns the patient toward the examination table. With your helper, gradually lower the patient onto the table. Work together to avoid jolting the patient unnecessarily.

12. After the patient is comfortable and safely positioned on the examination table, unlock the wheels on the wheelchair and move it back from the table to an area where it won't get in the way.

13. Provide the patient with a gown and drape. If necessary, help the patient disrobe.

Hands On

ASSISTING WITH PREGNANT PATIENTS

3-4

1. Wash your hands.

2. Greet the patient by name, and escort her to the prepared examining room. Identifying the patient by name helps to prevent errors.

3. Prepare the patient for the examination as you would for any other adult patient (see the Hands On procedure *Preparing the Adult Patient for the Physical Examination*) by explaining the examination procedure and measuring and recording vital signs, height, and weight. The physician may require a urine sample.

4. Ask the patient if she has any specific questions regarding her pregnancy. Following the policies in your medical office, notify the physician of her specific questions. Provide the patient with patient education information, if available and appropriate.

5. Provide instructions for disrobing and explain how to put on the gown. Leave the room to give the patient privacy while disrobing, unless she asks for help.

6. Have the patient use a stool to step up to the examining table. Help her sit on the edge of the table. Cover her legs with a drape and provide additional drapes as needed for privacy.

7. During the examination, take care when asking the patient to move into different body positions. Some body positions may not be suitable for pregnant women.

8. Watch for signs that the patient is uncomfortable. Be especially vigilant during changes in body position. When a pregnant patient has been lying on the examination table for a length of time, blood may collect in the pelvic regions. Sitting up suddenly can cause dizziness or hyperventilation. Help the patient to sit up slowly and give her time to adjust to sitting before she stands up.

9. At the end of the examination, help the patient down from the examination table. Leave the room to give her privacy (unless she asks for help) while she dresses.

Hands On

ASSISTING WITH THE ADULT PHYSICAL EXAMINATION

3-5

1. Wash your hands and prepare the examination room and patient. When the physician is ready to begin the physical examination, you will assist by handing the physician the appropriate instruments and positioning the patient appropriately. Anticipating the physician's needs saves time and makes the procedure more efficient.

2. Begin by handing the physician the instruments necessary to examine different body areas. Although all physicians follow a systematic procedure, the order for examining different body areas may vary slightly depending on the physician.
   - head and neck—stethoscope
   - eyes—ophthalmoscope, penlight
   - ears—otoscope, tuning fork
   - nose—penlight, nasal speculum
   - sinuses—penlight
   - mouth—gloves, tongue blade, penlight. Pass the tongue blade by holding it in the middle. When it is returned to you, grasp it in the middle again so that you do not hold the end that was in the patient's mouth.
   - throat—glove, tongue blade, laryngeal mirror, penlight

3. Help the patient drop the gown to the waist for examination of the chest and upper back. Then hand the physician the stethoscope. Only the parts of the body being examined should be exposed. Preserve patients' privacy by keeping them covered as much as possible.

4. Help the patient pull up the gown and remove the drape from the legs. Hand the physician the reflex hammer to test patient reflexes.

5. Help the patient to lie supine. Open the gown at the top to expose the chest again. Place the drape to cover the waist, abdomen, and legs. Hand the physician the stethoscope.

6. Cover the patient's chest. Lower the drape to expose the abdomen. Hand the physician the stethoscope.

7. Assist with the genital and rectal examinations. After the examination of these areas, hand the patient tissues to wipe off any excess lubricant.

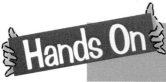

ASSISTING WITH THE ADULT PHYSICAL EXAMINATION (*continued*) 3-5

For females:
- Help the patient into the lithotomy position and drape appropriately.
- Provide the physician with appropriate supplies and instruments for examining genitalia and reproductive organs. These include a glove, lubricant, a speculum, microscope slides or prep solution, and a spatula or brush.
- For the rectal examination, provide a glove, lubricant, and a fecal occult blood test slide.

For males:
- Help the patient stand, if necessary. Have him bend over the examination table for a rectal and prostate examination.
- For a hernia examination, provide a glove.
- For a rectal examination, provide a glove, lubricant, and fecal occult blood test slide.
- For a prostate examination, provide a glove and lubricant.

After the examination of these areas, hand the patient tissues to wipe off any excess lubricant.

8. With the patient standing, the physician may assess legs, gait, coordination, and balance.

9. Help the patient sit on the edge of the examination table. The physician often discusses findings with the patient at this time. The physician may also provide instructions.

10. Perform any follow-up procedures or treatments.

11. Leave the room while the patient undresses unless the patient needs assistance. It's important to protect the patient's privacy.

12. Return to the examination room when the patient has dressed to answer any questions, reinforce instructions, and provide patient education. The patient's ability to follow the treatment plan depends on how well he understands it. Patient education is the responsibility of all health care workers, including medical assistants.

13. Escort the patient to the front desk. If necessary, you can help clarify any appointment scheduling or billing issues.

(*continued*)

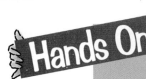

ASSISTING WITH THE ADULT PHYSICAL EXAMINATION (*continued*) 3-5

14. Properly clean or dispose of all used equipment and supplies. Any instruments, supplies, and equipment that came into direct contact with the patient must be decontaminated or disposed of appropriately.

15. Clean the room with a disinfectant and prepare for the next patient.

16. Wash your hands and record any instructions from the physician in the patient's record. Note any test results, specimens taken for testing, and the laboratory where the specimens are being sent. Remember that if procedures and instructions are not recorded, they are not considered to have been done.

Charting Example:
01/09/2007 1:30 P.M. CC: annual physical examination complete per Dr. Smith. ECG done; results given to Dr. Smith. Blood drawn and sent to Acme Lab for a CBC, electrolytes, and liver panel. Pt. instructed to return to office in 2 weeks to discuss results of laboratory tests. Pt. given written and verbal instructions regarding an 1800-calorie low-sodium diet to follow as ordered per Dr. Smith. Pt. verbalized understanding.
_____ J. Bohr, CMA

Hands On

MEASURING DISTANCE VISUAL ACUITY

3-6

1. Wash your hands and prepare the examination area. Make sure the area is well-lighted.
   - A distance marker must be exactly 20 feet from a Snellen Eye Chart. All distance visual acuity testing is done at 20 feet for consistency results.
   - The chart must be at eye level.

2. Identify the patient by name and explain the procedure. Patients who understand the procedure are more likely to have accurate test results.

3. Position the patient at the 20-foot mark. The patient may be standing or sitting, as long as the chart is at eye level.

4. Note whether the patient is wearing glasses. If not, ask about contact lenses and record the information. Patients usually wear their corrective lenses during the visual acuity examination. The patient record must indicate if contact lenses or glasses were worn.

5. Have the patient cover the left eye with an eye occluder.
   - For the sake of consistency, the test always starts with the left eye covered.
   - The patient's hand should not be used to cover the eye. Pressure against the eye or peeking can affect the results.
   - Instruct the patient to keep both eyes open, even though one is covered. Closing one eye can cause the other eye to squint, which can affect the results.

6. Stand beside the chart and point to each row as the patient reads it aloud. Begin with the first row, the 20/200 line. The line number is on the right side of the chart next to each line. If patient reads these lines easily, move down to smaller figures. If the patient has difficulty reading the larger lines, you'll need to notify the physician.

7. Record the smallest line the patient can read with either one or zero errors, depending on your office's policy. In the record, you need to include the eye tested, the line number, and the errors. Here's an example: Right eye 20/40—1.

8. Repeat the procedure with the right eye covered. Record the results as in step 7. Here's an example: Left eye: 20/20—0.

(continued)

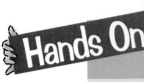

MEASURING DISTANCE VISUAL ACUITY *(continued)*

3-6

9. Repeat step 6 with both eyes uncovered. Record the results as in step 7. Here's an example: Both eyes 20/40—1.

10. Be sure to document the procedure in the patient's record. Procedures are not considered to have been done if they are not recorded.

Charting Example:
04/16/2007 4:40 P.M. Visual acuity: Right eye 20/40—1. Left eye 20/20—0. Both eyes 20/40—1. Both eyes with correction (contact lenses) 20/20. Dr. Smart aware. _____ J. Smith, RMA

Hands On

MEASURING COLOR PERCEPTION

3-7

1. Wash your hands. Then put on gloves and get the Ishihara color plate book and a cotton-tipped applicator. In this case, you wear gloves to protect the color plates. Oils from your hands can alter the colors and interfere with testing.

2. Identify the patient by name and explain the procedure. Make sure the patient is seated comfortably in a quiet, well-lighted room.
   - Indirect sunlight is best. Sunlight should not shine directly on the color plates. The colors fade with exposure to bright lights.
   - Patients who wear glasses or contact lenses should keep them on. Corrective lenses don't interfere with the color perception test.

3. Hold the first plate in the book about 15 to 30 inches from the patient. The first plate should be obvious to all patients and serve as an example. Ask the patient if she can see the number formed by the dots on the plate.

4. Record the patient's results by noting the number of the figure the patient reports for each plate. Write the plate number followed by the patient's response.
   - If the patient cannot see the pattern, record the plate number followed by the letter X.
   - The patient should not take more than three seconds to read the plate and should not squint or guess. These behaviors indicate that the patient was unsure and the plate should be recorded as X.

5. Continue showing plates and recording patient responses for plates 1–10. Plate 11 requires the patient to trace a winding bluish-green line between two X's using the cotton-tipped applicator. Patients with a color deficit will not be able to trace the line.
   - If 10 or more of the first 11 plates are read without difficulty, the patient does not have a color deficit. No additional testing is needed.
   - Plates 12, 13, and 14 are usually used to assess the degree of deficiency in patients with red-green color deficiencies.

(continued)

Hands On

MEASURING COLOR PERCEPTION (*continued*)

3-7

6. Store the color plate book in a closed, protected area to protect the integrity of the colors. Remove your gloves and wash your hands.

Charting Example:

12/22/2007 10:30 A.M. Tested color vision using Ishihara color plates 1–11. All read correctly and no deficiencies were noted.

_____ B. Cotton, CMA

Hands On   ASSISTING WITH THE PELVIC EXAMINATION

3-8

1. Wash your hands before you begin. Assemble all appropriate equipment and supplies. These may include: a gown and drape; the appropriate size vaginal speculum (The vaginal speculum can be warmed under running water, on a heating pad set on warm, or in a warming drawer found on some examination tables.); cotton-tipped applicators; materials for the Pap smear, such as an Ayre spatula or a histobrush; water-soluble lubricant; examination gloves; examination light; tissues; glass microscope slides and fixative solution; a laboratory request form; identification labels; a pencil; a basin or container for used instruments; and a biohazard waste container.

2. Label each slide with the date and type of specimen. Using a pencil, write on the frosted end of the slide. Each slide should be labeled *C* for cervical, *V* for vaginal, or *E* for endocervical (the region at the cervical opening into the uterus).

3. Greet the patient by name and explain the procedure. Identifying the patient by name prevents errors and may help put her at ease.

4. Ask the patient to empty her bladder and, if necessary, collect a urine specimen. An empty bladder makes the examination more comfortable.

5. Provide the patient with a gown and drape and ask her to disrobe. If she's also having a breast examination, she needs to disrobe completely. The gown should open to the front. If the patient is not having a breast exam, she need only disrobe from the waist down.

6. When the physician is ready, assist the patient into the lithotomy position. Her buttocks should be at the bottom edge of the table. This position may be embarrassing to the patient and may stress her back and legs. Explain that she won't need to stay in this position any longer than necessary for the examination.

7. Adjust the drape to cover the patient's abdomen and knees, exposing the genitalia. Adjust the light over the genitalia for maximum visibility.

(continued)

Hands On

ASSISTING WITH THE PELVIC EXAMINATION (*continued*)

3-8

8. Assist the physician with the examination by handing instruments and supplies as needed. Anticipating the physician's needs leads to a more thorough and efficient procedure.

9. After putting on examination gloves, hold the glass slides while the physician obtains and makes the smears.

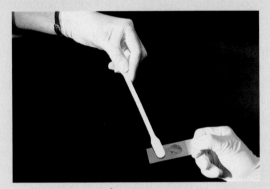

Hold the slide by the frosted edge to receive the smears.

10. Spray or cover each slide with fixative solution. Hold the slide four to six inches from the can and spray lightly once. Or carefully drop the fixative solution onto the slide.
    • The fixative preserves the cervical scrapings for analysis.
    • Spraying the solution too close may distort the cells or blow them off the slide.

11. When the physician removes the vaginal speculum, have a basin or other container ready to receive it.

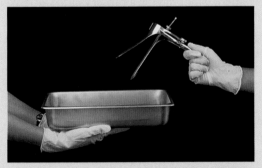

Using a basin to receive used instruments makes it easy to transfer them to a soaking solution for sanitizing.

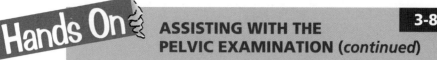

**ASSISTING WITH THE
PELVIC EXAMINATION (*continued*)**

3-8

12. Apply about one to two inches of lubricant across the physician's two fingers. Lubricant helps make the manual examination more comfortable. Don't place lubricant on the vaginal speculum before insertion. It can cause inaccurate Pap smear results!

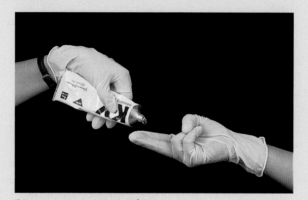

Take care not to touch the end of the lubricant container to the physician's gloves!

13. Encourage the patient to relax during the bimanual examination. Your support may help the patient feel less anxious.

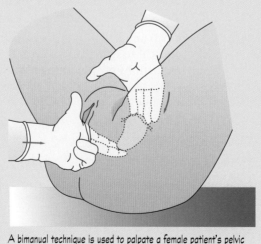

A bimanual technique is used to palpate a female patient's pelvic organs.

(*continued*)

Hands On

14. After the examination, help the patient slide to the far end of the examination table. Then remove both feet from the stirrups at the same time.
    - Moving the patient away from the stirrups helps prevent strain and possible injury while removing her feet from them.
    - Removing both feet at the same time also puts less strain on the patient.

15. Offer the patient tissues to remove excess lubricant. Help her sit up if necessary. Watch the patient for signs of vertigo. Some patients, especially if elderly, may be dizzy when they sit up.

16. Ask the patient to get dressed and assist if needed. Respect the patient's privacy as she dresses.

17. Reinforce any instructions from the physician regarding follow-up appointments. The patient also will appreciate knowing when and how to get laboratory results from the Pap smear.

18. After the patient leaves, properly care for and dispose of equipment. Clean the room and remove gloves. Wash your hands. Document your responsibilities during the procedure, such as routing the specimen, patient education, and so on.

Charting Example:
02/04/2007 3:00 P.M. Pt. pap and pelvic today per Dr. Todd. Cervical and vaginal slides sent to Acme lab for cytology. Pt. given written and oral instructions per obtaining results.
_____ B. Lewis, RMA

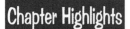
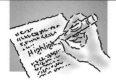

Chapter Highlights

- The purpose of the physical examination is to assess general health and detect signs and symptoms of disease.

- During a physical examination, the medical assistant's duties may involve taking a medical history, preparing the patient for the examination, assisting during the examination, and collecting specimens.

- Depending on office policies, the medical assistant may be asked to remain in the room during the physical examination to provide legal protection for the physician.

- Medical assistants must be familiar with the instruments and supplies used for a general physical examination or a specialty examination.

- In preparing the examination room, the medical assistant should check the examination table, the equipment, and the supplies.

- The medical assistant has an important role in preparing the patient for the examination. Duties may include obtaining the medical history and chief complaint, checking vital signs, and obtaining specimens. Patient privacy is a top priority.

- As the physician examines different parts of the body, the patient may be asked to assume different positions. The medical assistant needs to be familiar with different examination positions to assist the patient if needed.

- Elderly, disabled, and pregnant patients may need extra assistance before, during, and after the examination. The medical assistant must be sensitive to patient needs and feelings.

- The physician normally follows a systematic order in examining the patient. The examination typically begins with the head and neck and progresses to the legs and feet.

- The physician uses six different techniques to gather information during a physical examination—inspection, palpation, manipulation, percussion, auscultation, and mensuration.

- Besides assisting with the general examination, the medical assistant may need to help with specialty procedures such as measuring distance visual acuity, measuring color perception, or assisting with pelvic examinations.

- After the examination, the medical assistant may need to help the patient dress, give further instructions, or perform follow-up procedures. The medical assistant is also responsible for cleaning the examination room and preparing it for the next patient.

- It's important to watch for opportunities to teach patients about signs and signals that can indicate health problems. Medical assistants may teach patients procedures such as breast self-examination or testicular self-examination.

Chapter 4

ASSISTING WITH MINOR OFFICE SURGERY

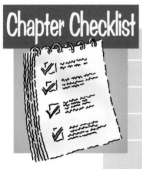

Chapter Checklist

- Explain the principles and practices of surgical asepsis

- Describe how to perform a surgical scrub

- Wrap items for autoclaving

- Perform sterilization techniques

- List some of the surgical instruments commonly used in the medical office

- Summarize how to care for and clean medical instruments

- Explain how to prepare a treatment room for a surgical procedure, including how to open a sterile surgical pack

- List possible indicators that a surgical pack has been contaminated

- Explain how to apply surgical gloves

- List strategies for maintaining a sterile field

- Prepare patient for and assist with procedures, treatments, and minor office surgeries

- Explain how to prepare the patient's skin for minor surgery

- Identify different methods for wound closure and the necessary supplies

- Outline the medical assistant's responsibilities in collecting specimens

- List the responsibilities of the medical assistant following minor surgical procedures

- Explain how to apply bandages and note the signs of impaired circulation

- Identify the phases of wound healing and their main characteristics

As a medical assistant, you may need to assist with minor surgeries performed in the medical office. The types of surgeries performed in a medical office will depend on its medical specialty. But typical office procedures in a general medical practice include:

- inserting or removing **sutures,** surgical stitches used to hold body tissues together

- making **incisions** for drainage, a surgical process of cutting into the body to remove fluids and discharge from wounds or cavities

- performing sebaceous cystectomy—the removal of a **cyst,** an abnormal sac under the skin that's filled with fluid or fatty matter

Minor Surgery and Surgical Asepsis

The process for preparing the patient and setting up supplies and equipment is much the same, no matter what surgery is being performed. For any surgical procedure, medical assistants practice **surgical asepsis,** otherwise known as "sterile technique."

> You already know how _medical_ asepsis stops microbes from spreading from one patient to another. _Surgical_ asepsis stops microbes from getting into the patient's body during an invasive procedure.

Surgical asepsis is a set of practices designed to keep areas or items free of microorganisms. Its purpose is to destroy organisms before they enter the body. Surgical asepsis is necessary:

- when handling sterile instruments that break the skin

- when performing or assisting with surgical procedures

- when changing wound dressings

WHAT'S DIFFERENT ABOUT SURGICAL ASEPSIS?

Surgical asepsis requires the absence of microorganisms on instruments, equipment, and supplies. The procedures you'll use for surgical asepsis are different from those you learned for medical asepsis. Even your hand-washing technique will be different. The following table shows the differences between medical and surgical asepsis.

Comparing Medical and Surgical Asepsis

	Medical Asepsis	Surgical Asepsis
Definition	Destroys microorganisms after they leave the body	Destroys microorganisms before they enter the body
Purpose	Prevents transmission of microorganisms from one person to another	Prevents entry of microorganisms into the body during invasive procedures
When to Use	During contact with a body part that is not normally sterile	During contact with normally sterile parts of the body
Hand-Washing Techniques	Hands and wrists are washed for 1–2 minutes	Hands and forearms are washed for 5–10 minutes with a brush
Cleaning Techniques	Typically use sanitation and disinfection	Need to use sterilization

THE SURGICAL SCRUB

The goal of the surgical scrub is to remove microbes from the hands, nails, and forearms. This will minimize the risk of infection to the patient. The process requires a sink that has a foot or arm control for the running water. You'll also need the following supplies:

- surgical soap in a dispenser
- an orange stick or nail brush
- a sterile brush
- sterile towels

The scrubbing procedure should take at least five minutes for each hand and arm. It's best to follow a systematic approach so you don't miss any areas.

PERFORMING A SURGICAL SCRUB

To perform a surgical scrub, follow these steps.

1. Remove any rings, watches, or bracelets. Jewelry provides hiding places for microbes. Don't let your clothing touch the sink.

2. Adjust the water to a comfortable temperature. If it's too hot, it can dry the skin, causing cracks and breaks. If it's too cold, the soap won't lather properly.

3. Hold your arms at or higher than waist level. (During surgical procedures, all areas below the waist are considered contaminated.) Keep your hands higher than your elbows. Otherwise, water may run down from unscrubbed areas of your arms and contaminate your hands.

4. Use an orange stick or nail brush to clean under each nail. Then discard the orange stick taking care not to touch the insides of the sink or the faucet.

5. Apply surgical soap and wash your hands thoroughly. Use a firm circular motion. Hold your fingers up and rub each side of each finger, between the fingers, and the back and front of each hand. This process should take about five minutes for each hand.

6. Keeping your hands higher than your elbows, wash your wrists and forearms thoroughly with soap. Rinse your arms and hands under running water without touching the sides of the sink or faucet.

7. Using more surgical soap and a sterile brush, scrub all the surfaces you just washed. As before, follow a systematic approach. Begin with your fingers, then scrub your hands, and finally your arms. Don't scrub too hard, as that could scratch your skin.

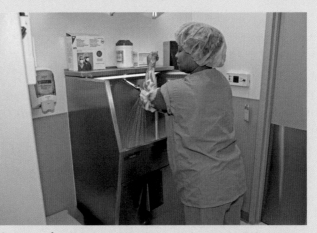

The process of scrubbing your hands and arms with the sterile brush should take at least five minutes.

8. Discard the sterile brush and rinse your hands and arms by passing them through the running water in one direction—from the hand to the elbow. Remember to keep your hands higher than your elbows.

9. Turn off the faucet using the foot or arm mechanism.

10. Dry your hands using a sterile towel. Using one end of the towel, dry one hand, then the arm, then the forearm. Use the other clean end of the towel to dry the other hand, arm, and forearm. Avoid touching your clean hands with the part of the towel that comes into contact with your arms.

Keep your hands higher than your elbows at all times!

Sterilization Techniques and Equipment

Sanitation and disinfection are the main ways medical assistants maintain medical asepsis. Sanitation is maintaining a healthful, disease-free environment. **Sanitizing** means reducing the microorganisms on a surface by using low-level disinfection practices.

Instruments and equipment used in surgical procedures must be sanitized first and then sterilized. **Sterilization** is the complete elimination or destruction of all microbes, including spores. Here are the most common sterilizing agents:

- steam under pressure (autoclaving)
- dry heat
- **ethylene oxide** (gas used in sterilization)
- liquid chemicals
- microwave process

Steam is the most common method of sterilization in medical offices. One of the newest methods combines microwave radiation with the steam to shorten the sterilization process. The method you use will depend on what must be sterilized and the types of microbes that must be destroyed. Several types of equipment are used for sterilizing items in the medical office. Here's what you'll need to know to sterilize things correctly in your office:

- how the equipment works
- what the equipment is used for
- when to schedule preventive maintenance
- how to schedule service, if necessary

- what supplies to order so the equipment can operate properly

The table below shows the basic information for each method of sterilization.

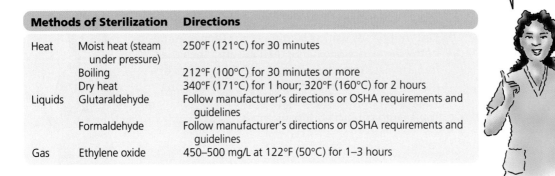

For instruments and equipment used in surgical procedures, sanitize before you sterilize.

Methods of Sterilization		Directions
Heat	Moist heat (steam under pressure)	250°F (121°C) for 30 minutes
	Boiling	212°F (100°C) for 30 minutes or more
	Dry heat	340°F (171°C) for 1 hour; 320°F (160°C) for 2 hours
Liquids	Glutaraldehyde	Follow manufacturer's directions or OSHA requirements and guidelines
	Formaldehyde	Follow manufacturer's directions or OSHA requirements and guidelines
Gas	Ethylene oxide	450–500 mg/L at 122°F (50°C) for 1–3 hours

SANITIZING COMES FIRST

Sanitization or disinfection is the first step in preparing instruments for sterilization. Two different methods are commonly used for sanitization.

- *Cleaning by hand* is especially appropriate for delicate instruments that can be damaged easily.

- *Mechanical washing* uses a machine. Mechanical washers can be used for cleaning most instruments. They're useful for cleaning sharp instruments that can cause injury when cleaned by hand.

SANITIZING INSTRUMENTS

Before cleaning instruments by hand, be sure to put on heavy duty utility gloves, a gown, and eye protection. You need to protect yourself and your clothes from contaminants that might splash up during the procedure. Follow these key guidelines for sanitizing instruments:

1. Take any removable sections of an instrument or equipment apart. If the item can't be sanitized right away, soak the instrument or equipment in a solution of cold water and detergent so blood and other substances don't dry on the instrument.

2. Before you begin cleaning an instrument, check to make sure it works properly. Equipment that's broken

should be repaired or discarded, according to office policy.

3. Rinse the instrument with cool water. Hot water can cause some contaminants to stick to the instrument. This will make it harder to clean.

4. Force streams of hot soapy water through any tubular or grooved instruments. You need to clean the inside as well as the outside.

5. Use a hot, soapy solution to dissolve fats or lubricants.

6. Next, place the instruments in a soaking solution, according to office policy. After soaking them 5 to 10 minutes, use friction to clean them. Use a soft brush or gauze to wipe each instrument and loosen microorganisms. Don't use abrasive materials on delicate instruments and equipment. A soft brush works well on grooves and joints.

7. While cleaning, keep instruments immersed in the cleaning solution to avoid spreading microorganisms through the air.

8. Open and close the jaws of moveable instruments, such as forceps or scissors, several times to make sure all contaminants have been removed.

9. Rinse instruments well to remove soap residue and any remaining microorganisms.

10. Dry instruments thoroughly before sterilization. Excess moisture can interfere with the sterilization process. It also can cause instruments to rust or become dull.

Be sure to discard used brushes, gauze, and solution after sanitizing instruments and equipment. These items are considered grossly contaminated and cannot be reused.

THE AUTOCLAVE

The **autoclave** is the most commonly used piece of equipment for sterilization. It's a device that uses steam heat under high pressure to sterilize objects. The autoclave consists of two chambers and a vent. Here's how it works.

- The outer chamber is the place where pressure builds. Distilled water is added to a reservoir. It's converted to steam when a preset temperature is reached.

Closer Look | ULTRASONIC CLEANING

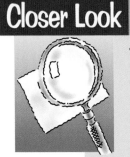

The ultrasonic cleaning unit is a method of machine washing that sanitizes items using high-frequency sound waves. Items are submerged in a tank of water and cleaning solution. Vibrations from sound waves create bubbles. Scrubbing action from the bubbles loosens soil from instruments. After the recommended amount of time, items are rinsed and dried in the unit. When they're removed, they're ready for sterilization.

- The inner chamber is where sterilization occurs. Steam is forced into the inner chamber. As the pressure inside the chamber increases, the temperature rises to 250°F or higher. This is much higher than the normal boiling point of water, which is 212°F or 100°C. The high temperature of the steam destroys all organisms, including viruses and spores.

- The air exhaust vent is located on the bottom of the autoclave. It allows air in the inner chamber to be pushed out and replaced by steam. When no air is present, the chamber seals and the temperature gauge starts rising.

Most autoclaves can be set to vent, time, turn off, and exhaust at preset times and levels. With older models, you may need to do this manually.

All manufacturers provide instructions for operating the machine. They also recommend the time needed to sterilize different types of loads. The autoclave instructions should be posted near the machine in a place where everyone can see them.

WHEN TO USE THE AUTOCLAVE

The autoclave is commonly used to sterilize:

- minor surgical equipment and instruments
- surgical storage trays and containers
- some surgical equipment, such as bowls for holding sterile solutions

You'll find guidance on how to prepare instruments for sterilization in an autoclave in the Hands On procedure on page 224.

Autoclave Wrapping Material

Autoclave wrap may be double layers of cotton muslin, special sterilization paper, or plastic or paper pouches or bags. Many offices use a variety of materials. But whatever wrapping material you use, be sure it has these properties:

- permeable to steam but not contaminants
- resists tearing and puncturing during normal handling
- allows for easy opening to prevent contamination of the contents
- maintains the sterility of the contents during storage

> The autoclave can't be used for any equipment that can be damaged by water! These items can be sterilized with gas.

Special Indicators

Items to be sterilized in the autoclave are wrapped before they're placed inside. But it's the special indicators that help ensure the items are properly sterilized. These special indicators include autoclave indicator tape, sterilization indicators, and the culture test.

Autoclave Tape. Autoclave indicator tape is a special tape placed on the outside of the wrap used to package equipment that's going into the autoclave. As you wrap the equipment, you should write on the tape what's inside the package and the date it's being autoclaved.

Autoclave tape is designed to change color when it's exposed to steam. But the tape doesn't guarantee that items inside the package have been heated enough to be sterilized—only that the outside has been exposed to steam.

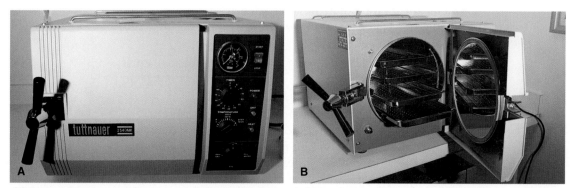

(A) This type of autoclave may be found in a medical office. Note its clearly marked dials and gauges. (B) This photo gives you a peek inside the autoclave.

Sterilization Indicators.

Sterilization indicators are placed inside the wrapped packs to show that proper temperature and pressure were reached during the sterilization process. They're placed inside the wrapping so you'll know the steam penetrated the inner parts of the pack.

There are several different kinds of sterilization indicators. Some change colors at high temperatures. Others are tubes containing wax pellets. If the pellets melt, it shows that the required temperature was reached.

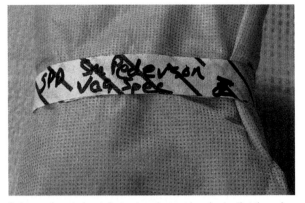

Stripes on the autoclave indicator tape change color, showing that the pack has been exposed to steam.

Only assume items have been sterilized if the indicators show the time and temperature at which the sterilization process was achieved. The color of the autoclave tape alone isn't good enough.

Culture Tests.

The culture test is the best method for checking the effectiveness of the sterilization. Strips with heat-resistant spores are placed between packages in the autoclave load. When the sterilization process is finished, the strips are removed from the packets and placed in a broth culture for incubating. At the end of the incubation period, the culture is compared with a control to see if all the spores have been killed.

Loading an Autoclave

For effective autoclaving, steam needs to reach everywhere! The location of items in an autoclave can make a big difference in where the steam goes. Follow these tips for loading the items to be sterilized.

- Load the autoclave loosely to allow steam to circulate. If too many items are put in, enough steam may not get to and penetrate the packs in the center.
- Place the packs on their sides for the best steam circulation. This applies to containers and bowls too. If a container or bowl is upright, air will settle into its interior. This will keep steam from circulating to the inner surfaces. Container lids should be wrapped separately.

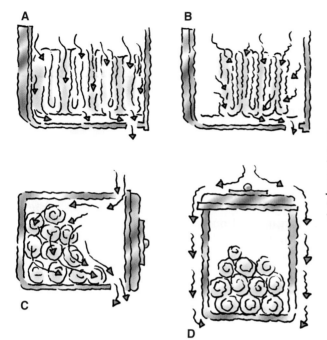

(A) When packages are properly placed in the autoclave, steam can circulate easily. (B) In this drawing, the packages are placed too close together which prevents proper steam sterilization. (C) When the dressings are properly placed in the autoclave, the jar should be able to lie on its side so the steam can circulate easily. (D) In this drawing, the dressings are packed too tightly which prevents proper steam sterilization.

FILLING THE RESERVOIR

Use only distilled water to fill the reservoir tank. Tap water contains chemicals and minerals that may coat the interior chamber and clog the exhaust valves. This can cause the autoclave to function improperly.

When filling the interior chamber with water from the reservoir, make sure the water level is up to the fill line. Adding too much water can make the steam saturated and less efficient. Too little water means there won't be enough steam produced. The sterilization process depends on getting the correct level of steam.

The Autoclave at Work

Besides steam, three other elements are critical for proper sterilization:

- temperature
- pressure
- time

- *Personal protective equipment.* When using the chemical solution, you need to protect yourself. Wear heavy duty utility gloves, protective goggles, and an apron to cover your clothing. If the chemical comes into contact with your skin, eyes, or mucous membranes, it can cause irritation or burns.
- *Vent hood.* The vent hood is used to remove unwanted fumes the chemicals may release into the air. For safety reasons, you need to use the vent hood when working with any chemical solutions.

The Hands On procedure on page 229 details the steps you need to follow in performing chemical sterilization. The chemicals used are sometimes similar to those used for sanitizing. A key difference is the exposure time. The exposure time for the sterilization process varies for different chemicals.

Always check the instructions provided by the chemical manufacturer to find out the correct exposure time for sterilization. Also, you'll need to make sure the chemical solution hasn't expired. The instructions should advise you on how long you can expect the chemical to remain effective.

After Chemical Sterilization

When the instruments have soaked in the chemical solution for the proper length of time, they can be removed. Because the items are now sterile, you must wear sterile gloves or use sterile transfer **forceps** to remove items from the solution. (Forceps are a tool that allows you to hold and grasp objects. You'll learn more information about this tool later in the chapter.)

You'll need to rinse the chemical solution from each instrument before it comes into contact with the patient. Rinse each item thoroughly using sterile water. Dry the item with a sterile towel.

Surgical Instruments

To assist the physician with minor surgical procedures, you must be familiar with the surgical instruments. You also must know how to care for each instrument.

As a clinical medical assistant, you'll need to know how to set up instruments and equipment for surgical procedures. You may be the one to pass instruments to the physician during the procedure as well.

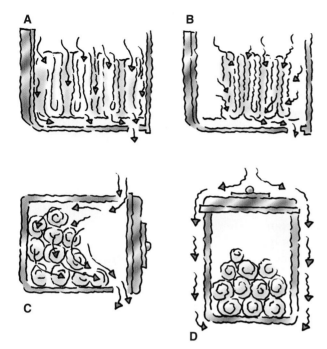

(A) When packages are properly placed in the autoclave, steam can circulate easily. (B) In this drawing, the packages are placed too close together which prevents proper steam sterilization. (C) When the dressings are properly placed in the autoclave, the jar should be able to lie on its side so the steam can circulate easily. (D) In this drawing, the dressings are packed too tightly which prevents proper steam sterilization.

FILLING THE RESERVOIR

Use only distilled water to fill the reservoir tank. Tap water contains chemicals and minerals that may coat the interior chamber and clog the exhaust valves. This can cause the autoclave to function improperly.

When filling the interior chamber with water from the reservoir, make sure the water level is up to the fill line. Adding too much water can make the steam saturated and less efficient. Too little water means there won't be enough steam produced. The sterilization process depends on getting the correct level of steam.

The Autoclave at Work

Besides steam, three other elements are critical for proper sterilization:

- temperature
- pressure
- time

You'll find information about these levels in the instruction manual for your office's autoclave. In general, 250°F at 15 pounds of pressure for 20 to 30 minutes is sufficient. However, the temperature, pressure, and time may vary depending on the items being sterilized. Solid or metal loads may take a little less time than soft, bulky loads.

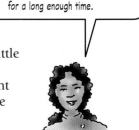

> Don't set the timer until the proper temperature has been reached. Some microbes are only killed if they're exposed to high enough temperatures for a long enough time.

When the items have been in the autoclave at the right temperature for enough time, the timer will ring. Be sure to vent the autoclave to allow the temperature to drop safely. Newer autoclaves vent automatically.

Don't handle or remove items until they're dry. If the coverings are still moist, microorganisms from your hands might be drawn inside. For more details on how to use the autoclave, read the Hands On procedure on page 227.

Storing Autoclaved Items

Once the items are dry, remove the packages. Store them in a clean, dry, and dust-free area. Packs that are sterilized on-site in an autoclave are considered sterile for 30 days. After 30 days, they must be sterilized again. You can avoid unnecessary work by placing recently autoclaved items toward the back of the cabinet. Move items that were previously autoclaved up to the front.

MAINTAINING THE AUTOCLAVE

You're responsible for performing routine maintenance on the autoclave. A schedule, or log, for maintenance should be posted near the machine. The log should include spaces for initials or a signature after the maintenance has been performed. Routine maintenance includes:

- cleaning the lint trap
- washing the interior of the chamber with a soft brush or cloth
- checking the functioning of all components, especially the rubber seal for cracks or wear

The following steps should be taken at least once a week:

1. Drain the water from the autoclave and replace it with a cleaning solution.

2. Run the cleaning solution through a heat cycle for at least 20 minutes, then drain it and replace with a distilled-water rinse.

3. Run the rinse through a heat cycle for at least 20 minutes and drain.

4. Remove the shelves from the autoclave and scrub them. Also wipe the inside clean.

5. Refill the autoclave with distilled water.

From time to time, you also may need to check the performance of the autoclave using culture tests or other controls. It's important to keep good records of any tests done to check the autoclave's performance—and the results. If they show the sterilization process wasn't effective, you must report this fact in the log. Your report should include information about the problem and how it was resolved.

COLD CHEMICAL STERILIZATION

Not all items can be sterilized in the autoclave. Those that are sensitive to heat, too large, or very delicate are usually sterilized using a cold chemical solution. For example, one instrument commonly sterilized this way is an **endoscope.** Endoscopes are long flexible tubes with an optical system that allows the physician to look inside body cavities.

Equipment and Supplies

Here's a list of items needed for chemical sterilization.

- *A large container.* The container must be large enough to submerge the items in the chemical solution. It should be used only for the sterilization process. Also, it should have a lid that can be closed tightly. By covering the container, you ensure that the chemical solution will not evaporate during the process. The lid also prevents airborne microorganisms from entering the solution.

- *Appropriate chemical solution.* The sterilizing solution you'll use depends on what your medical office prefers. It also may depend on the type of items being sterilized. Some chemicals, such as hydrogen peroxide or bleach, will corrode metal instruments. No matter what chemical is used, it's important to follow the manufacturer's instructions carefully when mixing the solution. If it's too diluted, the instruments won't be sterilized properly.

If you put soaking wet items into the chemical solution, you'll be adding extra water. You need to dry them first.

- *Personal protective equipment.* When using the chemical solution, you need to protect yourself. Wear heavy duty utility gloves, protective goggles, and an apron to cover your clothing. If the chemical comes into contact with your skin, eyes, or mucous membranes, it can cause irritation or burns.

- *Vent hood.* The vent hood is used to remove unwanted fumes the chemicals may release into the air. For safety reasons, you need to use the vent hood when working with any chemical solutions.

The Hands On procedure on page 229 details the steps you need to follow in performing chemical sterilization. The chemicals used are sometimes similar to those used for sanitizing. A key difference is the exposure time. The exposure time for the sterilization process varies for different chemicals.

Always check the instructions provided by the chemical manufacturer to find out the correct exposure time for sterilization. Also, you'll need to make sure the chemical solution hasn't expired. The instructions should advise you on how long you can expect the chemical to remain effective.

After Chemical Sterilization

When the instruments have soaked in the chemical solution for the proper length of time, they can be removed. Because the items are now sterile, you must wear sterile gloves or use sterile transfer **forceps** to remove items from the solution. (Forceps are a tool that allows you to hold and grasp objects. You'll learn more information about this tool later in the chapter.)

You'll need to rinse the chemical solution from each instrument before it comes into contact with the patient. Rinse each item thoroughly using sterile water. Dry the item with a sterile towel.

Surgical Instruments

To assist the physician with minor surgical procedures, you must be familiar with the surgical instruments. You also must know how to care for each instrument.

As a clinical medical assistant, you'll need to know how to set up instruments and equipment for surgical procedures. You may be the one to pass instruments to the physician during the procedure as well.

The tools used in minor surgery all have specific functions. The main functions are:

- cutting
- dissecting
- grasping
- holding
- **retracting** (pulling back body tissues to expose other areas)
- **suturing** (the process of using stitches to close cuts made in body tissues)

Surgical instruments are designed with different shapes to suit their functions. They can be curved, straight, sharp, blunt, serrated (grooved), toothed, or smooth. Many are made of stainless steel and are reusable. But some are disposable.

COMMON SURGICAL INSTRUMENTS

The most widely used surgical instruments are:

- *Forceps and clamps.* These tools generally have two clamping blades and a handle. They're used for grasping and holding things.
- *Scissors.* Like common household scissors, surgical scissors consist of two cutting blades joined by a small screw.
- *Scalpel.* This small surgical knife has a straight handle and a straight or curved cutting blade.

You'll read about these instruments, along with some others, in more detail.

Forceps and Clamps

Forceps and clamps form the largest group of surgical instruments. Both are used for the same tasks—to grasp, handle, compress, pull, or join tissue, equipment, or supplies.

They come in many kinds and sizes. Some have teeth or **serrations.** (A serration is a groove cut into the blade of an instrument to improve its grasp.) They can have curved or straight blades. Some have sharp tips. Others have ring tips or blunt tips.

Many forceps have **ratchets** in the handles. Ratchets are notched mechanisms that click into position to maintain tension. They work to hold the tips of the forceps tightly together. Some forceps have spring handles that are compressed between thumb and index finger to grasp objects.

You need to learn the names and purposes of the basic types of forceps. This will help you know which instrument is needed when the physician asks for it. Here are some of the more common ones.

Hemostats. A **hemostat** is a surgical instrument with slender, straight or curved jaws. Usually, it's used to grasp and clamp blood vessels to establish **hemostasis** (the stopping of blood flow or bleeding).

Kelly Hemostats. Kelly hemostats are larger than many other hemostats and they have serrations only on the tips of their blades. Those with long handles are used for grasping blood vessels. Like other hemostats, their blades can be straight or curved.

Sterile Transfer Forceps. Sterile transfer forceps are used to transfer sterile supplies, equipment, and other surgical instruments to a **sterile field.** A sterile field is a specific area that is considered free of microbes.

Needle Holder. A **needle holder** is used to hold and pass a needle through tissue during suturing. It's sometimes called a suture forceps.

Spring or Thumb Forceps. *Spring or thumb forceps* help the user grasp tissue for dissection or suturing. Tissue forceps and splinter forceps are types of spring forceps.

Towel Clamps. Towel clamps are used to hold sterile drapes in place. Sterile drapes are placed around the operative site to protect it from microbes. They expose only the part of the body where surgery is being performed. This helps maintain the sterile field. In some surgeries, such as during vasectomies, towel clamps are also used to clamp tissue.

Scissors

Surgical scissors are used for cutting sutures and bandages. Physicians also use them to **dissect** (cut apart) superficial, deep, or delicate tissues. The points on surgical scissors may be blunt, sharp, or both, depending on the function of the instrument. There are several kinds of scissors.

- *Straight scissors* cut deep or delicate tissue and sutures.
- *Curved scissors* dissect superficial and delicate tissues.
- *Suture scissors* have a straight top blade. The blunt bottom blade is curved out or hooked to fit under, lift, and grasp sutures for snipping.

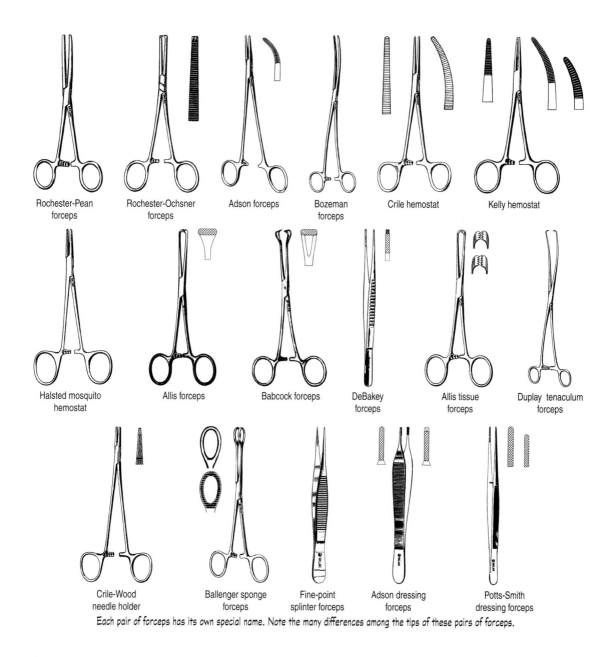

Rochester-Pean forceps

Rochester-Ochsner forceps

Adson forceps

Bozeman forceps

Crile hemostat

Kelly hemostat

Halsted mosquito hemostat

Allis forceps

Babcock forceps

DeBakey forceps

Allis tissue forceps

Duplay tenaculum forceps

Crile-Wood needle holder

Ballenger sponge forceps

Fine-point splinter forceps

Adson dressing forceps

Potts-Smith dressing forceps

Each pair of forceps has its own special name. Note the many differences among the tips of these pairs of forceps.

- *Bandage scissors* are used for removing bandages. The bottom blade is flattened, blunt, and longer than the top blade. The longer blade fits safely under bandages. The most common type is Lister bandage scissors.

Scalpels

Scalpels are another type of cutting tool. They consist of a reusable steel handle and a disposable blade. The handle can hold different blades for different surgical procedures. Many offices use scalpels with disposable handles and blades that are packaged as a one-piece sterile unit.

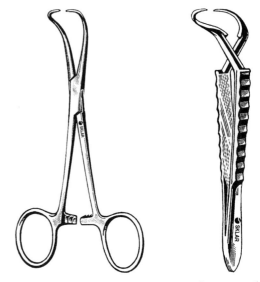

Backhaus towel clamp

Jones cross-action towel clamp

Towel clamps are essential for keeping sterile drapes in place.

Secrets for Success LEARNING SURGICAL TERMS

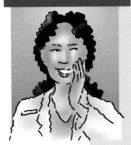

Learning the terms for surgical procedures can be challenging. Even if the procedure isn't done in the medical office, you may encounter the term during patient care. It's useful to keep in mind that root words (usually body parts) are often combined with suffixes or endings that indicate some kind of surgical action. Here are some common suffixes:

- *-ectomy* refers to excision or removal. For example, a cyst*ectomy* is the removal of a cyst.

- *-otomy* refers to incision or cutting. A trache*otomy* is a procedure for cutting into the trachea, or windpipe, to create an airway.

- *-plasty* means repair. A rhino*plasty* is surgical reconstruction of the nose.

- *-ostomy* is forming an opening. A col*ostomy* is a surgical procedure to create a new opening for waste to pass from the colon.

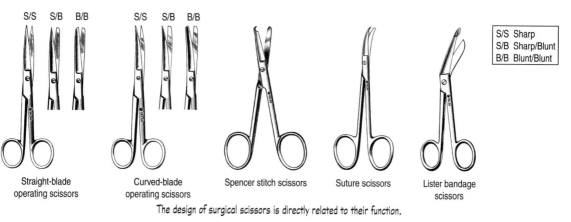

S/S	Sharp
S/B	Sharp/Blunt
B/B	Blunt/Blunt

Straight-blade operating scissors

Curved-blade operating scissors

Spencer stitch scissors

Suture scissors

Lister bandage scissors

The design of surgical scissors is directly related to their function.

Scalpels have different uses.

- Scalpels with straight or pointed blades are used for incision (cutting into tissue) and drainage procedures.
- Scalpels with curved blades are used to **excise,** or cut out, tissue.

Scalpel blades come in several sizes, with #10, #11, and #15 being the most common. Handles also come in different sizes. The larger the size number, the more delicate the handle. For example, a #3 handle would be a sturdier handle than a #7.

Scalpel blades must be handled carefully before use to avoid contamination and damaging the blade. You will need forceps or a needle holder to remove the scalpel blade from the packet and attach it to the scalpel handle. When you're finished, you should use forceps to remove the used blade to avoid injury.

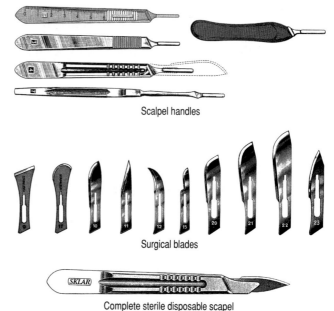

Scalpel handles

Surgical blades

Complete sterile disposable scapel

Scalpels have such varied uses that many types of handles and blades are available.

Probes, Directors, and Retractors

Before performing a procedure, the physician may first explore a cavity or wound with surgical tools including probes, directors, and retractors.

Probe. A probe is a thin, flexible instrument that can help the physician examine the angle and depth of the cavity or wound. There are many different kinds of probes. The physician's choice of probe depends on the area being explored.

Director. The director guides the knife or instrument once a procedure has begun. In surgical incisions, the director helps ensure correct depth and direction.

Retractor. Retractors are used to separate the edges of a wound and to hold open layers of tissue. Their main purpose is to expose areas beneath the surface tissues. Retractors come in different sizes and shapes. They may be plain or toothed. Toothed retractors may be sharp or blunt. Some retractors are designed to be held by an assistant during surgery. Self-retaining retractors can be screwed open and don't need to be held.

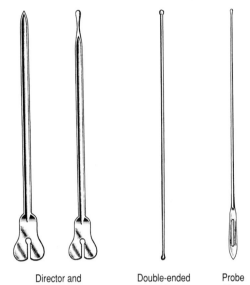

Director and tongue tie   Double-ended probe   Probe with eye

The director literally helps <u>direct</u> the knife or scalpel to limit its motion. The probe helps the physician see where an opening in the body goes.

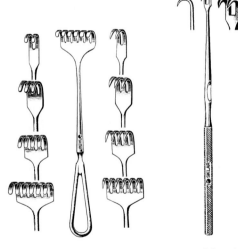

Volkman retractor   Lahey retractor   Senn retractor

Retractors are necessary so physicians can maintain the area on which they're operating more easily.

Other Surgical Instruments

Different medical specialties require different kinds of instruments for surgical procedures. The table below shows some of these surgical instruments and explains the use of each.

Commonly Used Instruments and Equipment Listed by Medical Specialty

Medical Specialty	Instruments	Use
Dermatology (disorders of the skin)	Keyes cutaneous punch	Remove a small circle of skin for microscopic study; available in different sizes (2–8 mm); disposable or reusable
	Schamberg comedone extractor	Remove blackheads or open pustules

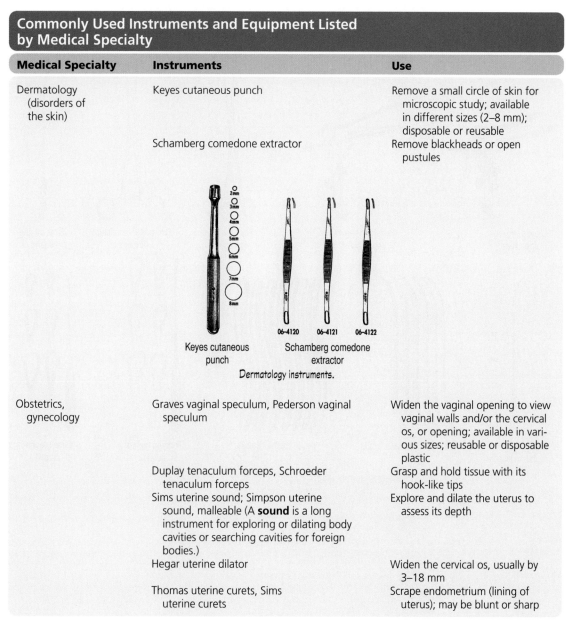

Keyes cutaneous punch

Schamberg comedone extractor

Dermatology instruments.

Medical Specialty	Instruments	Use
Obstetrics, gynecology	Graves vaginal speculum, Pederson vaginal speculum	Widen the vaginal opening to view vaginal walls and/or the cervical os, or opening; available in various sizes; reusable or disposable plastic
	Duplay tenaculum forceps, Schroeder tenaculum forceps	Grasp and hold tissue with its hook-like tips
	Sims uterine sound; Simpson uterine sound, malleable (A **sound** is a long instrument for exploring or dilating body cavities or searching cavities for foreign bodies.)	Explore and dilate the uterus to assess its depth
	Hegar uterine dilator	Widen the cervical os, usually by 3–18 mm
	Thomas uterine curets, Sims uterine curets	Scrape endometrium (lining of uterus); may be blunt or sharp

(continued)

Commonly Used Instruments and Equipment Listed by Medical Specialty (*continued*)

Medical Specialty	Instruments	Use
	Biopsy forceps	Secure pieces of tissue for microscopic study

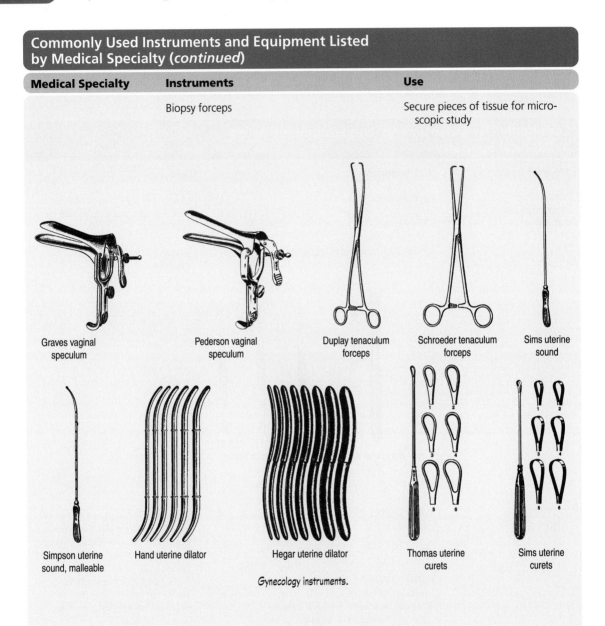

Graves vaginal speculum

Pederson vaginal speculum

Duplay tenaculum forceps

Schroeder tenaculum forceps

Sims uterine sound

Simpson uterine sound, malleable

Hand uterine dilator

Hegar uterine dilator

Thomas uterine curets

Sims uterine curets

Gynecology instruments.

Commonly Used Instruments and Equipment Listed by Medical Specialty (*continued*)

Medical Specialty	Instruments	Use
Ophthalmology	Desmarres lid retractor, Bailey foreign body remover	Hold eyelids open for removal of foreign bodies
	Schiotz tonometer	Measure intraocular pressure to diagnose glaucoma

Desmarres lid retractor

Bailey foreign body remover

Schiotz tonometer

Ophthalmology instruments.

Orthopedics (disorders of the skeletal system, including the bones, joints, and spine)	Oscillating plaster saw	Remove casts
	Stille plaster shears, Hennig plaster spreader	Remove casts

Oscillating plaster saw

Stille plaster shears

Henning plaster spreader

Orthopedic instruments.

(*continued*)

Commonly Used Instruments and Equipment Listed by Medical Specialty (*continued*)

Medical Specialty	Instruments	Use
Otology (disorders of the ear, a subspecialty of otolaryngology); rhinology (disorders of the nose, a subspecialty of otolaryngology)	Wilde ear forceps, Lucae bayonet forceps Vienna nasal speculum Buck ear curet	Insert or remove materials from ear or nose canal Open and extend nostrils for visualization of nasal passages Remove cerumen (ear wax) from deep ear canal

Wilde ear forceps	Lucae bayonet forceps	Buck ear curet	Vienna nasal speculum

Otology and rhinology instruments.

Medical Specialty	Instruments	Use
Proctology (disorders of the colon, rectum, and anus)	Hirschman anoscope, proctoscopes Sigmoidoscope Punch biopsy Alligator biopsy	Visualize lower intestinal tract; most have an **obturator** for ease of insertion. (An obturator is a smooth, rounded, removable inner portion of a hollow tube that allows for easier insertion.) Visualize lower sigmoid colon; may be rigid or flexible and has a fiber-optic light; some have a suction device Remove small, circular piece of tissue for study Grasp and excise tissue with jaws of instrument

Commonly Used Instruments and Equipment Listed by Medical Specialty (*continued*)

Medical Specialty	Instruments	Use

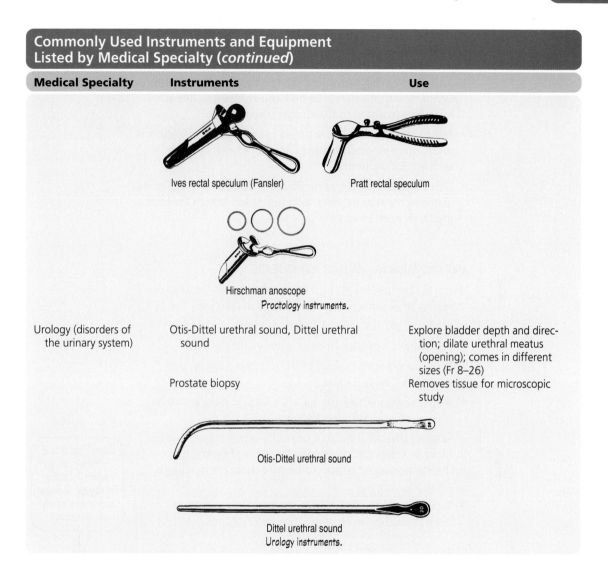

Ives rectal speculum (Fansler)   Pratt rectal speculum

Hirschman anoscope
Proctology instruments.

Medical Specialty	Instruments	Use
Urology (disorders of the urinary system)	Otis-Dittel urethral sound, Dittel urethral sound	Explore bladder depth and direction; dilate urethral meatus (opening); comes in different sizes (Fr 8–26)
	Prostate biopsy	Removes tissue for microscopic study

Otis-Dittel urethral sound

Dittel urethral sound
Urology instruments.

CARE AND CLEANING: IT'S YOUR RESPONSIBILITY

Taking good care of surgical instruments helps to ensure that they will function properly. Follow these guidelines to keep surgical instruments in good working order.

- *Rinse instruments as soon as possible.* Rinse instruments right after minor surgical procedures to remove obvious contamination. When substances dry or harden on instruments, they're harder to clean. Make sure you follow OSHA standards to prevent contact with blood or body fluids. This definitely includes wearing gloves.

- *Discard disposable instruments promptly.* Disposable scalpel blades should be removed from reusable handles and placed in sharps waste containers. If a disposable scalpel is used, the whole unit is placed in the sharps container. Syringes with needles attached and suture needles also must be discarded in the sharps container.

- *Sanitize instruments before they are sterilized.* Sterilization is more effective when instruments have been cleaned of visible contamination.

- *Check instruments before sterilization.* You need to make sure instruments stay in good working order. Watch for instruments in need of repair.

INSTRUMENTS—WHAT TO CHECK

Surgical instruments should be checked carefully to make sure they're working properly. Here's what to look for.

- Blades or points should be free of bends and nicks.
- Instrument tips should close evenly and tightly.
- Instruments with box locks should move freely, but should not be too loose.
- Instruments with spring handles should have enough tension to grasp objects tightly.
- Scissors should close in a smooth, even manner with no nicks or snags. (Scissors may be checked by cutting through gauze or cotton to be sure there are no rough areas.)
- Screws should be flush with the instrument surface. They should be freely workable, but not loose.

Oops! If you drop an instrument, always inspect it carefully for damage. Damaged instruments usually can be repaired.

Maintaining Surgical Equipment

You need to be familiar with the manufacturer's recommendations for each instrument or piece of equipment. Maintenance records should include any service provided by the manufacturer's representative. There also should be a place to record recommended or daily maintenance for keeping equipment in optimum working condition. Specific items in the maintenance record for each piece of equipment include:

- date of purchase
- model and serial number of equipment
- time of recommended service

Running Smoothly

REDUCING DAMAGE TO SURGICAL INSTRUMENTS

Surgical instruments are delicate! You can help minimize the chance of damage to instruments by following simple guidelines.

- Use instruments appropriately. Only use instruments for their specific purpose. For example, never use surgical scissors to cut paper or open packages. This could damage their cutting edges.

- Don't toss or drop instruments into a basin or sink. Blades or tips are easily damaged. Keep delicate instruments, such as tissue forceps or scissors, separate.

- Avoid stacking instruments in a pile. They may tangle and be damaged when separated.

- Always store sharp instruments separately. This helps prevent dulling or damaging sharp edges. It also helps prevent accidental injuries!

- Keep ratcheted instruments open when not in use. That way, the ratchet mechanism is less likely to be damaged.

- date service was requested
- reason for the service request
- name of the person requesting the service
- description of the service performed and any parts replaced
- name of the person performing the service and the date the work was completed
- signature and title of the person who acknowledged completion of the work

Warranties and guarantees should be kept with the equipment records, along with the name of the manufacturer's contact person. You need to know whom to call if there's a problem!

Maintaining Surgical Supplies

Clinical medical assistants need to keep an up-to-date master list of all supplies, including purchases and replacements. Parts and supplies that are vital to the operation of the facility

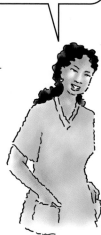

Ideally, one person is responsible for maintaining inventory, keeping maintenance schedules, and placing orders. If too many staff members are involved, some tasks can be overlooked or duplicated.

always should be kept on hand. Check instruction manuals for each piece of equipment when you order supplies for replacement or maintenance.

There are several factors to keep in mind when you decide which items to keep in inventory:

- shelf life of the item
- storage space available
- time required to order and receive the item

If a piece of equipment can't function without all of its components and some of the components have short lives, you need to have replacements on hand. For example, an ophthalmoscope without a light is basically useless.

Storage and Records

Clean and sterile supplies must be kept away from soiled items and waste. Sterile instruments, equipment, and supplies are usually kept in specific storage areas in the medical office. It's helpful if the storage area is near the rooms where the supplies will be used. The storage area should be kept neat and dust free.

Medical assistants are responsible for keeping accurate records of sterilized items and equipment. Typically, these records are kept in a log. The records include maintenance information about the equipment and load or sterilization information, including the following:

- date and time of the sterilization cycle
- general description of the load
- exposure time and temperature
- name or initials of the operator
- results of the sterilization indicator
- expiration date of the load (usually 30 days)

Getting Ready for Surgery

One of your responsibilities may be to prepare the treatment or examination room and the supplies needed for surgery. Many medical offices keep a box with index cards or a loose-leaf binder listing surgical procedures commonly performed in the office. It'll include the items you'll need to set up for the procedure.

Preparing the examination room and the supplies for surgery requires clean hands and careful technique to avoid contaminating the items inside the sterile area.

STERILE SURGICAL PACKS

Many of the basic supplies and equipment for a surgical procedure may be packaged together in a sterile surgical pack. Surgical packs may be prepared in the medical office or purchased from a commercial supplier.

Packs Prepared in the Medical Office

Sterile setups are wrapped in a suitable wrapper and prepared in the office using autoclave sterilization. Packs are labeled according to the type of procedure. Each pack contains the general instruments needed for the procedure. Some basic supplies, such as gauze, cotton balls, and towels also may be included before autoclaving.

Disposable Surgical Packs

Disposable surgical packs are popular because they're convenient and come with a variety of contents. They may contain one sterile item, such as a 4 × 4 sterile dressing, or a complete sterile surgical setup. Many are packaged with peel-apart wrappers. These wrappers have two loose flaps that can be pulled apart. They're designed to make it easy to drop the items carefully onto the operative field.

In some cases, the insides of the wrappers may be opened out and used as a sterile field. Some packages are enclosed in plastic and wrapped inside a barrier material that can be used as a sterile field.

Opening Surgical Packs

Labels for packs prepared in the office may only state the type of setup. However, labels on disposable sterile packs list the contents item by item. Disposable packs are generally more expensive than packages prepared in the office, so it's important to check that you have the right one for the procedure before you open it. You also need to check the expiration date on the package. If the pack has expired, don't use it. It may not be sterile!

Once a sterile pack has been opened, the procedure is similar whether the pack has been prepared commercially or in the office. Keep the following points in mind.

- Use clean hands to open the sterile items or packages.
- The outside surface of the outside wrapper is <u>not</u> sterile.
- Take care not to touch any sterile areas with your hands or other surfaces. The sterile area includes the inside surface of the outside wrapper, the inside wrapper (if any), and the contents of the package.

- If any sterile area or item does contact another surface, the pack is considered contaminated and must be replaced.
- Check the sterilization indicator inside the sterile pack. It indicates whether the items inside the package have been sterilized properly.

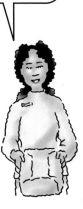

Read the directions for how to open the sterile package. If you open it incorrectly, the contents can become contaminated.

Watch for Contamination!

When you work with sterile surgical items, you need to know when items are considered contaminated—even if they haven't been used. Contaminated items must be repackaged and sterilized again if any of the following situations occur.

- *Moisture is present on the pack.* Microbes can be drawn into the package in liquid absorbed through its wrap. If a package sterilized in the medical office gets moist, it must be repackaged in a clean, dry wrapper and sterilized again. If a damp pack is disposable, it must be discarded.

- *Items are dropped outside the sterile field.* If an item touches a surface outside the sterile field, it's considered contaminated.

- *The pack's date has expired.* The date on the outside of the pack shouldn't be over 30 days old for packs prepared in the office. Commercially prepared packs shouldn't be used after the expiration date listed on the pack.

- *The wrapper is damaged or torn.* Damaged or torn wrappers could allow microbes into the package. Items should be discarded or rewrapped and sterilized again.

- *When any area is known or thought to have been touched by a contaminated item.*

APPLYING STERILE GLOVES

To move sterile items or place them on the sterile field, you must use sterile gloves. Be sure to choose gloves that are the right size for your hands. Follow these steps to apply them.

1. Before you put on the gloves, remove any rings or other jewelry. Rings may pierce the gloves and contaminate the procedure.

2. Wash your hands before applying gloves. Wearing gloves isn't a substitute for hand washing.

3. Place the glove package on a clean, dry, flat surface. The cuffed end of the glove should be facing you.

4. Pull the outer wrapping apart to expose the sterile, inner wrap.

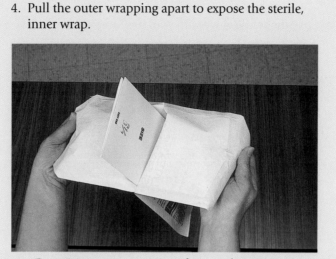

The sterile inner wrap is an extra layer of protection for sterile gloves.

5. With the cuffs toward you, fold back the inner wrap to expose the gloves.

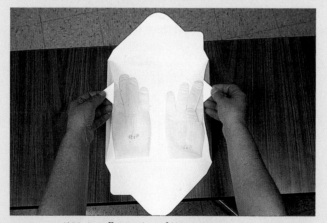

With the cuffs toward you, fold back the inner wrap.

6. Grasping the edges of the outer paper, open the package out to its fullest. Remember that the inner surface of the package is a sterile field.

7. Using your nondominant hand, pick up the dominant hand glove by grasping the folded edge of the cuff. Lift it up and away from the paper to avoid brushing an unsterile surface. (The folded edge of the cuff is contaminated as soon as it is touched with the ungloved

hand.) Be very careful not to touch the outside surface of the sterile glove with your ungloved hand.

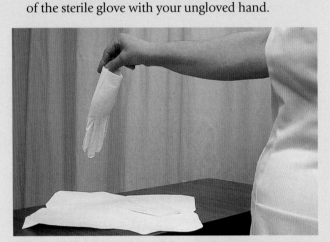

Using your nondominant hand, lift the cuff of the glove for the dominant hand. Touch only the inner surface of the cuff. To make this easier to do, curl your thumb inward as you insert your hand.

8. Curl your fingers and thumb together and insert them into the glove. This prevents you from accidentally touching the outside surface of the glove. Straighten your fingers and pull the glove on with your nondominant hand still grasping the cuff.

9. Unfold the cuff by pinching the inside surface that will be against your wrist and pulling it toward your wrist. Only the unsterile portions of the glove will be touched by your hands.

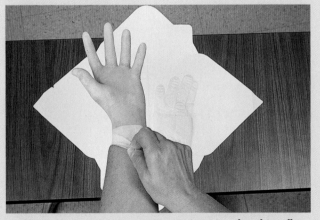

Pull the glove snugly into place, touching only the inside surface of the cuff.

10. Place the fingers of your gloved hand under the cuff of the remaining glove. Lift the glove up and away from the wrapper to prevent it from touching an unsterile surface. Slide your ungloved hand carefully into the glove with your fingers and thumb curled together.

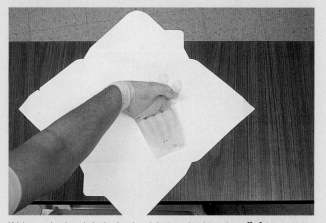

With your thumb curled, slip the gloved dominant hand into the cuff of the remaining glove.

11. Straighten your fingers and pull the glove up and over your wrist by carefully unfolding the glove. Folding the cuffs out to their fullest allows the greatest area of sterility.

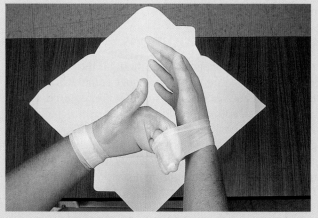

Unfold the cuff and pull the glove on snugly.

12. Settle the gloves comfortably onto your fingers by lacing your fingers together and adjusting the tension over your hands. The gloves should fit snugly without wrinkles or areas that bind the fingers.

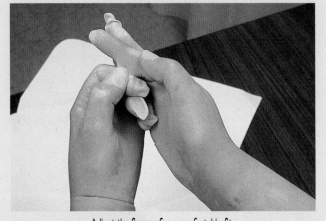

Adjust the fingers for a comfortable fit.

USING STERILE TRANSFER FORCEPS

One way to move sterile items or place them on the sterile field is to use sterile transfer forceps. When using sterile transfer forceps, the tips of the forceps and items being moved must stay sterile. The handles of the forceps are considered medically aseptic, but not sterile, because they are touched by the bare hands of the person using them. You'll find steps for using sterile forceps in the Hands On procedure on page 234.

Remove contaminated sterile gloves exactly as you would nonsterile gloves. For a review of how to do that, flip back to the Hands On procedure in Chapter 1.

PEEL-BACK PACKAGES AND SOLUTIONS

Sometimes, the sterile pack will contain all the supplies needed for a procedure, including gauze squares or cotton balls. In other cases, additional supplies are required.

Usually, small supplies are provided in commercially prepared, peel-apart packages. These packages contain small or single items to add to the sterile field. The packaging is designed with two flaps. The flaps allow the package to be opened without contaminating its sterile contents.

To open the package properly, you must use both hands. Here's how.

- Place your thumbs just inside the tops of the flaps' edges.
- Separate the flaps using a slow, outward motion of the thumbs and flaps.

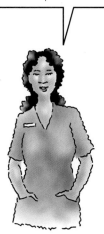

Closer Look

STORING STERILE TRANSFER FORCEPS

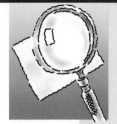

Sterile transfer forceps can be stored in one of three ways.

- *In a dry, sterile container.* The forceps and the container must be sanitized and autoclaved every day.
- *In a wrapped sterile package.* The wrapping protects the forceps from being exposed to microorganisms and maintains sterility.
- *In a sterile solution in a closed container system.* A closed container helps to protect tips of forceps from contamination. The forceps and the container must be sterilized every day. Fresh solution must be added daily.

- Keep in mind that the inside of the sealed package and its contents are sterile. They'll be contaminated if touched by anything that isn't sterile, such as a finger or airborne droplets from talking or sneezing when you open the pack.

Once the peel-back package is opened, there are three ways to add its contents to the sterile field.

- *Using sterile transfer forceps.* Once the package is opened, hold down the two edges. Lift the contents up and away with sterile forceps. This process often requires two people—one to hold the package open and the other to remove the contents with the sterile forceps.

- *Using a sterile gloved hand.* This method requires two people. The medical assistant opens the package and holds the edges carefully to avoid touching the physician's gloves. The physician uses a gloved hand to remove the contents.

- *Flipping the contents onto the sterile field.* To do this, you need to step back from the sterile field so that your hands and the outer wrapper of the package, which isn't sterile, don't cross the sterile

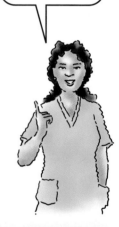

To reduce the chance of contamination, only one pair of forceps is stored in each container.

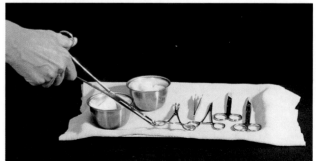

Sterile transfer forceps may be used to add or move items on the sterile field.

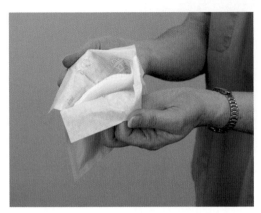

Open sterile packets by grasping the edges and rolling the thumbs outward.

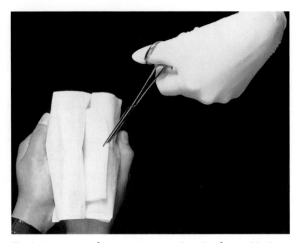

The physician may use forceps to remove small supplies from peel-back packages.

field. Pull the package edges down and away from the contents. Carefully drop or flip item onto the middle of the sterile field without touching the one-inch border around the edge of the sterile field.

Most items in peel-back packages are disposable items. This means they can't be resterilized after being opened. They must be discarded, even if they haven't been used. Because they're relatively expensive, sterile packs of disposable items shouldn't be opened until they're needed. You might place a small supply near the area where the procedure is being performed, to be opened only if necessary.

Small items aren't the only supplies not included in standard sterile packs. Solutions used during the surgical procedure must be added to the sterile field at the time of setup. Some procedures may require sterile water or saline. Some may require an antiseptic solution such as Betadine. Solutions need to be poured into sterile containers. To learn how to add solutions to the sterile field, read the Hands On procedure on page 235.

> Just inside the outer edge of every sterile field is a one-inch border that is considered not sterile.

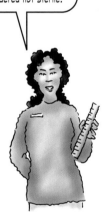

Preparing the Patient for Surgery

As a clinical medical assistant, you'll play an important role in preparing the patient before the physician performs minor surgery. You may need to:

- help obtain the patient's consent for the procedure
- answer questions about instructions to the patient

Running Smoothly   MAINTAINING A STERILE FIELD

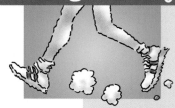

Even in minor surgery, it's important to prevent pathogens from entering the patient's body during the procedure. This requires that the surgical area or field remains sterile. Here's what to do—and what to avoid—to maintain a sterile field.

1. Always face a sterile field. That way, you can be sure it hasn't been contaminated. If you need to turn your back or leave the area, cover the field with a sterile drape. Make sure you use sterile techniques!

2. Hold all sterile items above waist level. When sterile items aren't where you can see them, you'll have to presume they've become contaminated.

3. Place sterile items in the middle of the sterile field. A one-inch border around the field is considered contaminated.

4. Don't spill any liquids, even sterile liquids, onto a sterile field. The surface below the field isn't sterile. Moisture can be wicked up into the field—along with microorganisms.

5. Don't cough, sneeze, or talk over the sterile field. Microbes from your respiratory tract can contaminate the field.

6. Never reach over the sterile field. Dust or lint from your clothing might enter the sterile field.

7. Don't pass soiled supplies, such as gauze or instruments, over the sterile field.

8. If you know or suspect the sterile field has been contaminated, alert the physician. Sterility must be established before the procedure can continue.

- position and drape the patient for the procedure
- prepare the patient's skin

INFORMED CONSENT

It's necessary to obtain **informed consent** from the patient before performing a surgical procedure in the medical office.

An informed consent form is a legal document that explains the course of treatment, including the risks and benefits to the patient. This form may be signed on a visit prior to the day of surgery or on the day of the surgery. The procedure can't go ahead unless the patient signs the form.

ANSWERING THE PATIENT'S QUESTIONS

Although the physician is responsible for obtaining informed consent, the patient may ask you questions about the procedure—for example:

- How long will it take?
- What preparations are needed?
- Is fasting necessary?

You may answer these questions after verifying the information with the physician.

Prior to the day of surgery, the patient may be given instructions about how to prepare for surgery. The physician may prescribe medication for the patient to take at home before the procedure. It's good practice to give the patient written instructions to take home.

You need to notify the physician if the patient seems confused or doesn't understand the instructions. Encourage the

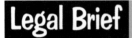

Legal Brief   INFORMED CONSENT

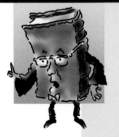

It's the physician's legal responsibility to give the patient a full explanation of any surgical procedure. By signing the informed consent document, the patient agrees that she has received this explanation. The document must state:

- the procedure
- the purpose of the procedure
- the expected results of the procedure
- any possible side effects, risks, and complications

The form should have spaces for the date and signatures of the patient, physician, and witness or witnesses. By signing the document, the patient voluntarily accepts the risks involved and agrees to the procedure. The medical assistant isn't responsible for informing the patient, but often acts as a witness.

SPECIAL CONSENT TO OPERATION OR OTHER PROCEDURE(S)

PATIENT _____   PATIENT NUMBER _____

DATE _____   TIME _____

1.   I HEREBY AUTHORIZE DOCTOR _____ AND/OR SUCH ASSIS-
     TANTS AS MAY BE SELECTED BY HIM, TO PERFORM THE FOLLOWING PROCEDURE(S):

     _____

     ON _____
          (NAME OF PATIENT OR MYSELF)

2.   THE PROCEDURE(S) LISTED ABOVE HAVE BEEN EXPLAINED TO ME BY DR. _____
     AND I UNDERSTAND THE NATURE AND THE CONSEQUENCES OF THE PROCEDURE(S).

3.   I RECOGNIZE THAT, DURING THE COURSE OF THE OPERATION, UNFORESEEN CONDI-
     TIONS MAY NECESSITATE ADDITIONAL OR DIFFERENT PROCEDURES THAN THOSE SET
     FORTH. I FURTHER AUTHORIZE AND REQUEST THAT THE ABOVE NAMED SURGEON, HIS
     ASSISTANTS, OR HIS DESIGNEES PERFORM SUCH PROCEDURES AS ARE IN HIS PRO-
     FESSIONAL JUDGMENT NECESSARY AND DESIRABLE, INCLUDING, BUT NOT LIMITED TO,
     PROCEDURES INVOLVING PATHOLOGY AND RADIOLOGY. THE AUTHORITY GRANTED
     UNDER THIS PARAGRAPH SHALL EXTEND TO REMEDYING CONDITIONS NOT KNOWN TO
     DR. _____ AT THE TIME THE OPERATION IS COMMENCED.

4.   I AM AWARE THAT THE PRACTICE OF MEDICINE AND SURGERY IS NOT AN EXACT SCI-
     ENCE AND I ACKNOWLEDGE THAT NO GUARANTEES HAVE BEEN MADE TO ME AS TO THE
     RESULTS OF THE OPERATION OR PROCEDURE.

5.   TISSUE REMOVED DURING SURGERY SHALL BE SENT TO PATHOLOGY TO BE EXAMINED
     AND DISPOSED OF IN ACCORDANCE WITH THE RULES AND REGULATIONS OF THE MED-
     ICAL STAFF OF THE SURGERY CENTER.

_____   _____
Procedure has been discussed with patient. (Surgeon's Signature)   SIGNATURE OF PATIENT

PATIENT IS UNABLE TO SIGN BECAUSE   ☐ HE (SHE) IS A MINOR _____ YEARS OF AGE

                                     ☐ OTHER (SPECIFY) _____

_____   _____
WITNESS   PERSON AUTHORIZED TO SIGN FOR PATIENT

                                              _____
                                              RELATIONSHIP OF ABOVE TO PATIENT

A consent form such as this one must be signed before the physician can perform a surgical procedure.

patient to call the office if he thinks of questions later. Of course, the instructions should be documented in the patient's medical record.

POSITIONING THE PATIENT

Before positioning the patient for a minor surgical procedure, ask the patient to void, or urinate, to help prevent discomfort during the procedure.

Here are some other ways you can make the patient more comfortable.

> Patients who didn't need help removing clothing before surgery often do need help afterward. Be sensitive and ready to assist if necessary.

- Offer to help the patient remove whatever clothing is necessary to expose the operative site.

- Provide the patient with extra sheets or a blanket. If the office is air conditioned, it may be uncomfortably cool for the patient's exposed skin.

- Help the patient into a comfortable position on the examining table. While waiting for the physician, there's no need for the patient to stay in an uncomfortable position, such as the lithotomy or the knee-chest position.

When the physician is ready to begin, help the patient into a position that exposes the operative site and makes it accessible to the physician. You may give the patient pillows for support or comfort.

Types of Drapes

The procedure and the patient's position determine the type of drapes used to expose the operative site and cover the patient. Disposable paper drapes are commonly used in the medical office. They come in many sizes and shapes, depending on their specific use. Paper drapes can be used alone or in combination with separate drape sheets and towels.

Fenestrated drapes have an opening to expose the operative site while covering other areas. They also come in various sizes. Small fenestrated drapes may be used for procedures such as inserting sutures. Large fenestrated drapes might be used to cover the legs and lower abdomen while exposing the perineal area—the area between the anus and the genital organs.

Some sterile drapes are combined with adhesive-backed clear plastic. The plastic sticks to the patient's skin and eliminates the need for towel clamps.

Draping the Patient

After the surgical scrub has been done, follow these steps for draping a patient with a sterile drape:

1. Pick up the drape on the one-inch border that's considered nonsterile. No gloves are needed.

2. Lift the drape over the surgical area without contaminating the drape.

3. Place the drape on the patient from his side farthest away to closest. This way you won't have to reach over the drape after you've placed it on the patient.

To remove contaminated drapes from the patient after the procedure, put on clean examination gloves. You need to follow standard precautions when removing soiled sheets, towels, or drapes after minor surgery. They could be contaminated with blood or body fluids. Carefully roll the items away from your body, keeping the contaminated edges inside. By surrounding the dirtier areas of the drape with the cleaner areas, your clothing is less likely to be contaminated.

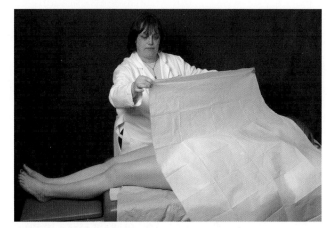

Notice how the medical assistant is holding only the border of the drape as she places it over the patient.

PREPARING SKIN

Before surgery, you need to remove as many microbes as possible from the patient's skin in the operative area. Preparing the skin decreases the chance of wound contamination and infection. Skin preparations may include:

- applying antiseptic solution
- removing gross contaminants and hair

You'll find steps for preparing a patient's skin for minor office surgery in the Hands On procedure on page 237. After the skin has been prepared, you can place the drape on the patient.

LAST-MINUTE QUESTIONS

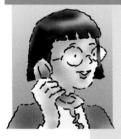

Q: *I was preparing a patient for surgery when he started asking lots of last-minute questions about his procedure. What's the best way to handle this?*

A: Because the procedure was already explained to the patient to obtain his consent, these last-minute questions may reflect his anxiety about the procedure. Remind the patient that it's normal to be concerned about a surgical procedure. Listen carefully to his concerns and take the time to answer his questions. Check to be sure he understands your responses. A calm and reassuring manner will help the patient feel more confident and less anxious about the procedure.

   If you're not sure of all the answers to his questions, and if he still seems anxious, notify the physician. The physician may need to take some time to talk to the patient before beginning the procedure.

Assisting with Surgery

During minor surgery, your role will be to assist the physician as needed. You may be asked to hold supplies for the physician, adjust the patient's drapes, pass instruments to the physician, or help collect specimens. As you become more experienced, you'll find it easier to anticipate what's needed and have instruments and supplies ready before the physician asks for them.

LOCAL ANESTHETICS

A **local anesthetic** is a substance that numbs the operative area to minimize pain or discomfort to the patient. Local anesthetic may be used occasionally if a wound contains embedded debris. The anesthetic is injected in the wound site to make the process of wound cleaning more comfortable for the patient.

   Many different kinds of anesthetics are used in the medical office. A few examples are:

- lidocaine (Xylocaine or Baylocaine)
- mepivacaine (Carbocaine)
- bupivacaine (Marcaine)

Sometimes, epinephrine is added to local anesthetics to cause vasoconstriction (the narrowing of blood vessels). It slows the absorption of the anesthetic by the body and lengthens its effectiveness. Epinephrine may be used when the physician expects a long procedure. But in some cases, vasoconstriction can damage body tissues. Anesthesia with epinephrine should never be used on the tips of fingers or toes, the nose, the ear, or the penis.

There are two methods for administering local anesthesia. The method used will depend on when the physician plans to administer the anesthesia.

Administering Anesthetic: Method 1

In the first method, you'll draw the anesthetic as the physician's assistant.

- When you draw the anesthetic for the physician into a syringe, it's important to keep the vial beside the syringe for the physician's approval.

- When you draw the anesthetic, the outside of the syringe and needle unit aren't sterile. The anesthetic is given to the patient before the physician puts on sterile gloves.

Administering Anesthetic: Method 2

In the second method, the physician draws the anesthetic. This method is used if the physician puts on sterile gloves before administering the anesthetic.

1. Include a sterile syringe and needle on the sterile field setup.

2. When the physician is ready to administer the anesthetic, show the physician the label on the vial. Then clean the rubber stopper of the vial with an alcohol swab.

3. You hold the vial while the physician draws the required amount into the syringe.

There are many ways to hold the vial securely while the physician draws the anesthetic. You and the physician will work together to develop a method that maintains surgical asepsis.

PASSING INSTRUMENTS

Passing instruments to the physician requires careful attention. You must maintain the integrity of the sterile field throughout the procedure. Tell the physician immediately if there's any possibility that the sterile field has been contaminated. Here are some tips for passing instruments during minor surgery:

- Watch the procedure closely so you can anticipate the physician's needs. For example, if the physician is making an incision, have sterile sponges ready to soak up any blood.
- The physician may ask for an instrument verbally, or show you what's needed with her hands. After you've worked together for a while, you'll learn what the physician is likely to ask for during different parts of the procedure.

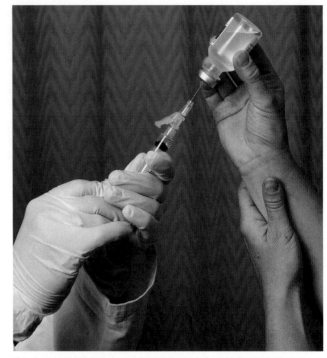

This photograph shows one way a medical assistant can hold the vial while the physician uses a syringe to withdraw the anesthetic.

- When passing an instrument to the physician, grip the instrument firmly by its tips. Hold blades or sharp edges down for safety. The handle end should be directed toward the physician.
- Place the instrument gently but firmly into the physician's palm or fingers.
- Wait until you feel the physician grasp the instrument before you let go. You don't want the instrument to drop onto the floor—or onto the patient!

WOUND CLOSURE

Many types of wounds need to be closed in order to heal rapidly, with minimal scarring. This is accomplished by **approximation,** or bringing the edges of the wound as close together as possible to their original position. There are several methods and materials for closing wounds. The most common ones are:

- sutures
- adhesives
- staples

Sutures

Sutures are sterile, surgical materials for connecting wounds and tissues. Sometimes, incisions are necessary to bring tissue layers into close approximation. Sutures are inserted:

- to bring tissues together after the removal of a cyst or tissue sample
- to close lacerations
- to help skin surfaces heal

Some sutures are absorbed by the body, while others must be removed.

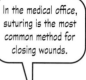

In the medical office, suturing is the most common method for closing wounds.

Adhesives

Adhesive skin closures may be used to approximate the edges of a small wound if sutures aren't needed. Strips are placed transversely across the line of the wound. In most cases, the strips are left in place until they fall off. In some cases, the physician may want them replaced or removed if they become soiled with drainage. Strips shouldn't be pulled away from the wound. Tension on the wound site may disrupt the healing process.

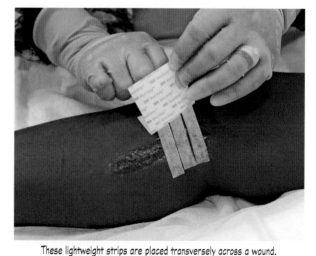

These lightweight strips are placed transversely across a wound.

Staples

Skin staples are sometimes used to close large incisions over areas where **dehiscence** can occur. Dehiscence is the separation of wound edges. Sterile skin staples are commonly made of stainless steel. Areas where staples might be used include the knee, hip, or abdomen. Specialized staples made of sterling silver may be used in neurosurgery. Staples usually aren't inserted in the medical office. They're removed when the wound is completely healed.

Suture Needles

The supplies used for suturing are needles and suture materials. There are several kinds of suture needles. Needles used for minor office surgery will depend on the type of surgery being performed.

Needles are classified in these ways: by shape, by point, or by eye.

Classified by Shape. Needles may be curved or straight. Curved needles usually are clamped in a needle holder before being handed to or used by the physician. Straight needles aren't clamped in a needle holder. They're handed to the physician with the point up. Straight needles rarely are used in medical offices.

Classified by Point. Needle points are cutting, or round and tapered. Cutting needles have sharp edges and are used to cut through tough tissues, such as skin. Straight cutting needles are called Keith needles. Noncutting tapered or round needles are used on **subcutaneous tissue.** Subcutaneous tissue is located below the skin. They also may be used on muscle, or on the peritoneum, a thin membrane lining the body cavity and covering some organs.

Classified by Eye. *Traumatic needles* have an eye and can be threaded with any length of suture material. *Atraumatic needles* are eyeless and come with a specific length of suture thread attached. Atraumatic needles are also called **swaged needles** because the suture material is swaged, or fused, to the needle in the manufacturing process.

Atraumatic needles cause less damage than traumatic needles when they pass through body tissues. Needles with eyes have a double thickness of suture where the suture passes through the eye. This double thickness makes a larger opening when pulled through tissues, compared to the single thickness of suture in eyeless needles.

Choosing a Needle. In medical offices, curved swaged needles are used far more often than any other type. Swaged needles are selected based on the size and length of the suture material and the needle **gauge.** The needle gauge, or needle diameter, is marked clearly on the packaging material. When a suture must be threaded through an eyed needle, both the needle gauge and the suture size must be selected.

Sutures, needles, and suture-needle combinations come in peel-apart packages. The packages are sterile on the inside. Sutures and needles can be added to the sterile field using sterile transfer forceps, a sterile gloved hand, or by carefully flipping them onto the field.

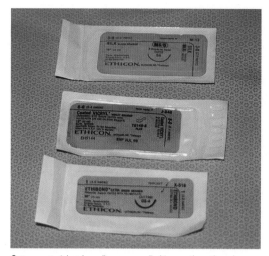

Suture material and needles are supplied in see-through packages with the size of the suture material and the type of needle listed on the packet. The inside of the packet is sterile.

> The physician usually selects the suture and the needle. Know your physician's preferences so you can have the right ones ready.

Suture Material. Suture material comes in various gauges and lengths. Very thick sutures are numbered from 0 to 7, where 7 is the thickest. Sutures smaller than size 0 are expressed with added zeros. Small sutures range from 11-0, the smallest, to 2-0. A fine 10-0 suture, about the diameter of a human hair, is used in **microsurgery,** or surgery performed with the aid of a microscope. Fine sutures also are used on places such as the face and neck because they decrease scarring.

TYPES OF SUTURES

There are two main types of sutures: *absorbable sutures* and *nonabsorbable sutures.*

Absorbable sutures are broken down by the body and don't have to be removed. Here are some other useful facts about these sutures.

- These sutures are referred to commonly as catgut. This suture material is made from the intestines of sheep or cattle.

- The two forms of absorbable gut suture are chromic and plain. Chromic means the suture is chemically treated to delay absorption by the body. Plain absorbable suture is not treated and is absorbed more quickly.

- Absorbable sutures are used most often in hospital settings to hold deep tissue.

Nonabsorbable sutures either remain in the body permanently or are removed after healing. Here are some other useful facts about these sutures.

- They're made of natural fibers such as silk or cotton; synthetics such as nylon, Dacron, or polypropylene, or stainless steel wire.
- Nonabsorbable sutures come in many different brands, lengths, sizes, and swaged needles, making them very versatile.
- They're used on the skin (where they can be removed), intestines, bone, or large blood vessels. They're also used to attach heart valves and in artificial and natural grafts.

COMMON OFFICE SURGICAL PROCEDURES

Two of the most frequently performed minor surgeries in a general medical office are:

- removing skin lesions
- draining abscesses

Biopsy is another procedure that's commonly performed in some medical offices. It is the removal of a tissue sample for diagnostic examination. You must follow standard precautions when you assist with any of these procedures.

Excision of a Lesion

A **lesion** is a local area of diseased or abnormal tissue. Some lesions that may be removed in a medical office include:

- mole
- skin tag
- **lentigine,** a small, flat, dark spot on the skin that resembles a freckle
- **keratosis,** a horny growth, such as a wart or callus

To excise something is to cut it out. Physicians use several techniques to excise lesions or remove them in other ways.

- *Standard method* refers to the process of excising the lesion using a scalpel.
- *Electrosurgery* is a process where high-frequency electric current is used to excise the lesion or else destroy it.
- *Laser surgery* uses focused, intense beams of light to penetrate and remove tissue.

- *Cryosurgery* is a method that uses extreme cold to either excise or destroy diseased or abnormal tissue.

Some lesions may be **desiccated** or **fulgurated** (destroyed by drying up) by using electrosurgical or cryosurgical methods. (You'll read more about electrosurgery shortly.) However, in many cases, samples are sent to a pathology laboratory for diagnosis. If samples are required, the lesion is excised using one of the above methods. The Hands On procedure on page 239 details the medical assistant's role in the excision of a lesion.

Tissue Biopsy

Excision also can be used to remove tissue for biopsy. The tissue is sent to the laboratory and examined under a microscope to assist in diagnosis. Typically, only small samples of tissue are needed for examination. When a lesion is biopsied, however, the entire lesion is generally excised for evaluation. In a **punch biopsy,** a small section is removed from the center of the abnormal tissue. Although some biopsies are performed in a hospital, skin biopsies can be performed in the medical office.

Cervical Biopsies

Another procedure that may be performed in the medical office is the cervical biopsy. This is a procedure in which a small piece of tissue is removed from a female patient's cervix. The physician removes the tissue during a colposcopy—a visual examination of the cervix using an instrument with a magnifying lens and a light (colposcope).

Physicians usually perform this procedure when a patient's Pap smear shows abnormal results, or when the physician sees an abnormal area on the cervix during a routine examination. You'll find steps for assisting with the colposcopy and cervical biopsy in the Hands On procedure on page 241.

Incision and Drainage

An abscess is a collection of pus that has formed in a cavity surrounded by inflamed tissue. An abscess is the body's response to an infection, when pathogens have entered through a break in the skin. Abscesses may be referred to as boils, furuncles (a single lesion), or carbuncles (several lesions grouped closely together). Abscesses are very painful for the patient. The site of the abscess must be **incised** (cut into) and the infected material drained before healing can take place. Learn how to assist with the incision and drainage procedure by reviewing the Hands On procedure on page 243.

Specimen Collection

Many minor office procedures yield specimens that must be sent to a laboratory for examination. Specimens include samples of tissue, foreign bodies, and samples of wound **exudate,** or drainage. It's your job to choose a proper container with an appropriate **preservative** for the procedure being performed. The preservative helps to prevent the sample from breaking down or decaying before it can be examined.

The laboratory where the specimen is sent usually provides the appropriate containers with preservative. There should be a stock of them on hand in the medical office. You'll need to assist the physician in collecting the specimen by holding the open container steady. The physician must drop the specimen directly into the preservative without touching the sides of the container.

You'll be responsible for attaching a label to the specimen. The label must contain the patient's name and the date. You'll also need to complete a laboratory request form to send with the specimen. Several pieces of information must be included on the form:

- the patient's name, age, and gender
- the patient's identification number or social security number
- the date the specimen was taken
- the type of specimen
- the location the specimen was taken from
- the type of examination requested
- the physician's name or laboratory contract number

Specimens collected during minor surgery must be sent to the pathology laboratory as quickly as possible!

ELECTROSURGERY

Medical offices often use electrosurgery to remove moles, cysts, warts, and certain types of skin and cervical cancers. In electrosurgery, high-frequency alternating current is used to destroy or cut and remove tissue. One advantage of this method is that the electricity seals small bleeding vessels and reduces the blood and cell fluid lost in the process.

Electrosurgical units use disposable **electrodes,** or devices that carry electricity. The tips on the electrodes have different shapes and sizes depending on their use. Electrode tips include blades, needles, loops, and balls. The following procedures are considered electrosurgery.

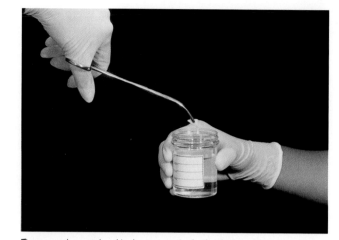

Tissue samples are placed in the preservative by the physician. You must hold the specimen container very steady.

- *Fulguration* destroys tissue with controlled electric sparks. The physician holds the electrode tip 1 to 2 mm from the operative site. A series of sparks destroys superficial cells at the site.

- *Electrodesiccation* dries and separates tissue with an electric current. The electrode is placed directly on the site.

- *Electrocautery* causes quick **coagulation** or clotting of small blood vessels with the heat created by electric current. This process is also called electrocoagulation.

- *Electrosection* is the incision or excision of tissue. Bleeding is minimal with this type of procedure. However, it may increase damage to the surrounding tissues.

During electrosurgery, you're responsible for the safety and comfort of the patient. You'll need to hand the electrode to the physician as needed. Always pass the electrode with the tip pointing down.

Electrosurgery Safety

The physician will power on and operate the electrosurgical unit. However, you could cause injuries to the patient, the physician, and yourself if you don't follow proper procedures. Pay close attention to these safety measures when assisting with electrosurgery.

- Make sure all working parts are in good repair. The electrical current is carefully regulated. If the machine is defective, the patient might be seriously injured.

- Make sure all metal is removed from the patient. You also need to ensure the patient doesn't have any metal implants or a cardiac pacemaker. Metal conducts electricity and can cause serious burns. Metal implants may become very hot, and pacemakers can malfunction.

- Be sure the patient is grounded with a pad supplied by the manufacturer. Attach the pad to the patient at a site recommended by the manufacturer. Some manufacturers advise placing the pad near the operative site. Others recommend placing it far away. Know what the recommendations are for the device in your office. Improper placement of the pad can lead to injury!
- Place the grounding pad firmly and completely against the patient's skin. With some pads, you must apply a conducting gel to the pad and to the patient. Adhesive-backed pads facilitate conduction through the grounding pad. If areas of the skin under the pad do not have good contact with the pad, hot spots may occur. Hot spots can burn the patient.

Maintaining the Electrosurgical Unit

Here are some hints to maintaining the electrosurgical unit properly.

- The electrode tips for the unit are usually disposable. They should be discarded after use.
- Some medical offices may still use reusable electrode tips. These should be disinfected and processed in the autoclave according to the manufacturer's directions. Reusable tips must be polished with steel wool if they become dull.
- The surfaces of the electrosurgical unit should be kept clean and dry.
- Machines should be covered when not in use.
- Electrosurgical machines must be inspected from time to time to ensure they are working properly. Check the operating manual for the regular maintenance to be performed by office staff. It also will contain information about how often routine inspections should be performed by trained technicians. A maintenance log should be kept as discussed in the beginning of the chapter.

LASER SURGERY

Lasers also can be used to cut tissue and coagulate small bleeding vessels. Lasers are devices that focus high-intensity light in a narrow beam to create extreme heat and energy. Light from a laser usually isn't visible. Colored filters illuminate the laser's target. This allows the physician to direct the laser beam to the surgical area.

There are many types of lasers, each with a specific medical use. The most common types of lasers used in the medical office are the:

- argon laser, used for coagulation
- carbon dioxide laser, used for cutting tissue
- Nd:YAG, used for coagulation and to separate warts and moles from surrounding tissues

You need to pay special attention when caring for and handling the laser. It's important to read and follow the maintenance schedules and procedures in the instruction manual. It's recommended that health care workers complete a training program before assisting with laser procedures.

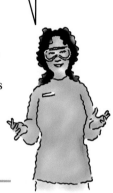

During a laser procedure, everyone in the room must wear goggles to protect their eyes—including the patient.

After Surgical Procedures

The medical assistant has several other important responsibilities once the surgery is complete.

- Applying **dressings** and **bandages** to surgical wounds. A dressing is a sterile material or cloth used to cover a wound and stop bleeding. A bandage is a material used to secure a dressing.
- Instructing the patient about postoperative wound care. This care includes observing the wound for changes that indicate infection or other problems with healing.
- Assisting with postoperative instructions such as prescriptions, medications, and scheduling return visits.
- Removing and caring for instruments, equipment, and supplies. You need to dispose properly of waste, including disposable items, sharps, and contaminated or unused supplies.
- Preparing the room for the next patient.

WOUND CARE

Sterile dressings and bandages protect wounds during the healing process. Sterile dressings have several purposes in wound care:

- to protect the wound from contamination
- to exert pressure on an open wound to control bleeding
- to absorb drainage such as blood, pus, or **serum** (a clear, sticky part of blood that remains after coagulation)

- to hold medications against the wound and facilitate healing
- to hide temporary disfigurement

Bandages are strips of woven material typically used with sterile dressings. The purposes of bandages are:

- to hold dressings in place
- to provide additional pressure to control bleeding
- to provide protection from contamination
- to keep an injured body part immobile during healing
- to support an injured body part
- to improve circulation

> A sterile dressing is considered contaminated if it's damp or outdated, if the wrapper is damaged, or if it's been improperly removed from the wrapper.

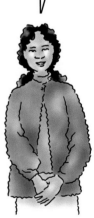

Sterile Dressings

Sterile dressings are items such as 4 × 4-inch absorbent gauze sponges and nonadhering dressings that are made for use on open wounds. They typically are prepackaged in small numbers. They come in various sizes and shapes, each for a specific use. You'll choose the dressing to use based on the size of the wound and the amount of drainage.

You must use sterile technique when handling dressings. A sterile dressing may be held in place by different kinds of bandages. You'll find out more about applying sterile dressings in the Hands On procedure on page 244.

Changing Sterile Dressings

When you remove a sterile dressing or change an existing one, always wear clean examination gloves. Observe the wound carefully for any drainage or exudates. Note the characteristics of the wound drainage in the patient's chart.

It's normal to see serum or bloody drainage in small or moderate amounts immediately following the closure of a wound. If you notice **purulent** drainage—that is, drainage with a color other than pink—notify the physician while the wound is still uncovered. The physician can then examine the wound and make a decision about how well healing is progressing. Look for specific steps on how to change an existing dressing in the Hands On procedure on page 247.

Types of Bandages

There are several different types of bandages, including roller, elastic, or tubular gauze. The type of bandage used depends on the nature of the wound or injury.

Closer Look — WOUND DRAINAGE

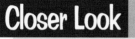

When observing wound drainage and documenting it in the patient's chart, be sure to note the color and amount as described below.

Color

- Serous drainage is clear.
- Sanguineous drainage is blood-tinged.
- Serosanguineous drainage is pinkish, or a mixture of clear and red.
- Purulent drainage is white, green, or yellow-tinged. It's usually accompanied by an unpleasant odor. This type of drainage is a sign of infection.

Amount

- *Copious* is a large amount.
- *Medium* describes a moderate amount.
- *Scant* refers to a small amount.

You also can quantify the amount by noting the size of the drainage (for example, 2-inch diameter, entire 4 × 4 dressing saturated) or the size of the dressing.

Roller Bandages. These bandages are soft, woven materials packaged in a roll. They're available in various lengths and widths, from one inch to six or more inches. The bandage size used depends on:

- the part being bandaged
- the desired thickness of the completed bandage

Most bandages are made of a porous, lightweight material. Some may be sterile. Others are just clean. Gauze bandages conform easily to body surfaces. Stretchy gauze is made to adjust to body contours. It resists unrolling much better than plain types of gauze. Kling and Conform are two frequently used brands.

Elastic Bandages. These are special bandage rolls with elastic woven through the fabric. They're generally brownish tan in color. Unlike other types of roller gauze, elastic bandages can be given to the patient to take home to be washed and reused many times. Ace is one brand of elastic bandage that's widely available.

Elastic bandages should be applied without wrinkling in partly overlapping layers. Some elastic bandages have adhesive backing, which helps keep the layers in place and provides a secure, snug, and comfortable fit. Adjust the bandage if it seems too loose or if the patient says it's uncomfortable or tight.

You must take care in applying this type of bandage because of the elastic fibers. The bandage must be applied snugly to give support to the injured part. But a bandage that's too tight can slow or cut off blood circulation. The bandage should be wrapped in the direction of blood flow.

Ask the patient how tight the bandage feels as it's being applied. Instruct the patient on signs of impaired circulation. The patient should check an extremity (a limb such as an arm or leg) distal (farthest away) from the bandage for these signs:

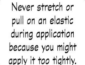

Never stretch or pull on an elastic during application because you might apply it too tightly.

- increased swelling or pain
- pale skin
- cool skin when compared to the other extremity
- bluish coloring to toenails or fingernails

Tubular Gauze Bandages. Tubular gauze bandages are used to enclose rounded body parts. The bandage looks like a hollow tube and is very stretchy. These bandages come in various widths from 0.672 inch to 7 inches. They can be used to enclose the fingers, toes, arms, legs, and even the head and torso.

Tubular gauze is applied using a tubular, framelike applicator. The applicator is made of metal or plastic and is available in various sizes. The size of the applicator should be slightly larger than the body part to be covered. This allows the gauze to slide easily over the body part. Applicators are marked according to a size number that corresponds to different sizes of tubular gauze.

Applying Bandages

When properly applied, bandages should feel comfortably snug. They should be fastened securely enough to remain in place until they're removed. Bandages may be fastened using safety pins, adhesive tape, or clips.

Here are the basic techniques to use when wrapping a gauze or elastic roller bandage.

- *Circular turn.* This technique is used mainly to anchor the bandage or to provide extra support. The bandage is wrapped around the body part two or more times, with each turn completely overlapping the previous turn.

- *Spiral turn.* After the circular turn anchors the bandage, the wrapping continues in a spiral manner up the body part. Each turn overlaps the previous one by one-half to two-thirds the width of the bandage. The spiral turn is a useful technique for bandaging parts like the wrist, fingers, and trunk.

- *Reverse spiral turn.* This wrapping technique also begins with a circular turn. Then each time the bandage is spiral-wrapped around the limb, it is twisted once. This method helps to fit limbs like forearms or lower legs that get larger as the bandaging continues.

- *Figure-eight turn.* This technique involves making slanting, overlapping turns that alternate moving up and down the limb in a crisscross pattern that looks like a figure eight. This is an effective method for bandaging joints, such as a knee, elbow, ankle, or wrist.

> You'll gain a patient's confidence when the bandage you apply is comfortable, looks neat, and stays in place.

STEPS FOR APPLYING BANDAGES

Here are some other important guidelines for applying bandages:

1. Observe the principles of medical asepsis. Surgical asepsis isn't necessary. The bandage may be used to cover a sterile dressing or may be used alone if there's no open wound.

2. Keep the area to be bandaged and the bandage itself dry and clean. Moisture could wick bacteria into the wound. A moist bandage encourages the growth of pathogens.

3. Never place a bandage directly over an open wound. Apply a sterile dressing first. The bandage should extend approximately one to two inches beyond the edge of the dressing.

4. Never allow the skin surfaces of two body parts to touch each other under a bandage. Wound healing can cause opposing surfaces to stick together. This would lead to the formation of scar tissue. For example, burned fingers must be dressed separately, then bandaged together.

5. Pad joints and any bony prominences to help prevent skin irritation. Without padding, the bandage may rub against the skin over a bony area.

6. Bandage the affected body part in the normal position. Joints should be slightly flexed to avoid muscle strain, discomfort, or pain. Muscle spasms may occur if the part is bandaged in an unnatural position.

7. Apply bandages by beginning at the distal part and extending to the proximal part of the body. Bandage turns that extend distal to proximal (farthest to nearest) help to return venous blood to the heart. They also help to make the bandage more secure.

8. Always talk to the patient during bandaging. If the patient complains that the bandage is too tight or too loose, adjust the bandage. Instruct the patient to do the same at home. The bandage should fit snugly but not too tightly.

9. When bandaging hands and feet, leave the fingers and toes exposed whenever possible. Visible fingers and toes make it easier to check for impaired circulation. If the skin feels or looks cold or pale, the nail beds look cyanotic (bluish), or the patient complains of swelling, numbness, or tingling in the toes and fingers, remove the bandage immediately. Reapply it correctly.

Suture and Staple Removal

As a medical assistant, you may be the one who removes sutures from a wound. Keep the following points in mind if you're removing sutures.

- Explain to the patient that it's normal to feel a pulling sensation during suture removal, but there shouldn't be pain.

- Cleanse the area with an antiseptic solution. Wear sterile gloves or use sterile transfer forceps. Clean the area using circular motions away from the wound or in straight wipes away from the suture line. The wipe should be discarded after each sweep. Use a new one for the next sweep across the area.

- Use a disposable suture removal kit or sterile reusable equipment.

You'll find specific steps for removing sutures in the Hands On procedure on page 249.

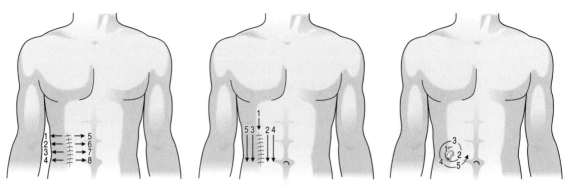

Clean a wound outward from the site following any of the numbered patterns.

Metal staples may be used to close some incisions after hospital surgery. Patients often leave the hospital before the staples can be removed safely. They return later to the physician's office to have the staples removed.

Frequently, it will be your responsibility to remove staples. Most medical offices use staple removal kits that

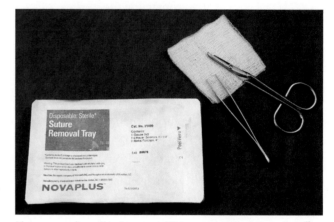

You may use a disposable suture removal kit to remove sutures in the medical office.

are similar to the kits supplied for suture removal. Instead of suture scissors, the kit will include a special instrument for removing staples. The Hands On procedure on page 251 will show you how to remove staples.

THE HEALING PROCESS

How a wound heals can depend on the type of wound and how it is treated. The illustrations on page 222 show how the nature of a wound is related to its healing.

Healing by Primary Intention

Healing by primary intention *is* the simplest form of healing. It occurs in wounds with edges that are closely approximated. Little or no bacteria enter the wound to complicate the healing process. Because the edges of the wound lie close together, new

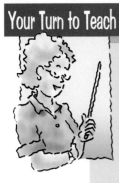

Your Turn to Teach | **POSTOPERATIVE INSTRUCTIONS**

After any surgical procedure, the patient should receive written and verbal instructions. They should include information about:

- caring for the postoperative wound
- taking prescribed medications correctly
- returning to the office for follow-up visits, dressing changes, and suture removal
- recognizing signs and symptoms of infection
- contacting the medical office if there are any problems, including an after-hours number

The patient should be informed of the signs and symptoms of infections. You need to make sure the patient understands these warning signs:

- excessive bleeding from the wound
- throbbing pain, or tenderness in the wound area
- pus or watery discharge collecting under the skin or draining from the wound
- drainage that is yellow, green, or foul-smelling
- a foul odor from the wound
- redness, red streaks, or excessive swelling around the area
- tender lumps or swelling in the armpit, groin, or neck
- chills or fever

Patients also should be on the lookout for abnormal flushing of the skin, general pain or tenderness, heat in the area of the wound, and any loss of function or mobility.

Tell the patient to call the medical office if these symptoms occur. Also teach patients about how to stop any excessive bleeding by applying direct pressure or elevating the body area.

Patients who require follow-up care will need additional information about several things.

- *Dressing and bandage changes.* Tell the patient, per the physician's instructions, when to return to the office to have dressings or bandages changed, or how and when to change the dressings and bandages at home.

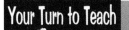

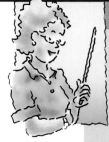

POSTOPERATIVE INSTRUCTIONS (*continued*)

- *Follow-up visits.* Remind the patient to schedule follow-up appointments before leaving and provide a reminder card for each appointment.
- *Showering or bathing.* After consulting with the physician, tell the patient when she can take a shower or bath. Advise the patient on whether the surgical wound can get wet. This depends on the location and depth of the wound and the physician's preference.
- *Laboratory results.* If a specimen was taken for analysis, tell the patient when the results will be available and how he will be informed.
- *Patient concerns.* Answer any questions about postoperative experiences. Encourage the patient to call the office at any time if there's a problem.

It may be necessary to ask permission to bring a caregiver into the room to hear these instructions, too. Some patients may not understand all of the directions immediately after the procedure.

cells form quickly to bind the edges. Capillaries or tiny blood vessels grow across the tissue break to restore circulation to the tissues. Scarring is usually minimal.

Healing by Secondary Intention

In wounds where skin edges are not closely approximated, the edges of the wound cannot join directly. Rough, pink tissue forms between the wound edges. This process is called granulation. The tissue contains new cells and capillaries. Nerves may not rejoin across the wound, which results in decreased nerve stimulus in the area. A large scab forms to protect the area while healing occurs below it. Scarring is more severe than with primary intention healing.

Healing by Tertiary Intention

A wound may be left open at first if there's a possibility that it's already contaminated with microorganisms. Closing it would only trap microorganisms and increase the likelihood of infection. Eventually, the open wound fills in with granular tissue. There's considerable scarring.

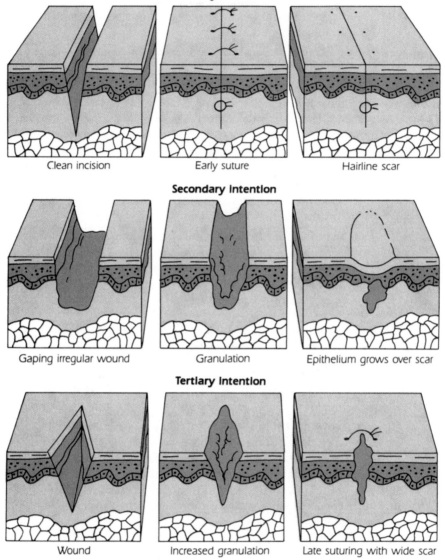

Primary Intention

Clean incision   Early suture   Hairline scar

Secondary Intention

Gaping irregular wound   Granulation   Epithelium grows over scar

Tertiary Intention

Wound   Increased granulation   Late suturing with wide scar

There are three types of wound healing: primary intention, secondary intention, and tertiary intention.

PHASES OF WOUND HEALING

Wound healing occurs in three main stages. The length of each phase may be different for different patients and different types of incisions.

1. *Phase I (inflammatory, lag,* or *exudative phase).* This phase usually lasts from one to four days.
   - The body attempts to heal itself by increasing circulation to the part and by beginning to repair or reroute blood vessels that supply the tissues.
   - The increased circulation brings more white blood cells to defend against pathogens.
   - Serum and red blood cells brought by the extra blood form a glue-like **fibrin,** a type of protein that works to block the wound.
   - As the fibrin dries, it pulls the edges of the wound closer together and forms a scab.

   Signs that this phase is working include:
   - **edema,** or swelling from the tissue fluid
   - warmth from the extra blood
   - redness from the vasodilation
   - pain from the pressure on the nerve endings caused by the edema

2. *Phase II (proliferative, healing,* or *granulation phase).* This phase may last from several days to several weeks.
   - The blood vessels continue to repair themselves. If the damage is severe, they may reroute.
   - The scab from phase I continues to dry and pull the edges of the wound closely together.

3. *Phase III (remodeling, maturation,* or *scarring phase).* This phase may take from weeks to years, depending on how severe the wound is.
   - Fibroblasts, the cells that produce body tissues, build scar tissue to protect the area.

Hands On

WRAPPING INSTRUMENTS FOR STERILIZATION IN AN AUTOCLAVE

4-1

This procedure should take ten minutes.

1. First, wash your hands and put on gloves. Then, gather the instruments to be sterilized and the necessary supplies, including autoclave wrapping material, autoclave tape, sterilization indicators, and a black or blue ink pen.

2. Check the instruments being wrapped to be sure they've been sanitized and disinfected and are dry. Also check that they're in working order. Instruments that are defective, broken, or in need of repair, sanitization, or disinfection shouldn't be wrapped or autoclaved.

3. Autoclave wrap may be double layers of cotton muslin, special paper, or appropriately sized instrument pouches. Be sure that the wrapping material has these properties:
   - permeable to steam but not contaminants
   - resists tearing and puncturing during normal handling
   - allows for easy opening to prevent contamination of the contents
   - maintains the sterility of the contents during storage

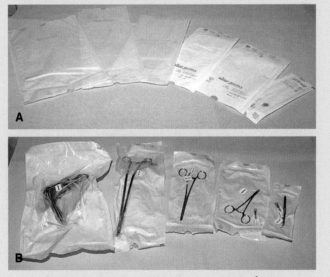

Autoclave pouches are convenient and come in a variety of sizes.

Hands On

WRAPPING INSTRUMENTS FOR STERILIZATION IN AN AUTOCLAVE (continued)

4-1

4. Tear off one piece of autoclave tape. Write the date, your initials, and the contents of the pack or the name of the instrument that will be wrapped. (After the item is wrapped, you can't see what's inside.) The date is necessary so it can be determined later if the contents are still considered sterile.

5. Lay the wrapping material diagonally on a flat, clean, dry surface. Place the instrument in the center of the wrapping material.
   - Ratchets or handles should be open to allow steam to penetrate all surfaces.
   - Include a sterilization indicator.

6. Fold the flap at the bottom of the diagonal wrap up. Fold back the corner to make a tab. The tab allows the pack to be opened easily without contaminating the contents.

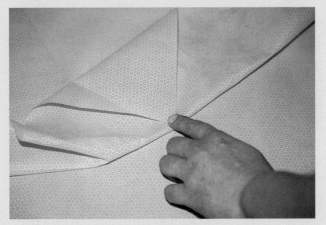

Make a tab with the corner.

7. Fold the left corner of the wrap in to the center. Again, fold back the corner to make a tab. Do the same for the right corner of the wrap.

8. Fold the top corner down, tucking the tab under the material.

9. Secure the wrapped instrument package with the labeled autoclave tape.

(continued)

Hands On

WRAPPING INSTRUMENTS FOR STERILIZATION IN AN AUTOCLAVE (continued)

4-1

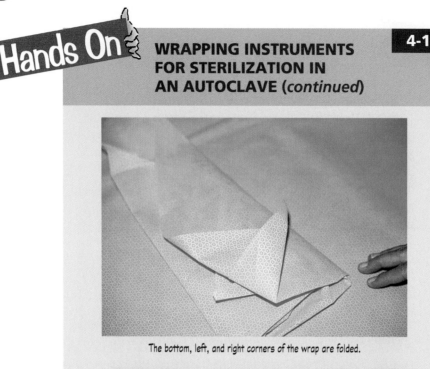

The bottom, left, and right corners of the wrap are folded.

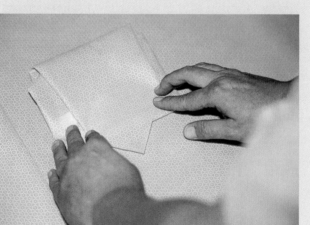

The top corner of the wrap is folded down. The tab will then be tucked under the fold in the material.

Hands On — OPERATING AN AUTOCLAVE   4-2

The autoclave procedure takes about one hour.

1. Gather the items wrapped for autoclaving, distilled water, and the autoclave operating manual.
   - Some medical offices will want you to include a separate, wrapped sterilization indicator with the autoclave load.
   - This allows you to check that the procedure was performed properly without opening a sterilized pack.

2. Check the water level in the autoclave reservoir. Add more distilled water if necessary.

3. Add water to the internal chamber of the autoclave. Make sure the water level is at the fill line.
   - Too little water means not enough steam will be produced.
   - Too much water can cause saturated steam, which extends drying time.

4. Load the autoclave, following these guidelines:
   - Place trays and packs on their sides, one to three inches apart. Air cannot circulate if items are too tightly packed. Placing them vertically stops air from pooling in containers.
   - Put containers on their sides with lids off. Removing lids and placing containers on their sides improves air circulation.
   - In mixed loads, place hard objects on the bottom shelf and softer packs on the top racks. Otherwise, hard objects may form condensation, which can drip onto softer items.

5. Read the instructions for closing and operating the machine. Most machines require similar procedures, such as in the list below.
   - Close the door and secure or lock it.
   - Turn on the machine.
   - When the temperature gauge reaches the required level (usually 250°F), set the timer. Many autoclaves can be programmed for the required time.
   - When the timer indicates the cycle is over, vent the chamber.
   - After releasing the pressure to a safe level, crack the door of the autoclave slightly to allow additional drying. Most loads dry in 5 to 20 minutes. Hard items dry faster than soft ones.

(continued)

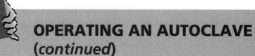

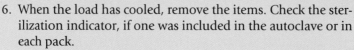

OPERATING AN AUTOCLAVE 4-2
(*continued*)

6. When the load has cooled, remove the items. Check the sterilization indicator, if one was included in the autoclave or in each pack.
   - If the indicator registers that the load or pack was properly processed, the items are considered sterile.
   - If not, the items are considered unsterile. They must be rewrapped and processed again.

7. Store the items in a clean, dry, dust-free area for 30 days. After 30 days, reprocessing is necessary. The pack must be rewrapped, taped with new tape with the current date, and autoclaved again.

8. Clean the autoclave according to the manufacturer's directions. Typically, cleaning involves scrubbing the interior chamber with a soft brush and mild detergent.
   - Pay attention to the exhaust valve. It can become blocked with lint accumulation.
   - Rinse the machine thoroughly and allow it to dry.
   - Record your maintenance procedures and the date they were performed in the maintenance and quality control logs.

Hands On

PERFORMING CHEMICAL STERILIZATION

4-3

The length of time required for this procedure will depend on the chemical being used.

1. Gather the following equipment and materials: the sterilization chemical, the material safety data sheet (MSDS) for the sterilization chemical, personal protective equipment (PPE), heavy-duty utility gloves, a stainless steel or glass container with airtight cover, sterile water, a sterile basin, sterile transfer forceps, sterile towels, and the items to be sterilized.

2. Put on disposable gloves, goggles, and other PPE. You need to protect your eyes, clothing, and exposed skin from possible harmful chemicals.

3. Scrub and sanitize the items to be sterilized to remove debris and body fluids.

4. Rinse and dry the items. They must be dry when placed in the chemical sterilization solution in order to avoid diluting the solution.

5. Check the expiration date on the container of the sterilization chemical. If the chemical is used past its expiration date, it may not be as effective.

6. Read the manufacturer's instructions on the container of the sterilization chemical and review the MSDS for the chemical being used. This step minimizes the risk of injury from mishandling of the chemical and provides first-aid information should an accident occur.

7. Put on the heavy-duty utility gloves over the disposable PPE gloves. These gloves will protect your disposable gloves from punctures by sharp instruments and exposure to harsh chemicals that might damage your skin.

8. Mix or prepare the solution according to the manufacturer's directions on the label. This will ensure that the solution used is the correct strength.

9. Pour the solution into a glass or stainless steel container with an airtight lid. The solution should be left covered in order to avoid loss of potency through evaporation or injury from splashes or inhalation of fumes.

(continued)

Hands On

PERFORMING CHEMICAL STERILIZATION (continued)

4-3

10. Carefully place the dry sanitized items into the container in order to avoid splashing, making sure they are completely covered by the solution. Replace the container's airtight lid.

11. Label the lid with the name of the chemical, the date and time, and the length of time required for sterilization.

12. Leave the items in the solution for the required time. This may be from 20 minutes to 3 hours or more, depending on the chemical being used. Do not open the container or add more items during this time.

13. After the recommended processing time has expired, open the container and remove each item from the solution using sterile transfer forceps. With the sterile forceps, hold the item over a sterile basin and pour large amounts of sterile water over and through it. This will remove all traces of the chemical solution from the item.

14. Continue to hold the item over the sterile basin for a moment to allow the excess water to drain off. Then place the item on a sterile towel.

15. After all the items have been removed from the container, rinsed, and transferred onto sterile towels, dry them with another sterile towel. Take care to avoid touching the instruments or the side of the towel being used to dry them.

16. Use the sterile transfer forceps to place the items in storage for future use according to your office's procedures.

Note: Change the solution in the sterilization container every day or according to the manufacturer's instructions.

Hands On

OPENING STERILE PACKS

4-4

This procedure should take ten minutes.

1. Verify the procedure to be performed and remove the appropriate surgical pack (tray or item) from the storage area. Check the label for the contents and expiration date. Packs that are past the expiration date should not be used.

2. Check the package for tears, stains, and moisture, which would suggest contamination.

3. Place the package, with the label facing up, on a clean, dry, flat surface, such as a Mayo or surgical stand. Although the field will be protected by the barrier below it, using a clean surface keeps microorganisms to a minimum. The surgical stand makes it easy to move the field as needed.

4. Wash your hands. Carefully remove the sealing tape. Take care not to tear the wrapper. For commercial packages, carefully remove the outer wrapper. Many disposable packages are wrapped in clear plastic film that will become the sterile field when properly opened.

5. Loosen the first flap of the folded wrapper by pulling it up, out, and away from you. Let it fall over the far side of the table or stand. Then you won't need to reach across the sterile field again.

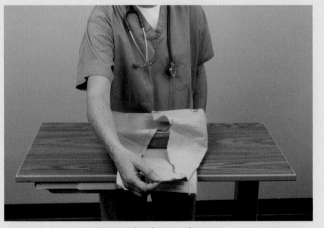

Open the first flap away from you.

(continued)

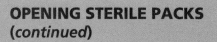

OPENING STERILE PACKS
(*continued*)

4-4

6. Open the side flaps in a similar manner to minimize your movements over the sterile field. Use your left hand for the left flap and your right hand for the right flap. Touch only the outer surface (which is not sterile). Do not touch the sterile inner surface.

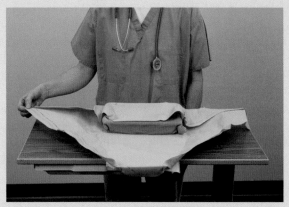

Open the side flaps.

7. Grasp the outer surface of the remaining flap. Pull it down and toward you. The outer surface of the wrapper should now be against the surgical stand. The sterile inside of the wrapper forms the sterile field.

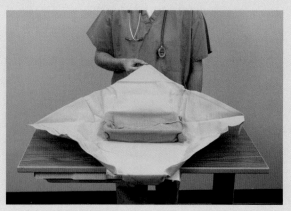

Pull the remaining flap down and toward you.

Hands On

OPENING STERILE PACKS (*continued*)

4-4

8. Some packages have a second inside wrapper. Repeat steps 5–7 to open the second wrapper. It also will provide a sterile field.

9. If you need to leave the area after opening the sterile field, cover the tray and its contents with a sterile drape. Here's how.
   - Without leaving or turning your back on the sterile area, open the sterile drape.
   - Carefully lift it out of the package by the edges. Take care not to touch the drape to any surfaces.
   - Place the drape over the sterile field working from your body outward so that your arms don't cross the uncovered sterile field. Your arms can cross the drape that is covering the tray.

Hands On

USING STERILE TRANSFER FORCEPS

4-5

This procedure should take ten minutes.

1. Sterile forceps often are stored in a container with sterilization solution. When you need to use them, slowly lift the forceps straight up and out of the container. Don't touch the outside of the container or the inside of the container above the level of the solution. These areas are not considered sterile.

2. Hold the forceps with the tips down at all times. This prevents contamination by preventing the solution from running up toward the unsterile handles and then down to the grasping blades and tips. Keep the forceps above waist level to avoid accidental or unnoticed contamination.

3. Use the forceps to pick up items to be transferred onto the sterile field. Drop the items carefully onto the field.
   - Don't let the forceps contact the sterile field. They may be moist from the soaking solution. Drops of solution on the sterile field could wick microorganisms from below.
   - Transfer forceps that have been wrapped and autoclaved may be placed with their tips on the sterile field and their handles extending beyond the one-inch border that is considered contaminated. This allows you to move objects easily around the sterile field.

4. When finished moving items, carefully place the forceps back into the sterilization solution. The solution keeps the tips of the forceps sterile for future use. The solution should be changed at least daily, or according to office policy.

Hands On   ADDING STERILE SOLUTION   4-6

This procedure should take ten minutes.

1. Place a sterile bowl or cup on the sterile field using sterile transfer forceps. Identify the correct solution by carefully reading the label. The label should be checked three times to prevent errors. Check the label:
   - when taking the container from the shelf
   - before pouring the solution
   - when returning the container to the shelf

2. Check the expiration date on the solution label. Don't use the solution if:
   - the solution is out of date
   - the label can't be read
   - the solution appears abnormal

   Out of date solutions may have changed chemically or deteriorated. They are not considered sterile.
   - Sterile water and saline bottles must be dated when opened.
   - If not used within 48 hours, they should be discarded.

3. If you're adding medication, such as lidocaine, to the solution, show the medication label to the physician. This allows the contents to be verified.

4. Remove the cap or stopper on the bottle. Hold the cap with your fingertips, with the opening facing down to prevent contamination.
   - If you must put the cap down, place it on a side table (not the sterile field) with the open end up.
   - If you'll be pouring the entire contents of the bottle into the sterile bowl or cup, you can discard the cap.
   - Keep the bottle so you can note the amount added to the field and for charting later.

5. Grasp the container with the label against the palm of your hand (known as palming the label). That way, if solution runs down the side of the bottle, it won't obscure the label.

6. Pour a small amount of the solution into a separate container or waste receptacle. The lip of the bottle is considered contaminated. Pouring off this small amount cleanses the lip.

7. Without reaching across the sterile field, carefully and slowly pour the desired amount of solution into the sterile container.

(continued)

Hands On

ADDING STERILE SOLUTION (continued)

4-6

- Pouring slowly reduces the chances of splashing and overfilling.
- Hold the bottle no more than six inches and no less than four inches above the container. The bottle of solution should never touch the sterile container or tray.
- Solution poured too quickly from an improper height may splash. Spilled solution may lead to wicking of contaminants from the field below.

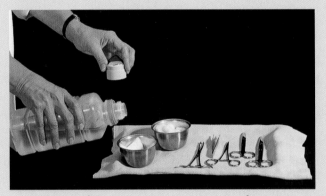

Hold the cap facing downward to prevent contamination of the inside.

8. After pouring the solution, recheck the label for the contents and expiration date. Replace the cap carefully, without touching the bottle rim with any unsterile surface of the cap. This ensures the contents will remain sterile.

9. Return the solution to its proper storage area or discard the container after checking the label again.

Hands On

PERFORMING HAIR REMOVAL AND SKIN PREPARATION

4-7

This procedure should take ten minutes.

1. Wash your hands.

2. Gather the equipment: nonsterile gloves; shaving cream, lotion, or soap; a new disposable razor; gauze or cotton balls; warm water; antiseptic solution; and sponge forceps.
   - A new razor must be used for each patient to prevent the spread of microorganisms.
   - The new blade also will ensure the closest possible shave.

3. Greet the patient by name and explain the procedure. Answer any questions the patient may have.

4. Put on gloves. Standard precautions must be observed when contact with blood or body fluids is possible.

5. Prepare the patient's skin. If shaving is required:
   - Apply shaving cream or soapy lather to the area to reduce friction.
   - Pull the skin taut and shave by pulling the razor across the skin in the direction of hair growth. This gives the closest shave, while reducing the chance of nicking the skin.
   - When all hair is removed from the operative area, rinse to remove soap residue and hair.
   - Thoroughly dry the area by patting with a gauze square.
   - Using gauze squares picks up stray hairs that might have been left behind during rinsing.

6. If shaving isn't necessary, wash and rinse the patient's skin with soap and water. Dry the skin thoroughly.

7. Apply antiseptic solution of the physician's choice to the skin surrounding the operative area. Here's how it should be done.
   - Use sterile gauze sponges or sterile cotton balls to apply the solution, or use antiseptic wipes.
   - Hold the gauze or cotton ball in sterile sponge forceps.
   - Wipe the skin in circular motions, beginning at the operative site and working outward. Discard each sponge after a complete sweep has been made to prevent contamination.

(continued)

Hands On

PERFORMING HAIR REMOVAL AND SKIN PREPARATION (*continued*)

4-7

- If the area is large or circles are not appropriate, the sponge may be wiped straight outward from the operative site. Use a fresh sponge after every pass over the skin. Repeat the procedure until the entire area has been thoroughly cleaned.
- A wipe that has been passed over the skin should never be returned to the cleaned area or to the antiseptic solution.

8. Holding dry sterile sponges in the sponge forceps, thoroughly pat the area dry. In some instances, the area may be allowed to air dry. Moist skin may moisten the sterile drapes, causing wicking and contamination.

9. Tell the patient not to touch or cover the prepared area to avoid contaminating the operative site.

10. Inform the physician that the patient is ready for the procedure. Drape the prepared area with a sterile drape if the physician will be delayed for more than 10 or 15 minutes.

Hands On

ASSISTING WITH EXCISIONAL SURGERY

4-8

This procedure should take 15 minutes.

1. Wash your hands and gather the equipment as described below.
   - *On the sterile field*, you'll need a basin for solutions, gauze sponges and cotton balls, antiseptic solution, a sterile drape, sterile syringes and needles for local anesthetic, dissecting scissors, a disposable scalpel, a blade of the physician's choice, mosquito forceps, tissue forceps, a needle holder, and a suture and needle of the physician's choice.
   - *At the side*, you'll need sterile gloves, local anesthetic, antiseptic wipes, adhesive tape, sterile dressings, and a specimen container with a completed laboratory request form.

2. Greet the patient by name and explain the procedure. Answer any questions the patient may have.

3. Set up a sterile field on a surgical stand with the at-the-side supplies and equipment close at hand. Cover the field with a sterile drape until the physician arrives.

4. Position the patient appropriately to expose the operative site.

5. Put on sterile gloves or use sterile transfer forceps and cleanse the patient's skin as described in the Hands On procedure on page 234. When you're finished, remove your gloves and wash your hands. (Some physicians prefer to cleanse the skin themselves using supplies on the field. Always follow the preferences of the physician in your medical office.)

6. If the physician asks you, assist during the procedure.
   - You may need to add supplies, watch for opportunities to assist the physician, and comfort the patient.
   - You don't need to wear sterile gloves unless you'll be handling sterile instruments or supplies.

7. If the lesion is to be sent to pathology for analysis, you'll need to assist in specimen collection. Follow standard precautions and wear examination gloves when handling specimens. Have the container ready to receive the specimen.

(continued)

Hands On

ASSISTING WITH
EXCISIONAL SURGERY (continued)

4-8

8. At the end of the procedure, wash your hands and dress the wound using sterile technique, as described in the Hands On procedure on page 244. The wound must be covered to protect the incision from contamination.

9. Thank the patient and provide instructions for postoperative care, including dressing changes, postoperative medications, and follow-up visits.

10. Wearing gloves, clean the treatment room and prepare it for the next patient. Follow standard precautions.

11. Record the procedure. Documentation should include postoperative vital signs, care of the wound, instructions on postoperative care, and processing any specimens.

Charting Example:

09/19/2007 8:45 A.M. Mole to posterior (L) shoulder removed per Dr. Snider. Specimen sent to Acme lab. T 98.4 (O) P 96 R 20 BP 134/78 (R) sitting. 4 × 4 DSD applied to surgical incision; minimal sanguinous drainage noted. Pt. given verbal and written instructions on wound care, postop antibiotics, pain medication, and follow-up visits. Verbalized understanding. To RTO x 2 days for drsg change._____ B. Cole, CMA

Hands On

ASSISTING WITH COLPOSCOPY AND CERVICAL BIOPSY

4-9

This procedure should take 20 to 30 minutes.

1. Label a specimen container with the patient's name and date. Prepare a laboratory request. Verify that the patient has signed the consent form. Colposcopy with biopsy is an invasive procedure that requires written consent.

2. Wash your hands.

3. Gather the equipment and supplies: sterile gloves, a gown and drape, a vaginal speculum, a colposcope, a specimen container with preservative (10 percent formalin), sterile cotton-tipped applicators, sterile normal saline solution, sterile 3 percent acetic acid, sterile povidone-iodine (Betadine), silver nitrate sticks or ferric subsulfate (Monsel solution), sterile biopsy forceps or punch biopsy instrument, a sterile uterine curet, sterile uterine dressing forceps, sterile 4 × 4 gauze, a sterile towel, a sterile endocervical curet, a sterile uterine tenaculum, a sanitary napkin, examination gloves, an examination light, tissues, and biohazard container.

4. Check the light on the colposcope to make sure it's functioning properly.

5. Set up the sterile field using sterile technique. Items that can be placed on the sterile field include the sterile cotton-tipped applicators and sterile containers for the solutions.

6. Pour sterile normal saline and acetic acid into their sterile containers. Cover the field with a drape to maintain sterility as you prepare the patient.

7. Greet the patient by name and explain the procedure, answering any last-minute questions from the patient.

8. When the physician is ready, assist the patient into the dorsal lithotomy position. If you are going to be assisting the physician from the sterile field, put on sterile gloves after you position the patient.

9. Hand the physician the applicator immersed in normal saline followed by the applicator immersed in acetic acid. Acetic acid swabbed on the area improves visualization of abnormal tissue.

(continued)

Hands On

ASSISTING WITH COLPOSCOPY AND CERVICAL BIOPSY (*continued*)

10. Hand the physician the applicator with the antiseptic solution (Betadine). The area to be sampled for biopsy must be swabbed to reduce microorganisms and pathogens.

11. If you didn't apply sterile gloves to assist the physician, apply clean examination gloves. Receive the biopsy specimen into the container of ten percent formalin preservative.

12. If necessary, provide the physician with Monsel solution or silver nitrate sticks to stop any bleeding. Monsel solution and silver nitrate act as coagulants.

13. When the physician is finished, remove your gloves and wash your hands. Assist the patient from the stirrups and into a sitting position. Explain to the patient that a small amount of bleeding may occur (a small sanitary pad should be sufficient). Have a sanitary napkin available.

14. Ask the patient to get dressed and assist as needed. Allow the patient privacy for dressing.

15. Reinforce any instructions from the physician regarding follow-up appointments. Tell the patient how to obtain the biopsy findings.

16. Wearing gloves, properly care for or dispose of equipment and clean the examination room. Remove your gloves and wash your hands.

17. Document the procedure, including routing the specimen and patient education.

Charting Example:
10/15/2007 10:45 A.M. Colposcopy performed per Dr. Lyttle; cervical biopsy obtained and sent to Acme lab for cytology. Minimal bleeding post procedure; pt. given sanitary pad, verbal and written instructions on post-procedure care. Verbalized understanding. _____ J. Pratt, CMA

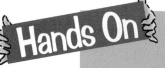 **ASSISTING WITH INCISION AND DRAINAGE (I & D)** 4-10

This procedure should take 15 minutes.

1. Wash your hands and gather the equipment as described below.
    *   *On the sterile field*, you'll need a basin for solutions, gauze sponges and cotton balls, antiseptic solution, a sterile drape, sterile syringes and sterile needles for local anesthetic, a commercial I & D sterile setup *or* scalpel, dissecting scissors, hemostats, tissue forceps, sterile 4 × 4 gauze sponges, and a probe (optional).
    *   *At the side*, you'll need sterile gloves, local anesthetic, antiseptic wipes, adhesive tape, sterile dressings, packing gauze, and a culture tube if the wound may be cultured.

2. The steps for this procedure are similar to those in the Hands On procedure for assisting with excisional surgery on page 239.
    *   You're expected to prepare the surgical field and the patient's surgical area as instructed or preferred by the physician.
    *   After the procedure, the wound must be covered to avoid further contamination and to absorb drainage.
    *   The exudate is a hazardous body fluid requiring standard precautions.
    *   Although a culture and sensitivity may be ordered on the drainage from the infected area, no other specimen is usually collected.
    *   Label the specimen container and prepare a laboratory request if a culture and sensitivity has been ordered.

Charting Example:
04/15/2007 11:30 A.M. Postop VS T 100.4 (O) P 88 R 24 BP 128/88 (R) sitting. 4 × 4 DSD applied to surgical wound on (L) posterior neck. Given verbal and written instructions on wound care, dressing changes, and follow-up. Verbalized understanding.
_____ E. Blake, CMA

Hands On

APPLYING A STERILE DRESSING

4-11

This procedure should take ten minutes.

1. Wash your hands and gather your supplies: sterile gloves, sterile gauze dressings, scissors, bandage tape, and any medication to be applied to the dressing, according to the physician's orders.

2. Greet the patient by name and ask about any tape allergies. Some patients are sensitive to certain tape adhesives. Hypoallergenic tape should be available.

3. Keeping in mind the size of the dressing, cut or tear lengths of tape to secure the dressing. Set the tape aside in a convenient place, such as affixing the end of each piece to a nearby countertop where it can be removed easily and applied. Having tape cut and prepared saves time and may prevent the dressing from slipping while tape is cut.

4. Explain the procedure and instruct the patient to remain still. The patient should avoid talking, sneezing, or coughing until the procedure is complete. You don't want droplets of moisture containing microorganisms to contaminate the sterile field or the wound.

5. Open the dressing pack to create a sterile field, leaving the sterile dressing on the inside of the opened package. Observe the principles of sterile asepsis!

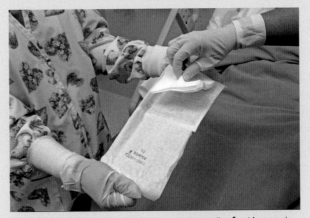

Sterile technique ensures that the dressing remains sterile after it's opened. Remember, packages of dressings are sterile on the inside.

Hands On

APPLYING A STERILE DRESSING (*continued*)

4-11

6. Use sterile technique to prevent wound contamination. Put on sterile gloves if you won't be using sterile transfer forceps to apply the dressing.

7. If a topical medication is needed, apply it to the sterile dressing that will cover the wound directly. Take care not to touch the medication bottle or tube to the dressing. The outside end of the medication container may not be sterile.

8. Using sterile technique, apply the number of dressings necessary to cover and protect the wound. Sterile dressings must be placed carefully on the wound. Dragging them over the skin can lead to contamination from microorganisms on the surrounding skin.

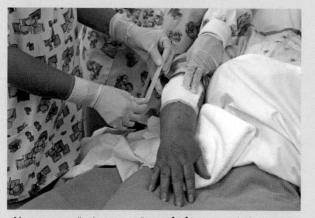

You can use sterile gloves or sterile transfer forceps to apply the dressing.

9. Apply the previously cut lengths of tape over the dressing to secure it. When the wound is completely covered, you may remove your gloves (discarding them appropriately) or keep them on to tape the dressing.

   • Avoid overuse of tape. Tape is used only to keep the dressing in place.

   • Too much tape can cause perspiration that will dampen the dressing and compromise its sterility. And keep in mind that too much tape may cause unnecessary discomfort to the patient when it has to be removed.

   • Tape shouldn't obstruct blood circulation.

(continued)

Hands On

APPLYING A STERILE DRESSING (*continued*)

4-11

10. Apply a bandage if necessary to hold the dressing in place, add support, or immobilize the area.

11. If the patient needs to change dressings at home, instruct the patient on how to do so.
    - Dressings should be kept clean and dry.
    - They need to be changed if they become wet or soiled, or as instructed by the physician.
    - Instruct the patient about wound care and signs of infection.

12. Return reusable supplies (unopened sterile gloves or dressings, tape) to their storage areas. Properly discard contaminated supplies or waste.

13. Record the procedure in the patient's chart.

Charting Example:

10/14/2007 4:45 P.M. DSD applied to surgical wound (L) anterior forearm. No bleeding from incision, edges well approximated with 4 sutures intact. Moderate amount of redness and swelling without discharge. Pt. given verbal and written instructions on dressing change and wound care at home. To RTO in 5 days for suture removal. _____ L. Hicks, CMA

Hands On

CHANGING AN EXISTING DRESSING

4-12

This procedure should take ten minutes.

1. Wash your hands and gather your supplies: sterile gloves, nonsterile gloves, sterile dressing, prepackaged skin antiseptic swabs or sterile antiseptic solution in a sterile basin and sterile cotton balls or gauze, tape, and biohazard waste containers.

2. Greet the patient by name and explain the procedure. Answer any questions the patient may have.

3. Prepare a sterile field, including opening sterile dressings. Follow the guidelines below when preparing the sterile field.
   - If using a sterile container and solution, open the package containing the sterile basin. Use the inside of the wrapper as the sterile field for the basin.
   - Flip the sterile gauze or cotton balls into the basin. Pour in the appropriate amount of antiseptic solution.
   - If using prepackaged antiseptic swabs, carefully open an adequate number for the size of the wound. Set them aside using sterile technique to avoid contamination.

4. Instruct the patient not to talk, cough, sneeze, laugh, or move during the procedure in order to prevent contamination of the sterile field.

5. Wearing clean gloves, carefully remove the tape from the wound by pulling it toward the wound. Pulling away from the direction of the wound may pull the healing edges of the wound apart.

6. Remove the old dressing. Never pull on a dressing that doesn't come off easily.
   - If the dressing is difficult to remove because of dried blood, soak it in sterile water or saline for a few minutes to loosen it.
   - Gently pull the edges of the dressing toward the center.
   - If this procedure doesn't loosen the dressing or causes undue discomfort to the patient, notify the physician.

7. Discard the soiled dressing in a biohazard waste container. Don't pass the dressing over the sterile field—it may shed microorganisms.

(continued)

Hands On

CHANGING AN EXISTING DRESSING (*continued*)

4-12

8. Before cleaning, inspect the wound for degree of healing, amount and type of drainage, and appearance of wound edges. If you inspect the wound after cleaning, most of the exudate will have been removed.

9. Remove and discard your gloves using medical aseptic practices.
   - The physician may want to inspect the wound before you remove exudates or drainage to assess the status of the healing process.
   - If a culture is ordered, the specimen must be taken before the wound is cleaned.

10. Using proper technique, put on sterile gloves. Clean the wound with the antiseptic solution ordered by the physician.
    - Clean in a straight motion with cotton or gauze and anti-septic solution or with prepackaged antiseptic swabs.
    - Discard the wipe after each stroke and use a fresh sterile one to continue.
    - Never return the wipe to the antiseptic solution or to the skin after one sweep across the area.

11. Remove your gloves and wash your hands. Change the dressing using the procedure for sterile dressing application in the Hands On procedure on page 244.

12. Record the procedure.

Charting Example:
11/23/2007 11:30 A.M. Wound to (R) lower leg changed, small amount of yellow purulent drainage noted—Dr. Blake aware. Wound culture for C&S obtained and sent to Acme laboratory. Wound cleansed with Betadine as ordered; DSD reapplied. Moderate amount of redness and swelling at wound site; edges well approximated. Instructed to RTO in 2 days for C&S results and dressing change._____ B. Lamont, CMA

Hands On   REMOVING SUTURES   4-13

This procedure should take ten minutes.

1. Wash your hands and apply clean examination gloves. Gather your supplies: skin antiseptic, sterile gloves, prepackaged suture removal kit *or* thumb forceps, suture scissors, and gauze.

2. Check the chart before you begin the procedure to see how many sutures or staples were applied. This way you can be certain that you have removed them all.

3. Greet the patient by name and explain the procedure. Answer any questions the patient may have.

4. If dressings are still in place, remove them and dispose of them in biohazard waste containers. Remove your gloves and wash your hands.

5. Wearing clean examination gloves, cleanse the wound with antiseptic, such as Betadine. Use a new antiseptic gauze for each swipe down the wound. The wound should be as free of pathogens as possible to prevent contamination.

6. Open the suture removal kit using sterile asepsis technique or set up a sterile field.

7. Put on sterile gloves. Suture removal is a sterile procedure.

8. The knots of the suture will be tied so that one tail of the knot is very close to the surface of the skin. The other will be closer to the area of suture that is looped over the incision. Here's how to cut and remove the sutures.

   - With the thumb forceps, grasp the end of the knot closest to the skin. Lift it slightly and gently up from the skin.

   - Cut the suture below the knot as close to the skin as possible. Cutting close to the skin frees the knot at an area that hasn't been exposed to the outside surface of the body. The only part of the suture that will pull through the tissues will be suture that was under the skin surface. This helps to avoid contamination by microorganisms from the outside skin surface.

   - Use the thumb forceps to pull the suture out of the skin with a smooth, continuous motion. Keep the forceps at a slight angle to the wound to prevent tension on the healing tissue.

(continued)

Hands On

REMOVING SUTURES
(*continued*)

4-13

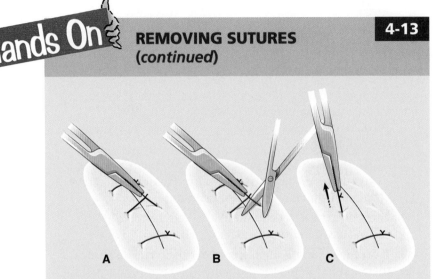

(A) With the hemostat or thumb forceps, lift the stitch up and away from the skin. This permits the blades of the scissors to slide under the stitch. (B) Cut the stitch near the skin. (C) Using the forceps, pull the freed stitch up and out.

9. Place the suture on the gauze sponge. Repeat the procedure for each suture to be removed. By setting the sutures on the gauze sponge, you can easily count the number removed. If six sutures were inserted and are to be removed, there should be six sutures on the gauze sponge at the end of the procedure.

10. Clean the site with an antiseptic solution. Cover it with a sterile dressing if the physician has directed you to do so. Some wounds still need to be protected; others have healed well enough to be left uncovered.

11. Thank the patient and properly dispose of equipment and supplies. Make sure you follow standard precautions. Clean the treatment area, remove your gloves, and wash your hands.

12. Record the procedure. Documentation must include the time, location of sutures, number removed, and the condition of the wound.

Charting Example:
06/29/2007 3:30 P.M. X6 sutures removed from (L) ring finger. Wound well approximated, no redness or drainage noted.
_____ J. Rose, RMA

Hands On   REMOVING STAPLES   4-14

This procedure should take ten minutes.

1. Wash your hands and gather your supplies: antiseptic solution or wipes, examination gloves, sterile gloves, sponge forceps, gauze squares, and prepackaged sterile staple removal instrument.

2. Greet the patient by name and explain the procedure. Answer any questions the patient may have.

3. If the dressing is still in place, put on clean examination gloves and remove it. Dispose of it in a biohazard waste container. Remove your gloves and wash your hands.

4. Clean the wound with antiseptic. Pat dry with sterile gauze sponges. The wound should be as free of pathogens as possible to prevent contamination.

5. Put on sterile gloves. Staple removal is a sterile procedure.

6. Gently slide the end of the staple remover under each staple to be removed.
   • Press the handles together to lift the ends of the staples out of the skin.
   • The remover is designed to open the staple so the ends will lift free with minimal discomfort to the patient.

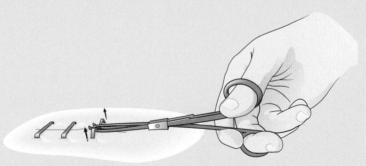

Slide the end of the staple remover under each staple. Press the handles together to lift the ends of the staple out of the skin.

7. Place each staple on a gauze square as it is removed. This helps in counting the staples at the end of the procedure.

8. When all the staples have been removed, gently clean the site with antiseptic solution.

(continued)

Hands On

REMOVING STAPLES
(*continued*)

4-14

- Pat dry and dress the site if the physician has ordered you to do so.
- The area must be dry before the new dressing is applied to avoid wicking microorganisms.
- The wound may be healed well enough to be left uncovered.

9. Thank the patient and properly dispose of equipment and supplies. Make sure you follow standard precautions. Clean the treatment area, remove your gloves, and wash your hands.

10. Record the procedure. Documentation must include the time, location of staples, number removed, and the condition of the wound.

Charting Example:
03/17/2007 10:30 A.M. X15 staples removed from (L) knee incision; edges well approximated; no redness or drainage noted. Wound left open to air as ordered by Dr. Perez. _____
_____ J. Daniels, CMA

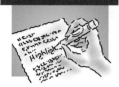

Chapter Highlights

- In assisting with minor surgical procedures, surgical asepsis is essential. Surgical aseptic techniques include sterilization and the surgical scrub. Before sterilization, equipment must be sanitized by hand or by using a mechanical washer. When caring for and cleaning medical instruments, handle them carefully. Check to ensure instruments are in good working order.

- The autoclave uses steam heat under high pressure to sterilize instruments. Items must be wrapped carefully before they're placed in the autoclave. Special indicators help to ensure the items are properly sterilized. Loading the autoclave requires careful attention to item positions so steam can penetrate. Time, pressure, and temperature are three factors that affect sterilization.

- Cold chemicals may be used to sterilize delicate instruments, instruments that are sensitive to heat, or instruments that are too large to fit into the autoclave.

- The medical assistant is responsible for setting up instruments and equipment for surgical procedures. It's important to learn the names of commonly used instruments. Some basic instruments are scissors, scalpels, forceps, and clamps. Different medical specialties have specialized instruments for surgical procedures.

- Supplies and equipment for specific surgical procedures are often packaged together in a sterile surgical pack. Surgical packs may be prepared in the medical office or purchased from a commercial supplier. Do not use surgical packs that show any signs of contamination.

- Careful attention is required to maintain the sterile field. Don't talk, cough, sneeze, or reach across the sterile field. Small supplies and solutions may be added using sterile techniques. Use sterile gloves or sterile transfer forceps to move sterile items. The physician must be informed if there is any possibility the sterile field has become contaminated.

- Before surgical procedures, the medical assistant may help to obtain informed consent and to reinforce preoperative instructions. When the patient is gowned, surgical drapes are provided to expose the operative area. The patient's skin is cleansed and shaved, if necessary.

- During minor surgery, the medical assistant may be asked to hold supplies for the physician, adjust the draping of the patient, pass instruments to the physician, and help collect specimens.

- Common surgical procedures performed in a medical office are excision of lesions and incision and drainage (I & D). If a specimen is collected, the medical assistant is responsible for providing an appropriately labeled container, preparing a laboratory request form, and sending the specimen to the laboratory.

- In the medical office, wounds usually are closed using sutures. The physician chooses atraumatic or traumatic needles in the appropriate size or gauge. Sutures may be absorbable or nonabsorbable. Nonabsorbable sutures need to be removed after healing.

- When the surgical procedures are complete, the medical assistant is responsible for applying dressings and bandages to surgical wounds. The medical assistant usually performs suture and staple removal as well. Sterile technique is necessary for infection control.

- The medical assistant reinforces the physician's instructions for postoperative wound care and tells the patient how to observe the wound for changes that indicate infection or problems with healing.

- After minor surgery, the medical assistant is responsible for removing and caring for instruments, equipment, and supplies. Standard precautions need to be followed in cleaning and disposing of waste.

Chapter 5

PHARMACOLOGY AND DRUG ADMINISTRATION

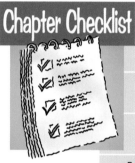

Chapter Checklist

- List the different ways patients receive medications from the physician

- Identify the three different names associated with most medications

- Describe the Schedule of Controlled Substances and provide an example of each

- Explain how to monitor the office inventory of controlled substances

- Maintain medication records

- Describe how to prepare a written prescription as directed by a physician

- Define what is meant by local effect and systemic effect for drug action

- Discuss the four general processes involved in pharmacokinetics

- Describe the main factors that influence a drug's effect on the body

- List resources for finding out more about medications

- List safety guidelines to follow when administering medications

- Identify three measuring systems used for medications and explain how to calculate adult and child medication doses

- Apply pharmacology principles to prepare and administer oral and parenteral (excluding IV) medications

- List the different types of injections, their appropriate needle lengths, and their sites of administration

- Describe problems that may occur when administering IV medication

- Explain what to do in the case of a medication error

- List the seven rights to check for reducing the risk of medication errors

Pharmacology is the study of drugs, their actions, dosages, and side effects. A **drug** is a chemical substance that affects how the body functions. Many drugs are used as medications. **Medications** are legal drugs that are used to treat illness according to established medical guidelines.

Pharmacology and the Medical Assistant

Patients receive medications in different ways. Medications may be:

- *Administered.* The medication is given to the patient in the office by an allied health professional or given by self or family member at home.
- *Dispensed.* The medication is supplied to the patient in the office for later use or given by a pharmacist at a pharmacy.
- *Prescribed.* A written order is given to the patient and taken to a pharmacist to be filled.

As a clinical medical assistant, you may be responsible for administering medications under the physician's supervision. You also may need to educate patients on how to use different kinds of medications that are dispensed or prescribed. It's important that you know different types of medications, their uses, and their potential abuses. For each medication, you'll need to be familiar with:

- the range of dosages
- the methods of administration
- any adverse, or unwanted, effects

TYPES OF MEDICATIONS

There are two general types of medications—over-the-counter (OTC) and prescription-only.

- *Over-the-counter medications* are usually available in pharmacies and supermarkets without any restrictions. Some drugs may be released as over-the-counter medications at a lower strength while a higher level of the drug requires a prescription. This can be confusing for patients, so you need to stay aware of the latest information about drug releases.

- *Prescription-only medications* must be prescribed or ordered by a physician, physician's assistant, or nurse practitioner. The prescription is a written order to the pharmacist. A physician, physician's assistant, or nurse practitioner must sign the prescription or it cannot be filled.

The Name Game

Most over-the-counter and prescription medications have three different names.

- **Chemical name.** This is the first name given to any medication. It identifies the chemical components of the drug. This name is used mainly by the researchers and will not be used in the medical office.

- **Generic name.** This name is assigned to the drug during research and development. It refers to the chemical ingredients that make up the drug. Generic drug names are usually made up of combinations of root words, prefixes, and suffixes that describe a certain type of drug or part of the body. Medical professionals often use the generic name in the medical office.

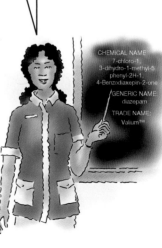

An example of the three different names for one drug.

CHEMICAL NAME:
7-chloro-1,
3-dihydro-1-methyl-5
phenyl-2H-1
4-Benzodiaxepin-2-one

GENERIC NAME:
diazepam

TRADE NAME:
Valium™

- **Trade name.** This is the name given the drug when it is ready for commercial use and distribution by the manufacturer. It's also known as the *brand name*. The trade name is registered by the U.S. Patent Office. After it is registered, the trademark symbol (™) must follow the name.

After the patent on a medication expires, other companies may manufacture generic versions and give them their own trade names.

The table on the next two pages gives you some basic information on common drugs, how they are classified, and their uses. The table includes prescription and over-the-counter drugs. It also provides their generic names and in some cases, common trade names.

> Here's a hint. Trade names always begin with a capital letter. Generic names are in all lowercase.

Sources of Drugs

Drugs come from many natural sources, such as plants, minerals, and animals. They also may be synthetic or prepared in the laboratory by artificial means. See the table on page 261 for more information.

LEGAL REGULATIONS

Federal laws and rules protect consumers by regulating the production, prescription, and dispensation of medications. Two government agencies in particular are involved with controlling drugs and their use.

- *Food and Drug Administration.* The Food and Drug Administration was established to regulate the manufacture and sale of drugs and food products. It ensures that the ingredients listed on the labels are accurate and that the drugs are safe to use.

> The DEA doesn't regulate all medications. It's only concerned with those that can be abused.

- *Drug Enforcement Agency.* Using some drugs may result in dependency or abuse. These drugs have been designated as **controlled substances.** The Drug Enforcement Agency (DEA) is a branch of the Department of Justice. Its mission is to control the use of all drugs listed as controlled substances by the Bureau of Narcotics and Dangerous Drugs (BNDD).

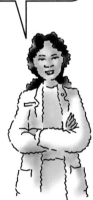

TIMELINE OF THE PURE FOOD AND DRUG ACT

The first federal law regulating medicine was the Pure Food and Drug Act. Here's a timeline of important milestones in the history of this law.

- The Pure Food and Drug Act was passed in 1906.
- In 1938, it was strengthened to require that a drug's safety be proved before being distributed to the public.
- In 1952, the Durham-Humphrey Amendment banned many drugs from being dispensed without a prescription.
- The Kefauver-Harris Amendment of 1962 required that prescription and nonprescription medications both be tested for their effectiveness before they are released for sale.

Common Drugs and Their Uses

Therapeutic Classification	Effect, Action, Uses	Common Examples
Adrenergic blocking agents	Affect alpha or beta receptors of adrenergic nerves	Metoprolol tartrate (Lopressor); propranolol hydrochloride (Inderal); Hytrin; Coreg
Adrenergic agents	Mimic activity of sympathetic nervous system (the part of the nervous system over which a person has no conscious control)	Epinephrine (Adrenaline); ephedrine sulfate
Analgesics	Relieve pain	Aspirin, acetaminophen (Tylenol), codeine
Antacids	Neutralize or reduce stomach acidity	Magnesia (Milk of Magnesia); calcium carbonate (Tums)
Anthelmintics	Kill parasitic worms	Piperazine citrate, mebendazole (Vermox)
Antianginal agents	Promote vasodilation	Nitroglycerine, diltiazem hydrochloride (Cardizem)
Antianxiety agents	Act on brain to relieve symptoms of anxiety	Alprazolam (Xanax); lorazepam (Ativan); chlordiazepoxide (Librium); diazepam (Valium)
Antiarrhythmics	Reduce or prevent irregular cardiac rhythms	Procainamide hydrochloride (Pronestyl); esmolol (Brevibloc); Lidocaine; Amiodarone
Antibiotics	Interfere with growth of or destroy microorganisms	Penicillin, lop cefaclor, tetracycline; Erythromycin; Levaquin
Anticoagulants and thrombolytics	Prevent or dissolve blood clots	Heparin sodium, Coumadin, streptokinase (Streptase); Lovenox; Plavix
Anticonvulsants	Reduce excitability of brain	Phenobarbital, phenytoin (Dilantin); Depakote; Neurontin
Antidepressants	Prevent or reduce symptoms of psychological depression	Amitriptyline hydrochloride (Elavil); fluoxetine hydrochloride (Prozac); Paxil; Zoloft; Wellbutrin
Antidiarrheals	Decrease intestinal peristalsis (contractions)	Loperamide hydrochloride (Imodium A-D); Lomotil
Antiemetic agents	Prevent nausea and/or vomiting	Dimenhydrinate (Dramamine); promethazine hydrochloride (Phenergan); Zofran
Antifungals	Destroy or slow the growth of fungi	Ketoconazole (Nizoral): miconazole nitrate (Monistat 3 or 7); Flagyl
Antihistamines	Counteract effects of histamine on organs and structures	Chlorpheniramine maleate (Chlor-Trimeton); diphenhydramine hydrochloride (Benadryl); loratadine (Allegra, Alavert)
Antihypertensives	Increase size of arteries	Methyldopate hydrochloride (Aldomet); prazosin (Minipress)
Anti-inflammatory agents	Reduce irritation and swelling of tissues	Aspirin, ibuprofen (Motrin); naproxen (Naprosyn)
Antilipemic agents	Reduce serum cholesterol	Zocor; Lopid; Zetia
Antineoplastic agents	Slow tumor growth	Cyclophosphamide (Cytoxan)

(continued)

Common Drugs and Their Uses (*continued*)

Therapeutic Classification	Effect, Action, Uses	Common Examples
Antipsychotics	Exact mechanism not understood; used to treat psychoses (mental state involving distorted perceptions of reality)	chlorpromazine (Thorazine); haloperidol (Haldol)
Antipyretics	Decrease body temperature	Aspirin, acetaminophen (Tylenol)
Antitussives, mucolytics, expectorants	Relieve cough, loosen respiratory secretions, aid removal of thick secretions	Codeine sulfate; dextromethorphan hydrobromide (Benylin); guaifenesin (Entex)
Antivirals	Inhibit viral replication	Acyclovir (Zovirax), AZT
Bronchodilators	Dilate bronchi (air passages leading from trachea to lungs)	Albuterol sulfate (Ventolin), Alupent
Cardiotonics	Increase force of myocardium (heart muscle)	Digoxin (Lanoxin), Primacor
Cholinergic blockers	Affect autonomic nervous system (the part of the nervous system that regulates automatic functions such as blood flow, digestion, and temperature)	Atropine sulfate, scopolamine hydrobromide
Cholinergics	Mimic activity of parasympathetic nervous system (the part of the nervous system that regulates automatic functions to conserve body energy, e.g., by slowing heart rate)	Neostigmine (Prostigmin); pilocarpine hydrochloride
Decongestants	Reduce swelling of nasal passages	Pseudoephedrine hydrochloride (Sudafed)
Diuretics	Increase secretion of urine by kidneys	Furosemide (Lasix); chlorothiazide (Diuril)
Emetics	Promote vomiting	Ipecacuanha (Ipecac syrup)
Histamine H_2 antagonists	Inhibit action of histamine at H_2 receptor cells of stomach	Cimetidine (Tagamet); ranitidine (Zantac); famotidine (Pepcid)
Hormones, female	Prevent symptoms of menopause	Estradiol (Estraderm, Premarin); medroxyprogesterone acetate (Provera)
Hormones, male	Therapy for testosterone deficiency	Androgen (Testamone)
Immunological agents	Simulate immune response to protect against disease	Vaccines against pneumococcus, influenza virus; diphtheria and tetanus toxoid
Insulin, oral hypoglycemics	Control diabetes	NPH, ultralente insulin; tolbutamide (Orinase); glipizide (Glucotrol)
Sedatives, hypnotics	Sedatives relax and calm; hypnotics induce sleep	Butabarbital sodium, Restoril
Stimulants	Increase activity of central nervous system	Doxapram hydrochloride (Dopram), amphetamine sulfate
Thyroid, antithyroid agents	Alter amount of thyroid hormone produced	Levothyroxine sodium (T4) (Levothroid)

Common Drugs and Their Sources

Source		Drug	Use
Plants	Cinchona bark	Quinidine	Antiarrhythmic
	Purple foxglove	Digitalis	Cardiotonic
	Opium poppy	Paregoric	Antidiarrheal
		Morphine	Analgesic
		Codeine	Antitussive, analgesic
Minerals	Magnesium	Milk of Magnesia	Antacid, laxative
	Silver	Silver nitrate	Placed in eyes of newborns to kill *Neisseria gonorrhoeae,* a bacteria that causes gonorrhea
	Gold	Solganal	Arthritis treatment
Animal proteins	Pork, beef pancreas	Insulin	Antidiabetic hormone
	Pork, beef stomach acids	Pepsin	Digestive hormone
	Animal thyroid glands	Thyroid, USP	Hypothyroidism
Synthetics		Demerol	Analgesic
		Lomotil	Antidiarrheal
		Gantrisin	Sulfonamide
Semisynthetics	*Escherichia coli* bacteria, altered DNA molecules	Humulin	Antidiabetic hormone

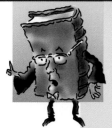

Legal Brief   THE CONTROLLED SUBSTANCES ACT

In 1970, the Controlled Substances Act was passed to regulate the manufacture and distribution of dangerous drugs. This act requires that anyone who manufactures, prescribes, administers, or dispenses controlled substances register with the U.S. government.

When a physician or practitioner registers, she receives a number that's called a DEA number. This registration limits which drugs that physician or practitioner can handle. The number is good for three years. It also must be updated if the office moves or opens another location. It's the physician or nurse practitioner's responsibility, not the DEA's, to make sure the registration is kept up to date. As a medical assistant, you may be responsible for maintaining or reminding the physician or practitioner about registration with the DEA.

Controlled Substances in the Medical Office

The DEA is responsible for revising the list of drugs in the Schedule of Controlled Substances. The table below tells you which drugs fall into each category. All the substances on the list have a potential for abuse and dependency. Drug dependence, also referred to as addiction, can be physical, psychological, or both.

Patients who take controlled substances must be monitored closely for signs of physical or psychological dependence.

- *Physical dependence.* A patient with a physical dependence on a drug will have mild to severe physiological symptoms. Symptoms gradually become more intense as the drug is stopped.
- *Psychological dependence.* A patient with a psychological dependence on a drug has developed a need for the feeling brought on by the drug.

Schedule of Controlled Substances

Schedule	Description	Examples
I	Highest potential for abuse; no accepted medicinal use in the U.S.; no accepted safety standards, although some are used in carefully controlled research projects.	Opium, marijuana, lysergic acid diethylamide (LSD), peyote, mescaline
II	High potential for abuse; accepted medicinal use in U.S. but with severe restrictions. Abuse can lead to psychological or physiological dependence. Requires written prescription; prescription cannot be refilled or called in to pharmacy by medical office. Only in extreme emergencies may physician call in prescription; handwritten prescription must be presented to pharmacist within 72 hours.	Morphine, codeine, cocaine, secobarbital (Seconal), amphetamines, hydromorphone (Dilaudid), methylphenidate (Ritalin)
III	Limited potential for psychological or physiological dependence. Prescription may be called in to pharmacy by physician and refilled up to six times in six months.	Paregoric, acetaminophen (Tylenol) with codeine, Fiorinal
IV	Lower potential for psychological or physiological dependence than those in schedules II and III. Prescription may be called into pharmacy by medical office employee; may be refilled up to five times in six months.	Chlordiazepoxide (Librium), diazepam (Valium), propoxyphene (Darvon), phenobarbital
V	Lower potential for abuse than those in schedules I to IV.	Buprenorphine (Buprenex), codeine in cough preparations

Monitoring Inventory

A medical office must order controlled substances from Schedule II using a federal order form (DEA Form 222). One copy of the form is filed with the DEA by the supplier. In most states, controlled substances from Schedule II may be ordered through the drug supplier for your office. Orders of substances from Schedules III to V don't require the form. However, the physician or practitioner's DEA number is still required.

When controlled substances are received in the medical office, the delivery receipt should be signed by two office employees. Each controlled substance is then tracked on a special inventory form. The receipts and inventory forms must be kept for two years. They also must be available for inspection by DEA officials. The illustration below shows an example of a controlled-substances inventory form.

Controlled Substance:	Meperidine (Demerol) 50-mg Injection					
Amount Ordered:	50-mg vials/ampules				Date:	

Date	Patient Name	Ordering Physician	Dose Given	Amount Discarded	Employee Signature

This is one example of a controlled-substances inventory form.

Controlled substances are kept in a safe or secure locked box. The number of people with keys or access should be limited. Careful records must be kept of how and when controlled substances leave the inventory. Controlled substances leave the inventory when they are:

- administered
- dispensed
- disposed of as waste

When a controlled substance is administered or dispensed, you need to record the following information:

- the drug's name
- the name of the patient who received the drug
- the dose given
- the date the drug was given
- the name of the physician who ordered the drug
- the name of the employee who handled the procedure

Federal law requires that every two years, the inventory of controlled substances must be checked. The amount of each drug on hand is compared to the amounts ordered and the amounts dispensed to patients. Many facilities also inventory their controlled substances whenever a different staff member assumes responsibility for the locked cabinet's key. Other facilities account for their controlled substances at the end of each day. You'll find exact steps for keeping records of controlled substances in the Hands On procedure on page 309.

If controlled substances are lost or stolen, notify local police immediately. It's the law!

Disposing of Controlled Substances

Sometimes, the physician may ask you to dispose of outdated medications or samples. You must follow federal, state, and local regulations when disposing of controlled substances. DEA Form 41 (Registrants Inventory of Drugs Surrendered) must be completed in quadruplicate and signed by the physician.

The information required for this form is similar to the information required for dispensing controlled substances. After completing the form, two copies are sent to the nearest DEA office. You'll then be notified about how to dispose of the drugs. Disposal methods may include incineration or shipping drugs to the DEA office by registered mail. Once the controlled substances are disposed of, the DEA will issue the physician a receipt. This receipt should be kept with the inventory records for controlled substances.

Prescribing Controlled Substances

In some cases, controlled substances are prescribed, not administered in the office. Some states require only that the prescription details be recorded in the patient's chart. Other states require that a separate file be kept in the medical office for copies of prescriptions for controlled substances.

Prescriptions for controlled substances must be written on special prescription forms. These forms are tamper-resistant and must be ordered from a government-approved security printer.

You must keep careful track of these forms so they are not lost or stolen. It's probably a good idea to keep them locked up until they're needed. Law enforcement officials recommend that the physician's DEA number *not* be preprinted on these prescription forms.

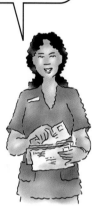

The DEA sends out information about changes in laws and procedures. Make sure your office is on the DEA's mailing list.

PRESCRIPTIONS IN THE OFFICE

The physician or nurse practitioner may ask you to fill out a prescription form for his signature. When you write a prescription, you must follow established guidelines. This includes using a traditional prescription form. There are several important pieces of information you must fill in on the form:

- *Date.* Prescriptions must be filled within six months of the date they are issued.
- *Patient's name and address.* The pharmacist needs this information to fill the prescription.
- *Inscription.* Just below or beside the symbol Rx, you write the name of the medication, the desired form (for example, liquid, tablet, capsule), and the strength (for example, 250 mg, 500 mL).

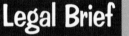 **Legal Brief** **ILLEGAL DRUG USE**

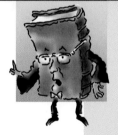

If you suspect that a physician or any health care professional is diverting controlled substances illegally, it's your legal and ethical duty to report your suspicions.

- Gather and document evidence to back up your suspicions. You'll need to present this evidence and the reasons for your suspicions when you report them to the proper authorities.
- In most instances, you'll be allowed to remain anonymous.
- In most cases, you should contact the local police.
- If a physician is involved, you'll need to report the evidence to the DEA and the American Medical Association (AMA) as well.
- If the suspected health care worker is not a physician or nurse practitioner, report the evidence to your supervisor.

Most states have programs to help health care professionals get help to deal with addiction or dependency issues.

- *Subscription.* This information tells the pharmacist how much of the drug to dispense. This could be the total number of tablets. For a liquid, it could be the total amount of the drug in milliliters.

- *Signature.* The signature section is not where the physician signs her name. It refers to the instructions for patients about taking the medication (for example, with meals, three times a day, four times a day). Sometimes the abbreviation *Sig.* may be used for this section.

- *Refills.* The number of times a prescription can be refilled should be indicated on the prescription. This is generally no more than five or six times within six months. If no refills are desired, the word *none* should be circled, or 0 should be written in.

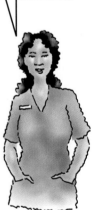

The symbol Rx is always found at the top left of the prescription pad. It's called the superscription, and means recipe, or "take thou."

- *Physician's signature.* The physician must sign the prescription. The physician is responsible for all prescriptions written in his office.

- *Generic.* Some physicians and insurance companies allow generic substitutes for some medications. You'll note on the prescription whether generic substitutions can be made. If the physician does not want a medication substituted with a generic version, write *DAW* on the prescription. This means "dispense as written."

- *DEA Number.* The physician's Drug Enforcement Administration (DEA) registration number should appear on every prescription as a way to track the delivery of controlled substances.

All prescription medications must be documented in the patient's medical record. This includes prescriptions that are called in or faxed to the pharmacist. The patient's chart is a legal document and may be called into court in the event of legal action. If the medication order isn't recorded, it will be presumed that the medication was never ordered. You'll find the exact steps for preparing a prescription in the Hands On procedure on page 311.

When prescribing, administering, or documenting patient prescriptions, you need to use appropriate medical terminology and abbreviations. The table on the next page lists common abbreviations and symbols you'll need to know.

Common Medical Abbreviations

Abbreviation	Meaning	Abbreviation	Meaning
aa	of each	os	mouth
amp	ampule	oz	ounce
amt	amount	p	after
aq	aqueous	pc	after meals
bid	twice a day	pm, PM	afternoon or evening
c̄	with		
cap	capsule	po, PO	by mouth
g, gm	gram	qt	quart
gr	grain	R	right, rectal
gt(t)	drop(s)	Rx	take, prescribe
h, hr	hour	s̄	without
Id, ID	intradermal	Sig	label
IM	intramuscular (into muscle)	SL	sublingual
		sol	solution
IV	intravenous	SOS	once if necessary
Kg	kilogram	sp	spirits
L, l	liter	ss	one-half
lb	pound	stat, STAT	immediately
m, min	minim	supp	suppository
mcg, µg	microgram	syr	syrup
mEq	milliequivalent	tab	tablet
ml, mL	milliliter	T, tb, tbs, tbsp	tablespoon
n	normal	t, tsp	teaspoon
NaCl	sodium chloride	tid	three times a day
NKA	no known allergies	tinc	tincture (a solution of a substance in alcohol)
noc	night		
NPO	nothing by mouth		
NS	normal saline	ung	ointment

Prescriptions by Phone

Sometimes, the physician may ask you to phone a prescription order to a patient's pharmacy. It may be a new prescription order or a renewal. You'll need to provide the pharmacist with information that is similar to the information on the written prescription. This includes:

- patient's name and address
- prescription information
- name of the prescribing physician
- number of refills

You can't phone in a prescription for a controlled substance. In an urgent situation, the physician may do so. The amount of the controlled substance must be limited to what is needed for the situation. A written prescription must be sent to the pharmacist within 72 hours to follow up the phone call.

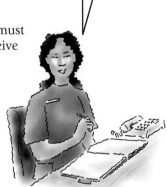

Document in the patient's chart any prescription renewals you make by phone. Remember, you also should document any phone conversations you have with the patient.

As a medical assistant, you also may need to deal with requests for prescription renewals that are phoned into the office from pharmacies and patients. These requests must be handled on the day they're made. Be sure you receive accurate information from the caller about the:

- patient's name, address, and phone number
- phone number of the pharmacy
- name of the medication, dosage, and amount

Once you have all the information, check it against the patient's medical record. Then, show the request and the patient's medical record to the physician. You must have the physician's approval before you phone in a renewal of a prescription. After you call it in, it's a good idea to call the patient to explain that the physician has renewed her prescription.

Patient Instructions

After patients receive a prescription in the office, you should provide verbal and written instructions for using the medication. Here's what they need to understand:

- how much medication to take
- when to take it
- instructions for how to take the medication (for example, with food or not)
- how the patient's body may react to the medication
- how long the medication should be taken for and why it's important to not stop taking some medications too soon
- side effects such as drowsiness or nausea
- when to report adverse reactions
- any safety precautions that should be taken, such as driving or operating machinery
- how the medicine should be stored
- how the medicine will react with alcohol and other medications, including over-the-counter drugs and herbs
- how to dispose of old and expired medicine

It's important to speak clearly and slowly while giving instructions about medications. Some elderly patients may have difficulty hearing you. You also should make sure the patient understands what you've said by watching for nonverbal cues and by having the patient repeat back the instructions.

Provide written instructions that include the name of the medication and directions for taking it. This helps to avoid confusion. Your medical office may have preprinted information sheets (from the American Medical Association) for common medications. Pharmacies also provide instruction sheets for patients. Encourage patients to call the medical office if they have any questions about taking their medication.

Drug Actions and Interactions

Every patient responds to drugs differently. To understand the actions and interactions of drugs and the human body, there are two main considerations.

- **Pharmacodynamics** refers to the ways drugs act on the body. This includes their actions on specific cells, tissues, and organs.

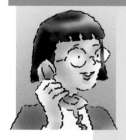

Ask the Professional   **CAN'T I JUST TAKE AN ASPIRIN?**

Q: *I gave a patient his prescription, but he said he prefers to use an herbal remedy or over-the-counter medication instead. How should I reply?*

A: Caution the patient that treating himself with an herbal remedy or over-the-counter medication isn't a substitute for the medication the physician has prescribed. OTC medications may not offer enough benefits to treat his illness. In some cases, they can cover up symptoms or even aggravate the problem. They might even interact with other medications that the patient is already taking.

Encourage the patient to follow the physician's instructions. Reassure him that if he has any questions while using the prescribed medication, he can call the office. You also should remind the patient not to mix OTC medications or herbal remedies with his prescription medications. Mixing medications can create a new set of problems, including unwanted drug effects.

If the patient still refuses to take the medication, tell the physician. Document the patient's refusal and reasons in the patient's medical record.

- **Pharmacokinetics** is how the drugs move through the body after they're swallowed or injected.

PHARMACODYNAMICS

Different drugs have different effects on the body. In pharmacodynamics, it's important to distinguish between the actions of drugs and the effects of those drugs.

- *Drug action* refers to the chemical changes the drug has on the body's cells. All drugs cause cellular change.
- *Drug effect* refers to the observable changes the drug has on the body. All drugs have some degree of physiological effect.

For example, the drug action of penicillin is to prevent bacteria from building up cell walls. The drug effect of penicillin is that it kills bacteria.

LOCAL OR SYSTEMIC EFFECTS

The effect of a drug may be either local or systemic (affecting an entire system). A **local effect** is limited to the area of the body where it's administered. When an ointment or lotion is applied to the skin, the drug action is limited to that area. The effect of the drug is local.

A **systemic effect** means that the drug is absorbed into the blood and carried to other parts of the body. Antibiotic therapy for a urinary tract infection produces a systemic effect. Antibiotic tablets are taken orally. Once the drug is absorbed into the bloodstream, it's carried to the urinary bladder. The drug acts on any microorganisms in the urinary bladder and destroys them.

A systemic effect can be obtained by administering drugs in several different ways:

- orally—by mouth and swallowed
- sublingually—under the tongue
- buccally—between the cheek and gum
- rectally—through the rectum
- by injection—into the bloodstream
- transdermally—through the skin
- by inhalation—through the lungs

PHARMACOKINETICS

The way the body reacts to the drug depends on:

- how it's administered
- how quickly it's absorbed
- how long it takes to act
- how quickly it's eliminated from the body

There are four general processes involved in pharmacokinetics.

- *Absorption* is the process of getting the drug into the bloodstream. The method of administration affects the absorption rate, or how fast the drug moves in the body. Two different drug products that contain the same active ingredients may be absorbed at different rates. Other ingredients in the product may affect the absorption rate.

- *Distribution* refers to the movement of the drug from the bloodstream into cells and tissues. Different drugs move into different types of body tissues at different speeds.

- *Metabolism* is the physical and chemical breakdown of drugs by the body. This often takes place in the liver. Patients with hepatic disease have problems with liver function and may not be able to break down a drug properly. This will affect the time it takes for the drug to act. It also may affect how long the drug will continue acting.

- *Excretion* is the process where byproducts of drugs are sent to kidneys to be removed from the body. Some drugs reach the kidneys largely unchanged. They can be detected in the patient's urine after excretion. But if the kidneys are compromised by disease, the medication may not be eliminated properly. Drugs that are not eliminated properly may build up in the body. This may lead to toxicity or poisoning.

Closer Look   FACTORS INFLUENCING DRUG ACTION

Many factors can influence a drug's action on the body. The table on page 272 lists some of the ways drugs may be affected by these factors.

Factors Influencing Drug Action

Factors	Effects on Drug Action
Age	Elderly people have slow metabolic processes. Age-related kidney and liver dysfunctions also extend breakdown and excretion times. You must monitor the cumulative effects of drugs in elderly patients. Children may have a more immediate response to drugs. Therefore, you should assess them frequently.
Weight	Many dosages of medications are calculated according to the patient's weight. As a general rule, the larger the patient, the greater the dose. However, you also need to take into account a person's sensitivity to a drug.
Gender	Women's reactions to certain drugs may be different from those of men because of the ratio of fat to body mass or differing hormone levels.
Time of day	The absorption of certain drugs is delayed by the presence of food in the stomach or small intestine. Other drugs may be better tolerated when there's food in the patient's stomach.
Psychological state	Nervous or highly excited patients may need larger or smaller amounts of certain drugs to achieve the desired effect than calmer patients require.
Existing pathology	If the body is compromised by a disease, then process, absorption, distribution, metabolism, and excretion may be affected.
Idiosyncratic and immune responses	Some people may have unexpected, abnormal, or allergic reactions to some drugs. The body must build an immune response, so first exposures may or may not indicate a problem. However, later reactions to the same drug may be more severe.
Cumulation	The rates at which the body absorbs, breaks down, or excretes some drugs can result in high concentrations and possible toxic effects if repeat doses are not adjusted for this factor.
Tolerance	Some medications given over a long period of time cause the body to become resistant to their effects. If this happens, larger doses may be required to get the desired result.

Pharmacokinetics may cause a drug to be **contraindicated,** or not recommended for use, if a patient has certain medical conditions. The drug's manufacturer lists contraindications, or situations when the drug should not be given, on the drug's box or an insert that comes with the drug.

DRUG INTERACTIONS

When two drugs are taken at the same time, the drugs may act on each other. When this happens, it's called an **interaction.** The drugs' effects may increase, decrease, or cancel each other out. Drug interactions can occur with prescribed drugs, over-the-counter medications, or herbal or other natural supplements. Alcohol consumption also can cause a drug interaction.

Types of interactions include **synergism, antagonism,** and **potentiation.**

- *Synergism* means that two drugs work together.
- *Antagonism* is an effect in which one drug makes the other less effective.
- *Potentiation* occurs when one drug extends or multiplies the effect of another drug.

Physicians and nurse practitioners sometimes may prescribe two or more drugs that interact to cause a specific effect. For example, a physician might prescribe both a muscle relaxant and a pain medication to treat an injury to a muscle or muscle group.

Some drug interactions produce unwanted effects. Here are two examples:

- Taking antacids to relieve symptoms of indigestion may prevent the absorption of antibiotics such as tetracycline (antagonism).
- Sedatives and barbiturates taken together can depress the nervous system (synergism).

Food-Drug Interactions

Patients take many prescription and over-the-counter medications by mouth, so the drugs are absorbed through the digestive system. Food in the digestive system can affect the absorption of the drug.

- Some medications are best absorbed when taken one to two hours after a meal. Examples are ampicillin or naf-cillin (Unipen), both antibiotics. The physician may rec-ommend that some drugs be taken an hour before or two hours after eating.
- Some medications should be taken with food to decrease the chance of stomach upset—for example, ibuprofen (Motrin), amoxicillin (an antibiotic), and verapamil (Calan, a heart medication).

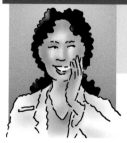

Secrets for Success   DRUG-RELATED TERMS

When working around drugs, you'll need to be familiar with specific terms related to pharmacology. The following table includes some basic terms you should know.

Drug-Related Terms

Term	Meaning
Therapeutic classification	States the purpose for the drug's use (for example, a *cardiotonic* drug strengthens the heart and blood vessels; an *anti-infective* drug fights infection)
Teratogenic category	The level of risk to fetal or maternal health, ranging from Category A to D (where D is most dangerous). Category X means that a drug should never be given during pregnancy.
Indications	Diseases and conditions for which the particular drug is prescribed
Contraindications	Conditions or instances when the particular drug should not be used
Adverse reaction	Undesirable side effects of a particular drug
Hypersensitivity	Excessive reaction (also known as a drug allergy); the body must build this response, so first exposures may or may not indicate a developing problem.
Idiosyncratic reaction	An abnormal or unexpected reaction to a drug that's peculiar to an individual patient; not technically an allergy

Other medications interact with specific types of food. Some nutrients in food can bind with drug ingredients and reduce absorption or decrease a drug's effectiveness. Here are some common medications that interact with food.

- *Atorvastatin (Lipitor).* This medication for reducing blood cholesterol levels interacts with grapefruit juice.
- *MAO inhibitors.* These medications for treating depression can interact with some foods such as cheese or alcohol. The interactions can result in severe headaches or dangerous increases in blood pressure.
- *Tetracycline.* The absorption of this antibiotic is less effective when taken with calcium or foods containing calcium.
- *Warfarin (Coumadin).* Green, leafy vegetables such as spinach or kale, which are high in vitamin K, may decrease the effectiveness of this blood thinner.

It's important to learn as much as you can about medications prescribed often in your medical office. You may need to educate patients on how to avoid food and drug interactions.

Allergic Reactions and Side Effects

When gathering information for the patient's medical history, it's important to ask about allergies of any sort, but especially allergies to medications. A drug **allergy** is a reaction such as hives, dyspnea (labored breathing), or wheezing. **Anaphylaxis** is a severe allergic reaction that can be life threatening. Allergic reactions can be immediate or delayed by two hours or longer.

If the medication is administered by injection, any allergic reaction usually occurs within minutes.

If the patient reports allergies to a medication, you need to interview the patient carefully about his symptoms. Medications that produce true allergic symptoms need to be noted in the patient's medical record. Drug allergies always should be noted prominently on the front of the patient's medical record and on each page of the medication record. Patients who've had an allergic reaction to a medication in the past shouldn't be given the medication again. It might cause an anaphylactic reaction.

If a patient is receiving allergy medication or any medication that has a high incidence of allergic reactions (such as penicillin for example), the patient should wait for 20 to 30 minutes and be rechecked before leaving the office. Some offices require that all patients who receive injections wait a specific amount of time (usually 15 to 20 minutes) before leaving. Once the patient is checked, be sure to document in the chart that there were no complaints or difficulties. Always follow the policies in your medical office regarding administering injections.

I don't see any drug allergies noted in your chart. Do you know if you have any?

SIDE EFFECT OR ALLERGY?

A patient may state she has an allergy to a medication, when the reaction was really a side effect. **Side effects** are predictable reactions to medications that occur in some patients. Manufacturers note expected side effects on the medication. Some common side effects include:

- nausea
- dryness of the mouth
- drowsiness

Side effects often are annoying, but they're not usually life threatening! They don't need to be noted on the patient's allergy list.

Closer Look

FOR MORE INFORMATION

There are several resources medical assistants can use to find out more about medications.

- *Physician's Desk Reference.* This resource includes the drug's chemical name, brand name or names, and generic name. It lists properties, indications, side effects, contraindications, dosages, and includes pictures of various medications. The physician must purchase this book.

- *United States Pharmacopeia Dispensing Information* (USPDI). Two paperback volumes provide information about drug sources, physical properties, tests for identity, storage, and dosage. The USPDI does not contain photographs of medications. The physician must purchase these books.

- *American Hospital Formulary Service* (AHFS). This is distributed to practicing physicians. It provides concise information arranged according to drug classifications.

- *Compendium of Drug Therapy.* This annual publication is distributed to physicians. It includes photographs of drugs and phone numbers of major pharmaceutical companies and poison control centers.

Administering Medications

You should be familiar with any medication the physician orders before you administer it. You also should know the procedures for administering the drug accurately and safely. If you're not familiar with a drug, look up its classification, usual dosage, and route of administration.

SAFETY GUIDELINES

As a medical assistant, you must follow important safety guidelines when administering medications. Following this list of guidelines will protect you and your patients.

1. Know your office's policies regarding the administration of medications.

2. Give only the medications the physician has ordered in writing. Don't accept verbal orders.

3. Check with the physician if you have any doubt about a medication or order.

4. Avoid conversation and other distractions while preparing and administering medications. Be attentive!

5. Work in a quiet, well-lighted area.

6. Check the label three times—once when taking the medication from the shelf, again when preparing the medication, and a third time when replacing the medication on the shelf or disposing of the empty container.

7. Place the order and the medication side by side to compare for accuracy.

8. Check the strength of the medication (for example, 250 as opposed to 500 mg) and the route of administration.

9. Read labels carefully. Don't scan labels or medication orders.

10. Check the patient's medical record for allergies to the medication or its components before giving it.

11. Check the medication's expiration date.

12. Be alert for color changes, precipitation, odor, or any indication that the medication's properties have changed. If the medication has changed in consistency, color, or odor, discard it appropriately.

13. Measure exactly. There should be no bubbles in liquid medication.

14. Stay with the patient while he takes oral medication. Watch for any reaction and record the patient's response.

15. Never return a medication to the container after it's been poured or removed.

16. Put on gloves for all procedures that might result in contact with blood or body fluids.

17. Never recap, bend, or break a used needle.

18. Have sharps containers as close as possible to the area of use.

19. Never give a medication that was poured or drawn up by someone else. Never prepare or draw up medication for someone else.

20. Always lock the medication cabinet when it's not in use.

21. Never give the keys for the medication cabinet to an unauthorized person. Limit access to the medication cabinet by limiting access to the cabinet keys.

SYSTEMS FOR MEASURING

The most common system of measurement used in the medical office is the metric system. But you may encounter other systems of measurement.

While working in the clinical setting, you may need to calculate a dose in one system of measurement using mathematical equations. Also, you may need to convert a measurement from one system to another. As you can imagine, it's important to understand the commonly used systems of measurement before trying to calculate doses.

Metric System

The **metric system** is used in the United States and throughout the world. Because it's based on multiples of ten, it uses decimals, not fractions. In the metric system:

- the base unit of length is the meter (m)
- the base unit of weight is the gram (g or gm)
- liter (L or l) is used to measure fluid volume

Prefixes are used in the metric system to show a fraction of the base unit or a multiple of it. The table on page 279 shows prefixes that are used most often.

With the base unit of a liter (1 L = approximately 1.06 quarts), fractional measurements are in milliliters (ml or mL). Other measures rarely are used in medication administration. Also, 1 cubic centimeter (cc), a solid, is equal to 1 mL. These measures are sometimes used interchangeably. Decagrams and centigrams are not used in medication administration.

Apothecary System

This older system of measurement is used less now than in the past. It's gradually being replaced by the metric system. However, some physicians may continue to use this system. In the **apothecary system of measurement,** liquid measurements include:

- drop (gt) or drops (gtt)
- minim (min or m)

Commonly Used Metric Prefixes

Prefix	Meaning	Value	Abbreviation	Example of Use	Example's Meaning
micro-	millionth of	0.000001	mc	8 mcg	8 micrograms (8 millionths of a gram) (0.000008 g)
milli-	thousandth of	0.001	m	3 mL	3 milliliters (3 thousandths of a liter) (0.003 L)
centi-	hundredth of	0.01	c	7 cm	7 centimeters (7 hundredths of a meter) (0.07 m)
deci-	tenth of	0.1	d	4 dL	4 deciliters (4 tenths of a liter) (0.4 L)
kilo-	thousand times	1000.0	k	5 kg	5 kilograms (5 thousand grams) (5000 g)

- fluid dram (fl dr)
- fluid ounce (fl oz)
- pint (pt)
- quart (qt)
- gallon (gal)

Some measurements for solid weights are:

- grain (gr)
- dram (dr)
- ounce (oz)
- pound (lb)

Roman numerals are used for smaller numbers. See the Roman numeral chart below for more information. For example, I = 1, V = 5, and X = 10. Fractions may be used when necessary, however, decimals aren't used in the apothecary system.

Roman Numeral	Arabic Number
I	1
V	5
X	10
L	50
C	100
D	500
M	1,000
V̄	5,000

Household System

The household system of measurement is used most often by patients. It includes measures commonly used for cooking, such as:

- teaspoon (tsp)
- tablespoon (tbsp)
- ounce (oz)
- cup (c)
- pint (pt)
- quart (qt)
- pound (lb)

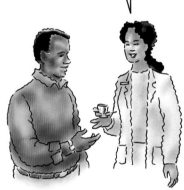

If you don't have a dosing cup, you may use standard measuring spoons and cups when you take medicine at home. These are much more accurate than silverware or regular cups.

Even though this system isn't used in the medical office for calculating doses, you may need to instruct patients on the proper household measurements for taking medications ordered in the metric system. For example, 5 mL is equal to 1 teaspoon (tsp).

COMMONLY USED EQUIVALENTS

It's a good idea to know similar measures for different systems of measurements. The table on page 281 provides the common equivalents for each system of measurement.

For example, you can see from the table that a teaspoon of liquid is about 5 mL in the metric system. So if the physician wants the patient to have 10 mL of a medicine every 4 hours, you can see from the table that you should tell the patient to take 2 teaspoons of it every 4 hours.

Converting Between Systems of Measurement

Sometimes, rather than using the table, you'll need to calculate the conversion from one system to another. Here are the medicine-related conversions you're most likely to need in a medical office.

1. Converting apothecary to metric:
   - To change grains to grams, divide the number of grains ordered by 15. Example: 30 gr ÷ 15 = 2 g
   - If the amount of grains is less than 1, change the grains to milligrams and multiply the grains by 60. Example: ¼ gr × 60 = 15 mg

Most Commonly Used Approximate Equivalents

Approximate Volume Equivalents

Metric	Apothecary	Household
0.06 mL	1 m	1 drop
1 mL	15 m	0.2 tsp
5 mL	1 fl dr	1 tsp (60 drops)
15 mL	0.5 fl oz (4 fl dr)	1 tbsp
30 mL	1 fl oz	2 tbsp
500 mL	16 fl oz	1 pt
1000 mL	32 fl oz	1 qt

Approximate Weight Equivalents

Metric	Apothecary	Household
1 gm	15 gr	
30 gm	1 oz	1 oz
450 gm	1 lb	1 lb
1 kg (1000 gm)	2.2 lb	2.2 lb

Approximate Length Equivalents

Metric	Apothecary	Household
1 cm (10 mm)		0.4 in
2.5 cm (25 mm)		1 in
30.5 cm (300 mm)		1 ft
90 cm (900 mm)		1 yd
1 m (100 cm)		3.25 ft (40 in)

2. Converting household to metric:
   - To change fluid ounces to milliliters, multiply the number of ounces by 30. Example: 4 oz × 30 = 120 mL
   - To change pounds to kilograms, divide the pounds by 2.2. Example: 44 lb ÷ 2.2 = 20 kg

3. Converting metric to household:
   - To change milliliters to fluid ounces, divide the number of mL by 30. Example: 150 mL ÷ 30 = 5 oz
   - To change kilograms to pounds, multiply the kilograms by 2.2. Example: 50 kg × 2.2 = 110 lbs

> Check your conversion calculations twice. It's better to take the time to check your answers than to make a mistake.

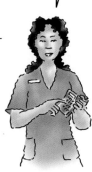

Converting Within the Metric System

In the metric system, it's sometimes necessary to convert measurements to the same unit. For example, the physician may order 0.5 g of medication, and the medication label may read 500 mg. These rules will help you make conversions within the metric system:

1. Milligrams and grams:
   - To change grams to milligrams, multiply the number of grams by 1000 (or move the decimal point three places to the right).
     Example: 0.5 g × 1000 = 500 mg
   - To change milligrams to grams, divide the number of milligrams by 1000 (or move the decimal point three places to the left).
     Example: 500 mg ÷ 1000 = 0.5 g

2. Milligrams and micrograms:
   - To change milligrams to micrograms, multiply the milligrams by 1000 (move the decimal three places to the right).
     Example: 5 mg × 1000 = 5000 micrograms
   - To change micrograms to milligrams, divide the micrograms by 1000 (move the decimal three places to the left).
     Example: 500 micrograms ÷ 1000 = 0.5 mg

3. Liters and milliliters:
   - To change liters to milliliters, multiply the liters by 1000 (move the decimal three places to the right).
     Example: 0.01 L × 1000 = 10 mL
   - To change milliliters to liters, divide the milliliters by 1000 (move the decimal three places to the left).
     Example: 100 mL ÷ 1000 = 0.1 L

CALCULATING ADULT DOSES

Administration of medication is an exact science. Calculation errors can kill patients. Although the physician is the one who orders the amount of medication to administer, you may be the one to calculate the amount to withdraw into a syringe or to pour into a medicine cup.

Before you can calculate the correct dosage, make sure the measurements are in the same system (metric, apothecary, household) and units. Here are some examples of when this could be a problem.

- The physician uses the apothecary system when ordering medication. But the medication is packaged according to the metric system. So, you'll need to convert the amount ordered by the physician to the metric system.

When using the metric system, be careful to keep the decimal point in the correct place.

- The physician orders a medication in grams. When the medication arrives, it's packaged in milligrams. You'll need to convert the physician's order to milligrams.

Once the measurement units are the same, there are two methods that can be used to calculate medication dosages for adults:

- ratio method
- formula method

The Ratio Method

In this method, two ratios are created using the information on the medication label and the desired dose in the physician's order. The proportion, or relationship between the ratios, should be the same. This allows you to calculate the amount of medication to administer. To calculate a dose using the ratio method, set up your problem like this:

$$\frac{\text{dose on label:}}{\text{quantity on label}} = \frac{\text{dose ordered:}}{\text{quantity to administer}}$$

OR

$$\frac{\text{dose on label (known)}}{\text{dose desired (known)}} = \frac{\text{quantity on label (known)}}{\text{quantity to administer (unknown)}}$$

Example 1: The physician orders erythromycin 250 mg. The label on the package reads erythromycin 100 mg/mL.

First, determine the proportion.

$$\frac{100 \text{ mg}}{250 \text{ mg}} = \frac{1 \text{ mL}}{x}$$

Follow these steps to calculate x (the amount to administer).

1. Cross multiply: $100 \times x = 100x$
2. Cross multiply: $250 \times 1 = 250$

3. The proportion is now: 100x = 250

4. Divide both sides by 100 to find x. So, x = 250 ÷ 100, x = 2.5.

   In this example, you need to administer 2.5 mL of the erythromycin for the patient to receive the dose (250 mg) ordered by the physician.

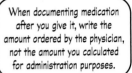

When documenting medication after you give it, write the amount ordered by the physician, not the amount you calculated for administration purposes.

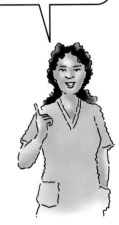

Example 2: The physician orders phenobarbital 25 mg. On hand are 12.5-mg tablets.
   First, determine the proportion.

$$\frac{12.5 \text{ mg}}{25 \text{ mg}} = \frac{1 \text{ tablet}}{x}$$

Then calculate the quantity to administer.

1. Cross multiply: $12.5 \times x = 12.5x$

2. Cross multiply: $25 \times 1 = 25$

3. Now write: $12.5x = 25$

4. To find x, divide both sides by 12.5.

5. $25 \div 12.5 = 2$, $x = 2$. Therefore, the quantity to administer is 2 tablets.

The Formula Method

Another way to calculate the dose to administer is to use this formula:

$$(\text{desired dose} \div \text{dose on label}) \times \text{quantity on label} = \frac{\text{quantity to}}{\text{administer}}$$

Example 1: The physician orders ampicillin 0.5 g. On hand, you have ampicillin 250-mg capsules. How much ampicillin should be administered?

1. Remember, both doses should be in the same unit of measure. First, convert grams to milligrams. Multiply the grams by 1000 (move the decimal point three places to the right). The result is 0.5 g = 500 mg. Therefore, the desired dose (0.5 g) is the same as 500 mg.

2. Put the information you know into the problem:

$$(500 \text{ mg} \div 250 \text{ mg}) \times 1 = \text{quantity to administer}$$

$$2 \times 1 = 2$$

3. The quantity to administer is 2 capsules.

Example 2: The physician orders 0.35 g of a medication and you have on hand a liquid of 700 mg/L. How many mL do you prepare to administer?

> You may use either the ratio method or the formula method to calculate the dose to administer. Just be sure to follow the exact calculations for whichever method you choose—and check your work!

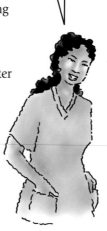

1. First, make sure both doses are in equal units. Change 0.35 g to milligrams by multiplying as in Example 1 ($0.35 \text{ g} \times 1000 = 350 \text{ mg}$).

2. Put the information you know into the problem:

$$(350 \text{ mg} \div 700 \text{ mg}) \times 1 = 0.5 \text{ mL} = \text{quantity to administer}$$

CALCULATING PEDIATRIC DOSES

Sometimes, you may know the adult dosage of a medication, but you need to know what the dosage would be for a child. Several formulas are used to calculate children's doses:

- body surface area (BSA) method
- Young's rule
- Clark's rule
- Fried's rule

The BSA Method

This is the most accurate method for children up to 12 years of age, and for adults who are below normal body weight. It requires a scale called a **nomogram.** This is a chart which uses the patient's height and weight to estimate the body surface area (BSA) in square meters. One is shown in the illustration on page 286.

A straight line is drawn from the patient's height in inches or centimeters (in the left column) to the patient's weight in kilograms or pounds (in the right column). The place where the line intersects the middle column is the patient's BSA, or body surface area. The nomogram on page 286 illustrates how it's used.

After you have determined the patient's estimated BSA, use this formula to calculate the child's dose:

$$(\text{BSA} \times \text{adult dose}) \div 1.7 = \text{child's dose}$$

Young's Rule

For this formula, you need the age of the child in years. It's used to calculate doses for children aged 12 months to 12 years.

Height		Surface Area	Weight	
Feet	Centimeters	Square Meters	Pounds	Kilograms

This nomogram can be used for estimating the surface area of infants and children up to 12.

$$\text{pediatric dose} = \frac{\text{child's age in years}}{(\text{child's age in years} + 12)} \times \text{adult dose}$$

Clark's Rule

Clark's rule is considered more accurate than Young's rule because it accounts for differences in body size and weight at different ages. In Clark's rule, the weight of the child in pounds is divided by 150 (the supposed weight of an average adult in pounds) and multiplied by the average adult dose to figure out the child's dose.

$$\text{pediatric dose} = \frac{\text{child's weight in pounds}}{150 \text{ pounds}} \times \text{adult dose}$$

Fried's Rule

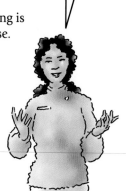

Fried's rule is used for calculating doses for infants less than 2 years of age. It bases the calculation on the child's age in months. The number 150, included in this formula, represents the age in months of a 12.5-year-old child. The thinking is that a 12.5-year-old child would be eligible for an adult dose.

$$\text{pediatric dose} = \frac{\text{child's age in months}}{150 \text{ months}} \times \text{adult dose}$$

Other Calibrations

Many medications that require careful calibration (adjustments) are dosed per kilogram of body weight. Instructions for calculating the amount to administer are included in the package insert that comes with the medication.

For example, the insert may state, "For adults and children over 25 kg (55 lb), give 500 mg. For children less than 25 kg, give 25 mg/kg." If the child who needs the medication weighs 20 lb, this weight must be converted to kg. Since 1 kg = 2.2 lb, this child weighs 9 kg. The equation for calculating the child's dosage is then:

$$25 \text{ mg} \times 9 \text{ kg} = 225 \text{ mg}$$

Administration Routes

There are many ways, or routes, for administering medication. The physician chooses the route of administration. The choice of the route can depend on three things:

- cost
- safety
- absorption rate

The many routes of administration can be divided into two main groups—**enteral** and **parenteral**. The enteral routes are all related to the digestive tract in some way. These routes include medications taken in the following ways:

- Orally chewed, swallowed whole, or dissolved sublingually or buccally
- Rectally (by insertion into the rectum)

- Nasogastrically (by tube placed through the nose into the stomach or small intestine)
- Gastrically (by tube placed through the mouth into the stomach or surgically implanted through the abdominal wall into the stomach)

Parenteral routes include any route other than the enteral ones—for example, injections, intravenous administration, and vaginal application.

There are many reasons to use parenteral methods of administration. Here are some of the most common ones:

- Some patients can't take oral medications.
- Some medications can't be absorbed through the gastrointestinal system.
- A patient's condition may require fast absorption of the drug.

Some drugs can be administered by one route only. This may be due to their form or chemical composition. Some may be toxic if given by a certain route. Some drugs may be absorbed only through one particular route. Others are effective when administered in a variety of ways. The different routes for drug administration are:

- oral (by mouth)
- under the tongue or beside the cheek
- injection
- intravenous (directly into a vein)
- inhalation
- topical (on the skin)
- through the eye, ear canal, or nose
- rectal
- vaginal
- intradermal

See the table on page 289 for advantages and disadvantages of oral and parenteral medications.

MEDICATION BY MOUTH

Patients often are given a medication to swallow in the form of a tablet, capsule, pill, or liquid. This method is preferred by many patients and is the easiest to administer. Drugs given orally in the medical office usually come in unit dose packs that contain a premeasured single dose of the

Oral Versus Parenteral Medication Administration

Oral Medications	Parenteral Medications
Advantages: • easily administered • economical to administer • administered with a high degree of safety	Advantages: • rapid response time to medication • accuracy of dosage • ability to concentrate the medication in a specific body area, such as a joint • ideal for patients who cannot take medication by mouth because of an illness or because the stomach acids would destroy the medication
Disadvantages: • objectionable taste and odor • discoloration of the teeth, mouth, and tongue • irritation to the stomach • poor absorption rate due to illness or nature of medicine • failure of patient to take medicine • less predictable effects on the body than when given by an injection • patient may be unable to swallow pill, tablet, or capsule	Disadvantages: • rapid allergic reactions • injury to bone, soft tissue, nerves, or blood vessel caused by needle • needle breakage in tissue • accidental injection into the vein instead of the soft tissue

drug. For more information about the different forms in which medications can be taken by mouth, study the table on page 290.

You'll find exact steps for administering oral medication in the Hands On procedure on page 313. Oral medications are absorbed through the walls of the gastrointestinal tract. However, medications taken this way usually are slow to take effect. Also, not every patient can take medications by this method. The oral route is not suitable for patients who:

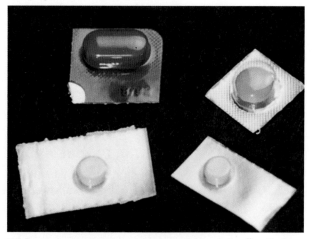

Unit dose packages make it easy to give oral medications in the office. They're labeled with the trade name, generic name, precautions, instructions for storage, and an expiration date.

- are unconscious

- have nausea and/or vomiting

- have been ordered to take nothing by mouth

Forms of Oral Medications

Form	Types	Description
Solids	Buffered caplet	Medication has an added agent to decrease stomach acidity and prevent stomach irritation.
	Capsule	Medication is powdered or granulated in a gelatin sheath. Sheath is designed to be dissolved by gastric enzymes or high in the small intestine.
	Enteric coated tablet	Dry, compressed medication is coated to withstand stomach acidity and dissolve in the intestines. Never crush or break enteric coated tablets.
	Gelcap	Oil-based medication in a soft gelatin capsule.
	Chewable	Tablet that's meant to be chewed completely before swallowing in order to release the medication more quickly into the system.
	Lozenge	Medication in a firm, compressed form, usually for a local effect in the mouth or throat. Caution patients to let lozenges dissolve slowly and avoid drinking fluids after taking a lozenge.
	Powder	Medication is in a finely ground form that may be difficult for some patients to swallow.
	Spansule, or time-release capsule	Medication is inside a gelatin capsule that will dissolve over time rather than all at once. Never open a time-release capsule unless recommended by the manufacturer.
	Tablet	Medication is shaped or colored for easy identification. Tablets usually dissolve high in the GI tract. They may be broken in half only if scored (marked with a line or groove) for that purpose.
Liquids	Syrup	A very sweet form of medication frequently used for children. It's usually flavored in addition to having a high sugar content.
	Elixir	Medication is dissolved in alcohol and flavored. It's less sweet than syrups and is usually preferred by adults. Not appropriate for alcoholics or diabetics.
	Emulsion	Medication is combined with water and oil. The emulsion must be shaken thoroughly to disperse the medication evenly.
	Extract	Highly concentrated form of medication made by evaporating volatile plant oils (oils that vaporize readily). It may be administered as drops and is usually given in a liquid to disguise the strong taste.
	Gel	Medication is suspended in a thin gelatin or paste.
	Suspension	Particles of medication are dissolved in a liquid. Must be shaken well before use.

UNDER THE TONGUE AND BESIDE THE CHEEK

Some medications may be placed in the mouth, but they aren't meant to be swallowed. They're absorbed into the body through the mucous membranes of the mouth rather than digested in the stomach.

- *Sublingual medication.* In the sublingual route, the medication is placed under the patient's tongue. It must not be swallowed. The drug is dissolved by the saliva in the patient's mouth. It's absorbed directly into the bloodstream through the mucous membranes covering the sublingual blood vessels. Caution the patient not to eat or drink until the medication is dissolved. One of the most common sublingual medications is nitroglycerin, taken by patients with heart-related chest pain.

- *Buccal medication.* In this method, the medication is placed between the patient's cheek and gum at the side of the mouth. The drug is then absorbed through the vascular oral mucosa. Not many medications are manufactured for this route. The patient should not chew or swallow the medication or eat or drink until it's absorbed. Many lozenges are designed to be absorbed buccally.

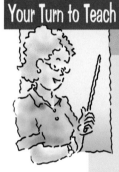

Your Turn to Teach

TEACHING PATIENTS HOW TO MANAGE PRESCRIPTION DRUGS

One of the roles of a medical assistant is to provide patients with verbal and written instructions about their medications. You'll need to explain how much to take, when to take it, and any potential side effects. You also should take the time to teach patients some general principles about how to manage their medications safely.

- Urge the patient to tell the physician about any and all drugs they use—both regularly and from time to time. This includes prescription drugs, OTC medications, and herbal supplements.

- Patients with more than one physician should inform each one about all the medications they are taking. Encourage patients to keep a list of all medications and dosages.

- For patients taking many medications, write out a chart or schedule to help them remember when and how to take each one.

- Explain that it's a good idea to ask the pharmacist how to store each medication. Many medications need to be stored in a cool, dry place, but some need to be refrigerated.

- Remind patients not to save old medications or share them with others. Out-of-date medications may lose their effectiveness or cause harmful effects.

INJECTIONS

Injection is the most efficient method of parenteral drug administration. However, it also can be the most hazardous. The effects are quite rapid, and the medication can't be retrieved once it's injected. Because the skin is broken, infections can develop if strict aseptic technique isn't followed.

Medications for injections are sometimes supplied in **ampules.** These are small glass containers that must be broken at the neck of the ampule. Once they're broken, the solution is aspirated or removed by suction. You must use a filter needle when getting medication from an ampule to prevent small pieces of glass from being drawn up. All medication inside must be either used or discarded.

Medications for injections also may be supplied as vials or prefilled cartridges. You can learn more about the steps for preparing an injection in the Hands On Procedure on page 316.

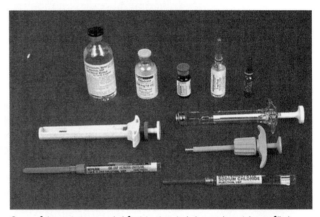

Some of the equipment needed for injections include ampules, vials, prefilled cartridges, and holders.

Vials

Vials are glass or plastic containers that are sealed at the top by a stopper. They may be single-dose or multiple-dose containers. The contents of vials may be in the form of a solution or a powder. Powders must be reconstituted— mixed with a specific amount and type of diluting agent. The **diluent,** or diluting agent, usually is sterile water or saline. Certain drugs, such as phenytoin (Dilantin), an anticonvulsant, require a special diluent supplied by the manufacturer.

When a powdered drug is reconstituted in a multiple-dose vial, you must write some information on the label:

- date of reconstitution
- initials of the person who reconstituted the drug
- diluent used
- strength of the medicine that was produced

Vials intended for multiple doses may hold up to 50 mL. They may be used repeatedly by inserting a needle through the self-sealing stopper to remove some of the solution. Unit dose vials usually contain 1 to 2 mL. All the solution is removed for a single injection.

RECONSTITUTING DRY MEDICATION

To reconstitute dry medication in a vial, follow these steps:

1. Check the vial label or manufacturer's instructions to find out how much diluent to add to the powder.

2. Wipe the top of the vial containing the diluent with an alcohol pad before inserting the needle. Then, withdraw the correct amount of diluent using aseptic technique.

3. Add the diluent to the vial containing the powder. Wipe the top of the vial with an alcohol pad before inserting the needle.

4. Replace the vial's stopper. Roll the vial between your palms until the powder is dissolved.

The concentration of the mixture will depend on how the medication will be given. The instructions from the drug's manufacturer usually tell how much diluent to add to the powder if the medication is to be given intravenously (IV), injected into the muscle (IM), or injected under the skin (SQ).

You must be sure that the concentration of the mixture is right for the method of administration. A dosage that's too strong for the way it's given may harm the patient's tissues. If the dose is too weak for the method of administration, the medicine may not have the proper effect.

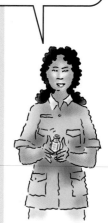

> Don't shake the vial. Shaking can cause unnecessary bubbles, which make it hard to measure the exact amount of medication needed.

Syringes and Needles

Your choice of syringe and needle depends on the type of injection and the size of the patient. The 3 mL hypodermic syringe is the most commonly used. In a medical office, syringes that hold 5 mL or more usually are used for **irrigation**—the process of flushing a wound, cavity, or medical instrument with water or other fluid to clean it.

Syringes have three main parts:

- the plunger
- the body or barrel
- the needle

The needle also has several parts. The illustration at right shows the different parts of a needle and syringe.

Needle lengths vary from 0.375 inch to 1.5 inch for standard injections. As

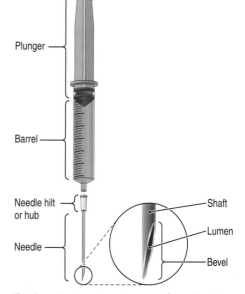

This illustration shows the various parts of a needle and syringe assembly.

you know from Chapter 4, the needle gauge refers to the needle gauge refers to the diameter of the needle lumen, or opening. Needle gauge varies from 10 (large) to 33 (small). Medical supply companies package hypodermic needles separately in color-coded packages or in color-coded envelopes with the syringe attached. The sizes are written on the package.

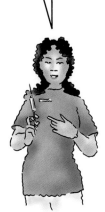

The syringe tip, inside of the barrel, shaft of the plunger, and the needle must be kept sterile!

Choosing a Needle. When choosing a needle, you need to select the right needle length and gauge for the route of the injection and the type of medication. The needle length depends on the route of the injection.

An adult **intramuscular injection,** or injection into muscle tissue, requires a needle length of 1 to 3 inches. Some factors that affect the choice of needle length are the size of the patient, the muscle being used, and the fat to muscle ratio. The gauge varies from 20 to 25, depending on the thickness of the medication to be administered. A small-gauge needle, such as 25 or 27, would make it difficult to draw thick medications into a syringe or inject them into a patient. Examples of thick medications are penicillin and hormones. A **subcutaneous injection** (injection into the fatty layer just below the skin) is usually given with a short, small-gauge needle, such as 25 gauge (0.625 inch) or 23 gauge (0.5 inch).

Types of Syringes. All hypodermic syringes are marked with calibrations showing milliliters and smaller divisions, depending on the size of the syringe. The other side of the syringe may be marked in minims (m), a very small fluid measure equaling about a drop.

Two special types of syringes used to administer medications are tuberculin syringes (1 mL) and insulin syringes.

- *Tuberculin (TB) syringes* are narrow and have a total capacity of 1 mL. Each syringe has 100 calibration lines. TB syringes are used for newborn and pediatric doses, for **intradermal** skin tests, and any time small amounts of medication are to be given.

- *Insulin syringes* are used only for administering insulin to diabetic patients. The insulin syringe has a

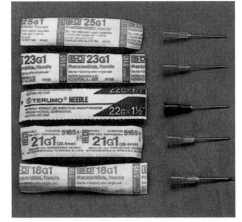

When considering needle gauges, remember, the higher the number, the thinner the needle.

total capacity of 1 mL but uses a different calibration system than other syringes. The 1-mL volume is marked as 100 units (U). The units represent the strength of the insulin per milliliter. Most of the insulin that is used today is U-100, which means that it has 100 units of insulin per milliliter. On the syringe, large lines mark each group of 10 units. Five smaller lines divide the 10 units into groups of 2. Each small line represents 2 units.

The prefix intra means into or within. Intradermal means "into the skin." Intramuscular means "into the muscle."

INTRA= into or within

Types of Injections

Different medications may be injected into different places in the body. The three main types of injections are:

- intradermal
- subcutaneous
- intramuscular

Intradermal Injections. These injections are administered into the dermis, or skin. The needle is inserted at angle of 10 to 15 degrees, almost parallel to the skin surface.

When administered correctly:

- the needle tip and lumen is slightly visible under the skin
- the bevel of needle must be up
- a small bubble known as a **wheal** is raised in the skin

Make sure the markings on the insulin syringe match the insulin being administered. For U-100 insulin, you need a 100 U syringe.

Closer Look   PREFILLED CARTRIDGES

Prefilled syringes contain a premeasured amount of medication in a disposable cartridge with a needle attached. The prefilled cartridge and needle are placed in a holder for administration. After a cartridge and holder are used, the cartridge should be discarded in a sharps biohazard container. The holder is reusable, but it must be cleaned first. This is often done by wiping it thoroughly with an alcohol swab. Some offices also have containers filled with alcohol into which the holder can be placed after use.

Recommended sites for intradermal injections are the anterior forearm and the back. You'll find exact steps for administering an intradermal injection in the Hands On procedure on page 321.

Intradermal injections are used to administer different kinds of skin tests for allergy testing and tuberculosis (TB) screening.

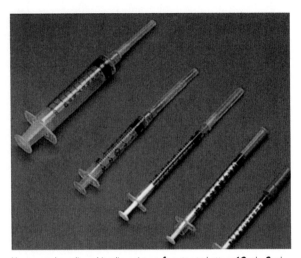

Here are tuberculin and insulin syringes; from top to bottom: 10 mL, 3 mL, tuberculin or 1 mL, insulin, and low-dose insulin.

TB TESTS

Two tests are used for the routine screening of TB—the tine test and the **Mantoux test.** Both use purified protein derivative (PPD) from a live tuberculin bacillus culture to test for tuberculin antibodies.

- *Tine test.* In the tine test, the applicator consists of small tines that contain PPD. After cleansing the forearm, press the applicator firmly into the intradermal layer of the skin. This test is not considered as useful for diagnostics as the Mantoux test. A positive tine test usually is followed by a Mantoux test.

- *Mantoux test.* An injection containing PPD is made into the intradermal layer of skin. A positive Mantoux test indicates only the possibility of exposure to TB. It does not indicate that the patient has TB. The CDC prefers the Mantoux test and considers it the most accurate TB test.

Both tests must be read within 48 to 72 hours. A positive Mantoux reaction has **induration** (a hard, raised area over the injection site) that is larger than 10 mm. A patient with a positive reaction will require a complete medical history and further testing, including a sputum culture and x-rays. Induration of less than 10 mm in a patient with no known risk factors is considered a negative result.

Subcutaneous Injections. Subcutaneous injections (SQ or SC) are given into the fatty layer of tissue below the skin. You should position the needle and syringe at a 45-degree angle. This method is chosen for drugs that may not be absorbed as rapidly through intramuscular or other routes. Common sites for subcutaneous injections include:

- upper arm
- thigh
- back
- abdomen

Check the Hands On procedure on page 324 for the exact steps in administering a subcutaneous injection.

Intramuscular Injections. To inject medication into muscles, you need to position the needle and syringe at a 90-degree angle to the skin. Absorption is fairly rapid because of the rich vascularity (blood supply) of muscle. If slower absorption is desired, the medication is mixed with an oil-based diluent rather than saline or water.

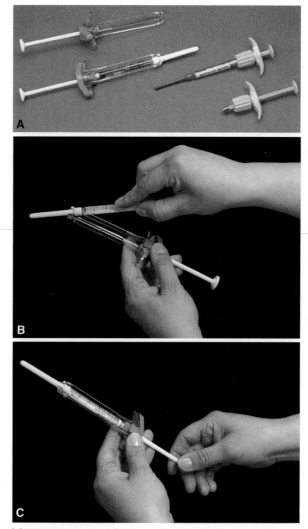

(A) This example shows prefilled medication cartridges and injector devices. (B) The prefilled cartridge is inserted into the injector device. (C) The medication is now ready for injection.

As previously noted, a one- to three-inch needle is needed to give an intramuscular (IM) injection to an adult. The length of the needle depends on the muscle chosen for the injection and the size of the patient.

The muscle chosen for the injection depends on the preferences of the medical assistant, the patient, and the amount of medication to be administered. Drug manufacturers also recommend sites for injecting specific drugs. You should try to follow their recommendations.

The table on pages 299–301 lists common injection sites and related precautions. The Hands On procedure on page 327 describes how to administer an IM injection.

Z-Track Method. In an IM injection, some medications may stain and discolor skin and irritate or damage tissues if they leak back along the line of injection. The Z-track method prevents leakage by sealing off layers of skin along the route of the needle.

In the Z-track method, the skin is pulled to one side, and the needle is inserted. After the solution is injected and the needle is withdrawn, the skin is allowed to return to its normal position. This blocks the solution from escaping from the muscle tissue.

Here are some precautions to keep in mind when using the Z-track method. If the medication is very caustic, the instructions may require that you change the needle after drawing up the solution. Follow the steps in the Hands On procedure on page 330 to learn how to use the Z-track method to administer an intramuscular injection.

THE INTRAVENOUS ROUTE

For the intravenous (IV) route, a sterile solution of a drug is injected through a

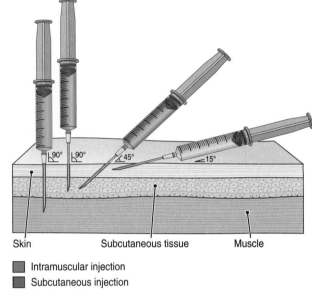

Skin   Subcutaneous tissue   Muscle

■ Intramuscular injection
■ Subcutaneous injection
☐ Intradermal injection

The angles of insertion are different depending on the kind of injection—intramuscular, subcutaneous, or intradermal.

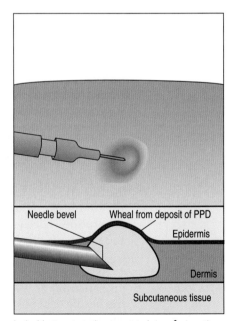

Needle bevel   Wheal from deposit of PPD

Epidermis

Dermis

Subcutaneous tissue

In the Mantoux test, the correct technique for inserting the needle involves depositing the PPD subcutaneously with the needle bevel facing upward.

Recommended Sites for Intramuscular Injections

Injection Site	Locating the Muscle	Cautions
Deltoid	The deltoid muscle is located by palpating the lower edge of the acromial process. At the midpoint, in line with the axilla on the lateral aspect of the upper arm, a triangle is formed. Medications are administered within the triangle.	No more than 1 mL should be injected into this muscle in an adult.

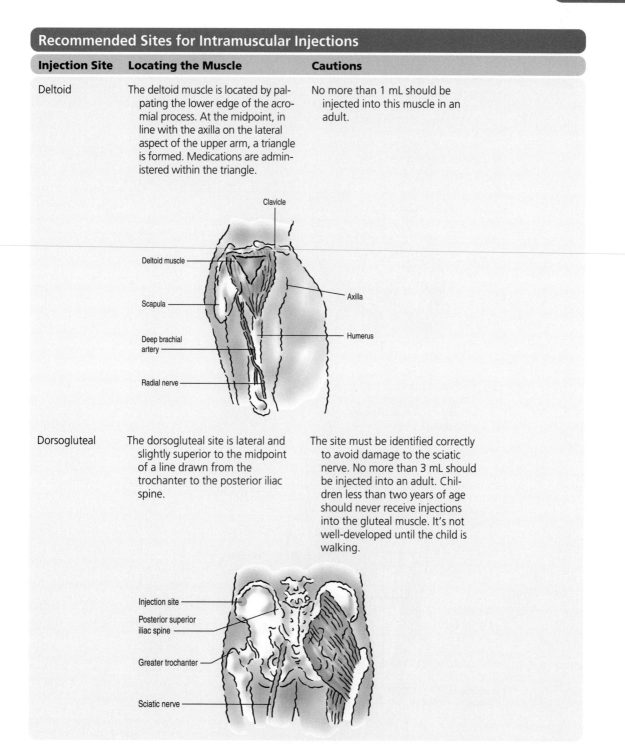

Dorsogluteal	The dorsogluteal site is lateral and slightly superior to the midpoint of a line drawn from the trochanter to the posterior iliac spine.	The site must be identified correctly to avoid damage to the sciatic nerve. No more than 3 mL should be injected into an adult. Children less than two years of age should never receive injections into the gluteal muscle. It's not well-developed until the child is walking.

(continued)

Recommended Sites for Intramuscular Injections (*continued*)

Injection Site	Locating the Muscle	Cautions
Ventrogluteal	The ventrogluteal site is located by placing the palm on the greater trochanter and the index finger toward the anterior superior iliac spine. The middle finger is then spread posteriorly away from the index finger as far as possible. A V or triangle is formed by this maneuver. Make the injection in the middle of the triangle.	No more than 3 mL should be injected into an adult.

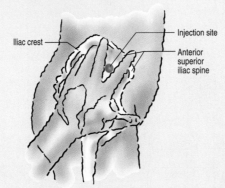

Iliac crest

Injection site

Anterior superior iliac spine

| Vastus lateralis | The vastus lateralis site is identified by dividing the thigh into thirds horizontally and vertically. The injection is given in the outer-most third. | No more than 3 mL should be injected into an adult. |

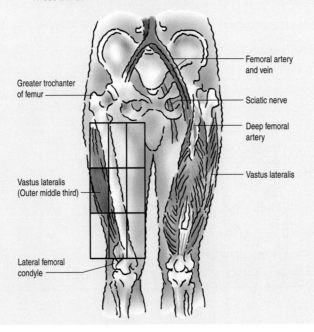

Femoral artery and vein

Greater trochanter of femur

Sciatic nerve

Deep femoral artery

Vastus lateralis (Outer middle third)

Vastus lateralis

Lateral femoral condyle

Recommended Sites for Intramuscular Injections (*continued*)

Injection Site	Locating the Muscle	Cautions
Rectus femoris	The rectus femoris site is located on the anterior of the thigh.	Use this site only when other sites are contraindicated.

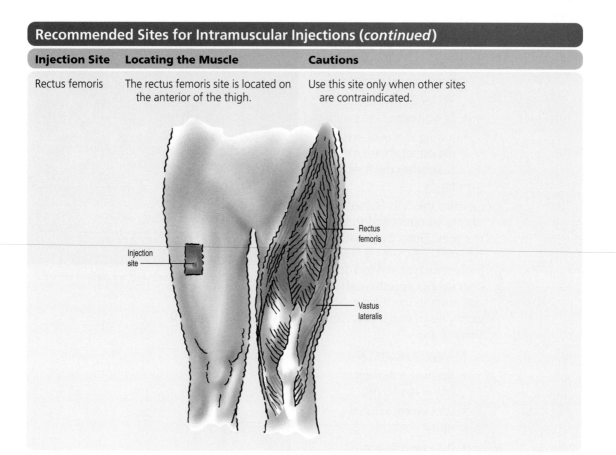

needle or **catheter** into a vein by **venipuncture**. A catheter is a thin, flexible tube that carries fluids into or out of the body. Venipuncture is the process of puncturing a vein with a needle.

Medication acts quickly when it's given by IV because it enters the bloodstream immediately. Only drugs intended for IV administration should be given using this route.

If the medication instructions recommend a specific site for injection, use that site.

Starting an IV

In most cases, the nurse administers IV medication. However, in some states, medical assistants in ambulatory care centers must set up equipment and fluids for an IV, perform the venipuncture, and regulate IV fluids as directed by a physician or nurse practitioner. You should not do this procedure unless you are registered with the state as state laws can prohibit medical assistants from administering IVs.

If you are permitted to start an IV, you need the following equipment:

- fluids, as determined by the physician
- IV catheter
- tubing that connects to the catheter with a valve to regulate the flow of fluids

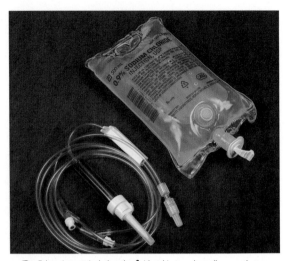

The IV equipment includes the fluid, tubing, and needle or catheter.

Once the IV is started, fluids are administered through the vein. These fluids either replace fluids lost by the patient or are used to administer medication through special ports in the tubing. Some examples of fluids that come prepackaged for use in IV therapy are:

- Ringer's lactate (RL)
- dextrose 5 percent and water (D_5W)
- 0.9 percent normal saline
- 0.45 percent normal saline
- combinations of the above (D_5NS, D_5RL)

The physician or nurse practitioner chooses the type and amount of fluid to be administered. An administration set (tubing) is used. The end of the tubing with the drip chamber is inserted into the IV fluid bag. The other end is inserted into the IV catheter after it's in the vein.

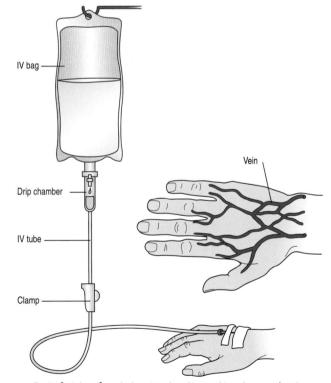

The IV fluid drips from the bag, into the tubing, and into the person's vein.

Setting the Rate

After securing the IV catheter and attaching the tubing, you need to adjust the flow of fluids. Adjust the roller clamp and watch the fluids drip into the drip chamber. Carefully count the drops per minute so you can adjust the flow of the fluid to the exact rate desired.

The amount of fluid to be administered is ordered by the physician or nurse practitioner in terms of milliliters per hour (e.g., 125 mL/hour). Here are the steps to follow in determining how fast to run the solution:

1. Determine the drop factor—the number of drops needed to deliver 1 mL of fluid. The drop factor should be listed on the tubing package. Macrodrop systems deliver 10 or 20 drops per milliliter. Microdrop systems deliver 60 drops per milliliter.

2. Check the physician or nurse practitioner order for the type of fluid (such as RL, D_5W), the amount (for example, 125 mL), and the time frame (usually per hour).

3. Use the following formula to calculate the number of drops per minute necessary to deliver the amount of fluid:

$$\text{drops per minute} = \text{volume in milliliters} \div \text{time in minutes} \times \text{drop factor (gtt/mL)}$$

4. Regulate the roller clamp so the correct number of drops flows into the drip chamber every minute.

CALCULATE DROPS PER MINUTE

Now you try. The physician order reads Ringer's lactate 100 mL/hour. The administration set delivers 10 gtt/mL (its drop factor). Using the formula, you can calculate the correct number of drops per minute.

$$\text{drops per minute} = 100 \text{ (milliliters)} \div 60 \text{ (minutes)} \times 10 \text{ (drop factor)} = 16.7$$

Decimals should be rounded up to the nearest tenth. So, the number of drops into the drip chamber should be 17 per minute. You need to regulate the roller clamp so 17 drops flow into the drip chamber every minute.

TKO and KVO Rates

Sometimes, the physician would like the patient to have an IV line, but not any specific fluids. The physician will order a to keep open (TKO) or a keep vein open (KVO) rate. Fluids flow at a slow rate, usually from 5 to 30 mL per hour, to keep the vein from clotting. The same formula is used to determine how many drops per minute it will take to achieve the KVO rate the physician orders (rate = volume ÷ time × drop factor).

For example, if the physician orders a KVO rate of 30 mL per hour and the administration set has a drop factor of 10 gtt/mL, here's how you'd figure the drop rate:

$$\text{drops per minute} = 30 \text{ (milliliters)} \div 60 \text{ (minutes)}$$
$$\times 10 \text{ (drop factor)} = 5$$

You would regulate the roller clamp so that 5 drops flow into the drip chamber every minute.

OTHER MEDICATION ROUTES

Besides orally, by injection, or intravenously, there are several more ways to administer medications to patients.

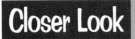 **Closer Look** **WATCHING FOR PROBLEMS WITH IVS**

You must watch the IV fluids and the site of venipuncture carefully. **Infiltration** occurs when IV fluid infuses into tissues surrounding the vein. This usually happens because the catheter has been displaced.

You usually can prevent this problem by carefully securing the IV catheter and IV tubing. If infiltration occurs, stop the flow of the fluids. Remove the catheter and notify the physician. Signs of infiltration are:

- swelling and pain at the IV site
- slow or absent flow rate into the drip chamber when the roller clamp is open
- no blood return or back up into the tubing when the fluid bag is placed below the level of the heart

If the physician or practitioner orders that the IV be reinserted, you must use the other arm or a site above the level of infiltration.

- by inhalation
- on or through the skin
- by instillation into the eyes, ears, and nose
- by insertion into the rectum or vagina

Inhalation

Some medications are administered through inspiration into the lungs. These medications are absorbed quickly through the alveolar walls into the capillaries. The alveolar walls are found in small sacs of tissue where air is exchanged in the lungs. The absorption rate for inhaled medications may be difficult to predict for patients with lung diseases.

Patients with chronic pulmonary disorders may self-administer medications. They use a handheld **nebulizer,** or inhaler. Both devices produce a spray of medicated mist that's inhaled directly into the lungs through the mouth or through the mouth and nose.

Most nasal medications are administered by sprays or nasal inhalers. Some nasal medications have a local effect, such as relieving nasal congestion or preventing allergy symptoms. Others have a systemic effect. For example, butorphanol (Stadol) is a nasal spray used to relieve moderate to severe pain.

Skin Medications

There are two general types of medications applied to the skin.

- **Topical medications** include creams, lotions, ointments, and sprays. They produce local effects.

- **Transdermal medications** typically are administered using a patch that's placed on the skin. They produce systemic effects. Medication administered transdermally is delivered to the body through absorption by the skin. Delivery is slow and a steady, stable level of medication is maintained in the body.

Never cut a transdermal patch—the rate of absorption of the medication would then be changed.

Transdermal patches may be placed in several locations:

- chest
- back
- upper arm
- behind the ear

The Hands On procedure on page 332 provides the exact steps for applying transdermal medications.

Eyes, Ears, and Nose

Some medications may be designed for administration through the eyes, ears, or nose. You may need to administer these medications in the office or instruct patients on how to administer them at home. A common method of administration for these medications is **instillation,** the administration of a liquid drop by drop.

- Ophthalmic medications are used to treat eye infections and to soothe eye irritation. They also may be used to dilate the pupils for diagnostic purposes. Eye medications usually are supplied as an ointment or a liquid and have a local effect. The label should state clearly that the medication is formulated for use in the eyes. You'll find exact steps for administering eye medications in the Hands On procedure on page 333.

- Otic medications, or ear medications, relieve ear pain and swelling, treat infections of the ear canal, or soften cerumen (ear wax). Ear medications typically come in the form of liquid drops and have a local effect. The Hands On procedure on page 335 provides steps for administering ear medications.

- Nasal medications can be administered by instillation. They usually are in the form of drops or sprays. Their most common use is to reduce swelling or drainage in nasal passages in patients suffering from colds or allergies. Some hormones also are administered nasally. Read the Hands On procedure on page 337 to learn how to instill nasal medications.

Suppositories have a cocoa butter or glycerin base that melts at body temperature. They need to be stored in the refrigerator.

Rectal Administration

Rectal medications are packaged in suppositories or liquid administered as an **enema**—a procedure where liquid is introduced into the bowel through a tube. Rectal medications can provide a local effect or be absorbed through the rectal mucosa for a systemic effect. Rectal medications may be used for patients who are NPO (allowed nothing by mouth) or who have nausea and vomiting. They are never used for patients who have diarrhea.

Rectal medications rarely are administered in the medical office. However, you may be asked to instruct patients on the proper technique for administering them at home. Both enemas and rectal suppositories should be retained by the patient for 20 to 30 minutes before elimination.

Vaginal Administration

Vaginal medications include creams, tablets, suppositories, and solutions for douches. Medications prescribed for the vaginal route typically have local effects. Examples include hormonal creams or antifungal preparations.

Instruct the patient to remain lying down for a while after the insertion of vaginal medications. For comfort, the patient may want to wear a light pad to absorb any drainage.

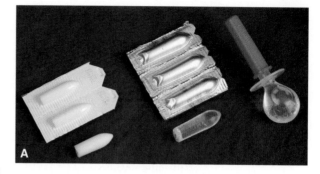

A

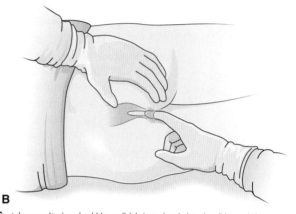

B

Rectal suppositories should be well-lubricated and placed well beyond the rectum's internal sphincter.

MEDICATION ERRORS

There are many steps for calculating, measuring, and administering medications. You need to perform each step carefully to avoid making errors that could harm your patients. Even so, all human beings occasionally make mistakes. If you notice that you've made a medication error, it's important that you report it to the physician as soon as possible.

Some medication errors might include:

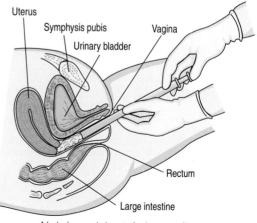

Uterus
Symphysis pubis
Urinary bladder
Vagina
Rectum
Large intestine

Vaginal cream is inserted using an applicator.

- giving the wrong medication to the patient
- giving a medication to the wrong patient
- giving the wrong amount of a medication

Medication errors and corrective actions must be documented in the patient's medical record. You'll also need to fill out an incident report to file in the office. The incident report verifies that all possible precautions were taken for the patient. It also can be reviewed to determine if steps can be taken to make sure similar errors don't happen in the future.

> After administering any medication, document it in the patient's medical record. Include the amount ordered by the physician and the route of administration.

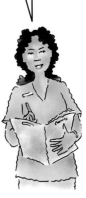

GETTING EVERYTHING RIGHT

You can avoid medication errors by preparing and administering medications carefully. By observing seven "rights" when giving any medication, you'll eliminate the possibility of many errors. Here's the "right" list to follow:

1. Right patient. Ask the patient to state her name. Some patients may answer to any name. So if you simply say the name, it won't ensure you have the right patient.

2. Right time. Medications ordered to be given in the office must be given before the patient leaves. Some patients may have to be told when the next dose is due.

3. Right dose. Check doses carefully. Many medications come in various strengths.

4. Right route. Medications are administered by a variety of routes. For example, is the proper route for a particular medication oral, intramuscular, or topical?

5. Right drug. Many medication names are very much alike. For instance, Orinase and Ornade may be confused if you're not careful. Always look up unfamiliar medications in a drug reference book such as the *Physician's Desk Reference* (PDR).

6. Right technique. Check how the medication needs to be given, such as orally with or without food. Intramuscular, subcutaneous, and intradermal injections should be given only after carefully choosing a site and using the right procedure.

7. Right documentation. The medical record is a legal document. Make sure the medication is documented *after* it's administered, not before. Check to be sure you're documenting it in the right medical record. All medications given in the medical office must be documented immediately with the name of the medication, dose, route, and site (if injected). Don't forget your signature. When appropriate, the patient's response should be charted as well.

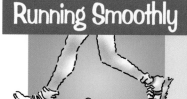

Running Smoothly

I MADE A MISTAKE!

You've been working hard all day. Suddenly, you realize you made an error in the medication you gave to a patient. What should you do?

Even if you're extremely careful, you may make an error when administering a medication. Don't try to hide the mistake or solve the problem on your own. Report the error to the physician right away! If you've given too much or given an incorrect medication, it might harm the patient.

If you report the error right away, immediate action can be taken to resolve the problem. For example, if you've given the wrong medication or the wrong amount, you may need to monitor the patient for adverse reactions. If the patient didn't receive the intended medication, you may need to administer it.

You'll need to document the error and all the actions taken to correct it in the patient's medical record. You also must complete an incident report. The report is kept on file in the medical office.

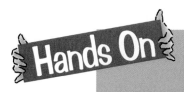

Hands On

ASSISTING WITH RECORD-KEEPING FOR CONTROLLED SUBSTANCES

5-1

1. Regularly check the inventory of the controlled substances kept in your medical office to ensure a minimal supply is in stock. Follow office policy and procedure. If supplies are running low, remind the physician and check to see if more should be reordered.

2. In most states, you may order Schedule II drugs from your regular supplier. Prepare DEA Form 222 to order Schedule II drugs. Be sure to include the physician's

(continued)

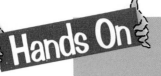

DEA registration number. The physician must sign the form.

- In some states, a copy of the purchase agreement (not the DEA form) must be sent to the state attorney general's office within 24 hours of placing the order.
- Drugs from Schedules III to V do not require DEA Form 222.

3. When you receive controlled substances, list them on the inventory form in the office. A copy of the purchasing invoice, shipping document, or packing slip must be kept on file as part of the purchasing record. Records for Schedule II drugs must be kept separate from other records.

4. When a Schedule II substance is dispensed to a patient, you must record it on a separate dispensing record *and* in the patient's medical record.
    - You must record the date, the patient's name and address, the drug, and the amount dispensed.
    - Dispensing records for drugs from Schedules III to V can just be kept in the patient's medical record.

5. When controlled substances are dropped on the floor or are spilled and cannot be given to the patient, you must record the loss on the inventory record. Have a witness verify what happened and sign the inventory document.

6. If you are asked to dispose of any outdated controlled substances, DEA Form 41 (Registrants Inventory of Drugs Surrendered) must be completed. The physician must sign the form. After the drugs have been destroyed, the physician will be issued a receipt. The receipt must be kept on file.

7. Every two years, the inventory of controlled substances must be checked. Check the inventory by counting the amount of each drug on hand. Compare the amount on hand to the amount of the drug ordered, and the amount dispensed to patients (and lost due to spills, etc.). Remember, controlled substances need to be stored in a locked cabinet.

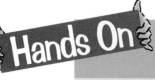

PREPARING PRESCRIPTIONS AS DIRECTED BY THE PHYSICIAN

5-2

1. Gather your supplies, including a prescription pad, the physician's written order, and the patient's medical chart. If the physician has given a verbal order, write it down. You need to be accurate in preparing the prescription.

2. If you're not familiar with the medication, look it up in a drug reference manual. You need to make sure you write the dose and other information correctly.

3. Ask the patient about any known allergies to the medication.

4. Be sure the physician's name, address, and telephone number are on the prescription form. Write the physician's DEA registration number (if not preprinted).

5. Write the patient's name, address, and date in the appropriate place on the form. The pharmacist needs this information to fill the prescription.

6. Just below or beside the superscription (Rx), write the name of the medication (inscription), the desired form (such as liquid, tablet, or capsule), and the strength—for example, *Tetracycline 250 mg*.

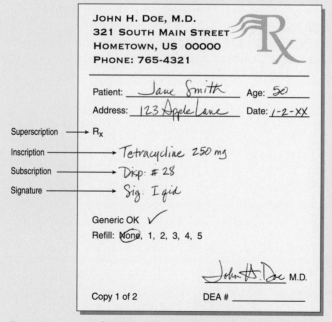

This sample prescription form shows where to write the essential information for a prescription.

(*continued*)

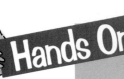

PREPARING PRESCRIPTIONS AS DIRECTED BY THE PHYSICIAN (*continued*)   5-2

7. On the next line (the subscription) write *Disp.* (dispense), along with the amount of the drug to be dispensed (for example, *#28* means 28 tablets).

8. The next line is the signature and should begin with *Sig.* This is where you write the instructions about how and when to take the medication.

9. If a generic substitute isn't acceptable, write *DAW* on the prescription or circle *No* on a preprinted form.

10. Indicate the number of refills (as directed by the physician) at the bottom of the prescription.

11. Once you've completed writing the prescription, take it to the physician to be signed. The physician must check and sign all prescriptions.

12. Put away the prescription pad in a locked cabinet or drawer. It shouldn't be accessible to patients.

13. Document the medication order on the patient's medical chart. Then, flag the order for the physician to sign.

Charting Example:
01/02/2007 10:00 A.M. Prescription for Tetracycline 250 mg, 4 x a day for 7 days as ordered by Dr. Doe._____ S. Campbell, CMA

Hands On

ADMINISTERING ORAL MEDICATIONS

5-3

This procedure should take five minutes.

1. Wash your hands and gather your supplies, including the physician's order, the correct oral medication, a disposable calibrated cup, a glass of water, and the patient's medical record.

2. Check the medication label and compare it to the physician's order. Note the expiration date. Remember to check the medication label three times—when taking it from the shelf, when measuring, and when returning it to the shelf.

3. If necessary, calculate the correct dose.

4. For a multidose container, remove the cap from the container. Touch only the outside of the lid to avoid contaminating the inside. Single, or unit dose, medications come individually wrapped. Packages may be opened by pushing the medication through the foil backing or by peeling back a tab on one corner.

5. According to your calculations and the label, remove the correct dose of medication.
   A. For solid medications:
      - Pour the correct dose into the bottle cap to prevent contamination.
      - Transfer the medication to a disposable cup.

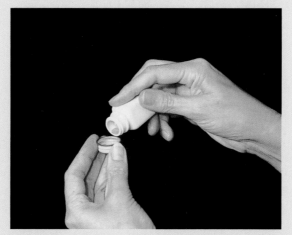

Pour the tablet into the bottle cap.

(continued)

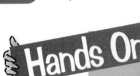

ADMINISTERING ORAL MEDICATIONS (*continued*)

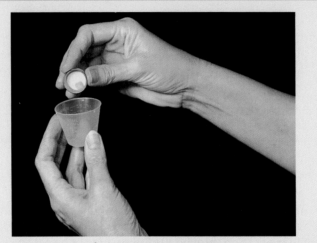

Transfer the medication to a disposable cup.

B. For liquid medications:
- Open the bottle and put the lid on a flat surface. The open end of the lid should face up to prevent contamination of the inside of the cap.
- Palm the label to prevent liquids from dripping onto the label. You don't want the label to become unreadable.
- With the opposite hand, place your thumbnail at the correct calibration on the cup. Holding the cup at eye level, pour the proper amount of medication into the cup. Use your thumbnail as a guide.

6. Greet and verify the patient's name to avoid errors. Explain the procedure. Ask the patient about any medication allergies that may not be noted on the chart.

7. Give the patient a glass of water to wash down the medication, unless contraindicated (as in the case of lozenges or cough syrup). Hand the patient the disposable cup containing the medication.

8. Remain with the patient to be sure all the medication is swallowed. Observe any unusual reactions and report them to the physician.

Hands On

ADMINISTERING ORAL MEDICATIONS (*continued*)

5-3

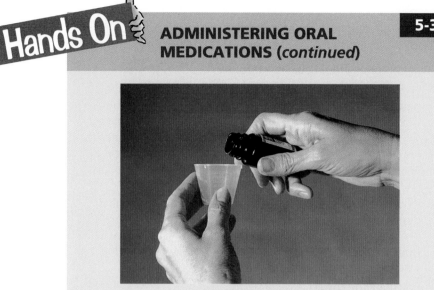

Palm the label of the container when pouring liquids.

9. Thank the patient and give any additional instructions as necessary.

10. Wash your hands and record the procedure in the patient's medical record.

Charting Example:

12/14/2007 8:45 A.M. Ampicillin 125 mg PO given to patient—NKA. _____T. Jones, CMA

Hands On PREPARING INJECTIONS 5-4

This procedure should take five minutes.

1. Wash your hands and gather your supplies, including the physician's order, medication for the injection in an ampule or vial, antiseptic wipes, a needle and syringe of appropriate size, a small gauze pad, a biohazard sharps container, and the patient's medical record. Choose the needle and syringe according to the route of administration, type of medication, and size of the patient.

2. Review the medication order and compare it to the label on the medication container. Check the expiration date. Remember to check the medication label three times—when taking it from the shelf, while drawing it up into the syringe, and when returning it to the shelf.

3. Calculate the correct dose, if necessary.

4. Open the needle and syringe package. Assemble if necessary. Make sure the needle is attached firmly to the syringe by grasping the needle at the hub and turning it clockwise on the syringe. A needle that isn't firmly attached may come off during the procedure.

5. Withdraw the correct amount of medication.
   A. From an ampule:
   - With the fingertips of one hand, tap the stem of the ampule lightly to remove any medication in or above the neck.
   - Wipe the neck of the ampule where the break will occur with an alcohol wipe. Wrap a piece of gauze around the neck to protect your fingers from broken glass. Snap the stem off the ampule with a quick downward movement of the gauze. Be sure to aim the break away from your face. Dispose of the ampule top in a biohazard sharps container.
   - After removing the needle guard, insert a filtered needle into the ampule. The needle lumen should be below the level of medication.
   - Withdraw the medication by pulling back on the plunger of the syringe. Take care not to touch the needle to the contaminated edge of the broken ampule. After you've withdrawn the correct amount, discard the ampule in the biohazard sharps container.

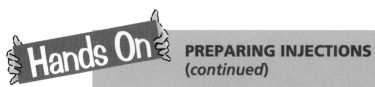

Hands On

PREPARING INJECTIONS (*continued*)

5-4

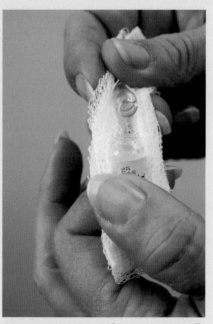

Grasp the gauze and ampule firmly when you snap off the top of the ampule.

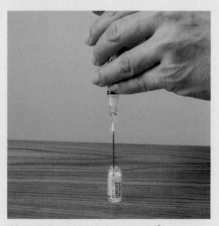

When withdrawing the medicine, be careful not to touch the edge of the broken ampule.

(*continued*)

Hands On

PREPARING INJECTIONS
(continued)

5-4

- Hold the syringe with the needle up. Remove any air bubbles by gently tapping the barrel of the syringe until the bubbles rise to the top. Draw back on the plunger to add a small amount of air. Then, gently push the plunger forward to eject the air from the syringe. Be careful not to eject any medication.

B. From a vial:
- Cleanse the stopper of the vial with an antiseptic wipe.
- Remove the needle guard. Pull back on the plunger to fill the syringe with a small amount of air equal to the amount of medication to be removed from the vial.
- Insert the needle into the vial through the center of the cleansed vial top. Inject the air from the syringe into the vial above the level of the medication so that you don't make bubbles or foam in the medication. Injecting air into the vial prevents a vacuum from forming in the vial, which would make it difficult to withdraw the medication.

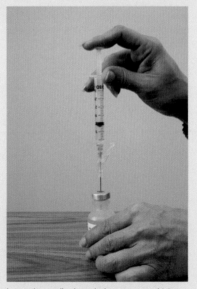

Insert the needle through the stopper and inject the air into the vial.

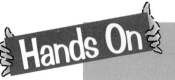

PREPARING INJECTIONS *(continued)*

5-4

- With the needle inside the vial, invert the vial, holding the syringe at eye level. Aspirate, or withdraw, the desired amount of medication into the syringe.
- Gently tap the barrel of the syringe with your fingertips to displace any air bubbles. Remove the air by pushing the plunger slowly and forcing the air into the vial.

6. Place the needle guard on a hard, flat surface. Without contaminating the needle, insert the needle into the cap and scoop up the cap with one hand. Recapping the needle protects the sterility of the needle until you administer the medication. You should use one hand to recap the needle to prevent needle sticks.

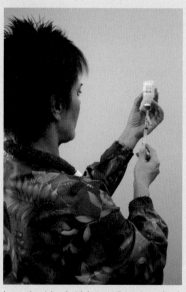

Invert the vial and withdraw medicine at eye level.

(continued)

Hands On

PREPARING INJECTIONS
(*continued*)

5-4

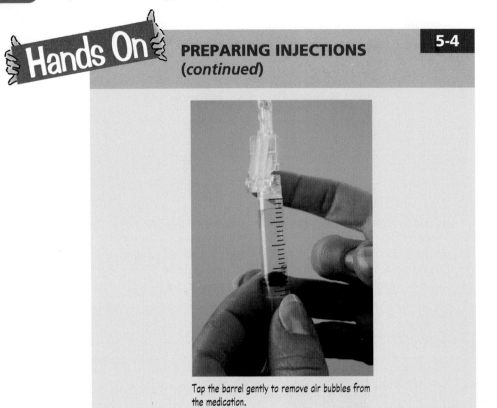

Tap the barrel gently to remove air bubbles from the medication.

Hands On

ADMINISTERING AN INTRADERMAL INJECTION

5-5

This procedure should take ten minutes.

1. Wash your hands and gather supplies, including the physician's order, medication for the injection in an ampule or vial, antiseptic wipes, a needle and syringe of appropriate size, a small gauze pad, a biohazard sharps container, clean examination gloves, and the patient's medical record. Choose the needle and syringe according to the route of administration and type of medication.

2. Review the physician's order and select the correct medication. Check the order carefully against the medication label. Make sure the expiration date hasn't passed. Remember to check the medication label three times—when taking it from the shelf, while drawing it up into the syringe, and when returning it to the shelf.

3. Prepare the injection according to the steps in the Hands On procedure on page 316.

4. Greet and identify the patient. Explain the procedure and ask the patient about any known medication allergies.

5. Select the appropriate site for the injection. Recommended sites are the anterior forearm and the middle of the back.

6. Prepare the site by cleansing with an antiseptic wipe. Use a circular motion, starting at the injection site and working toward the outside. The circular motion will carry microorganisms away from the site. Don't touch the site after cleansing.

7. Put on gloves. You must follow standard precautions for your protection.

8. Remove the needle guard. Using your nondominant hand, pull the patient's skin taut. Stretching the patient's skin allows the needle to enter with little resistance and secures the patient against movement.

9. With the bevel of the needle facing upward, insert the needle at a 10- to 15-degree angle into the upper layer of the skin. This angle ensures that penetration occurs within the dermal layer.
   - The bevel of the needle must be facing up for a wheal to form.

(continued)

Hands On

ADMINISTERING AN
INTRADERMAL INJECTION (*continued*)

- Stop inserting the needle when the bevel of the needle is under the skin. The needle should be slightly visible below the skin.

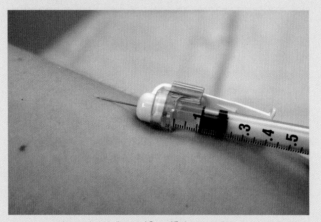

Insert the needle at a 10- to 15-degree angle.

10. Inject the medication slowly by depressing the plunger.
    - A wheal will form as the medication enters the dermal layer of the skin.
    - Hold the syringe steady! Moving the needle will be uncomfortable for the patient.

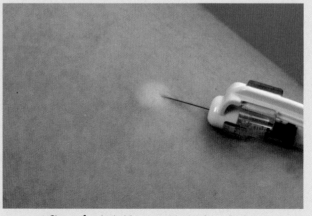

Observe for wheal while you are injecting the medication.

Hands On

ADMINISTERING AN INTRADERMAL INJECTION (*continued*)

11. Remove the needle from the skin at the angle of insertion.
    - Don't use an antiseptic wipe or gauze pad when withdrawing the needle.
    - Don't press or massage the site. Pressure on the wheal may press the medication into the tissues or out of the injection site.
    - Don't apply a bandage—it may cause redness or swelling that could result in an inaccurate reading of the test.

12. To reduce the risk of an accidental needle stick, don't recap the needle. Dispose of the needle and syringe in a biohazard sharps container.

13. Remove your gloves and wash your hands.

14. Depending upon the type of skin test administered, the length of time required for a reaction, and the policies of your medical office, perform one of the following:
    - Read the test results. Inspect and palpate the site for the presence and amount of induration.
    - Tell the patient when to return (date and time) to the office to have the results read.

15. Document the procedure, site, and results. Document any instructions to the patient.

Charting Example:
05/04/2007 10:35 A.M. Mantoux test, 0.1 mL PPD ID to (L) anterior forearm. Pt. given verbal and written instructions to return to office in 48–72 hours for reading the results— verbalized understanding. _____ P. King, CMA

Hands On

ADMINISTERING A SUBCUTANEOUS INJECTION

5-6

This procedure should take ten minutes.

1. Wash your hands and gather supplies, including the physician's order, medication for the injection in an ampule or vial, antiseptic wipes, a needle and syringe of appropriate size, a small gauze pad, a biohazard sharps container, clean examination gloves, an adhesive bandage, and the patient's medical record. Choose the needle and syringe according to the route of administration, type of medication, and size of the patient.

2. Review the medication order, select the correct medication, and compare it to the label on the medication container. Check the expiration date. Remember to check the medication label three times—when taking it from the shelf, while drawing it up into the syringe, and when returning it to the shelf.

3. Prepare the injection according to the steps in the Hands On procedure on page 316.

4. Greet and identify the patient. Explain the procedure and ask the patient about any known medication allergies.

5. Select the appropriate site for the injection. Recommended sites include the upper arm, thigh, back, and abdomen.

6. Prepare the site by cleansing with an antiseptic wipe. Use a circular motion starting at the intended injection site and working toward the outside. The circular motion will carry microorganisms away from the site. Don't touch the site after cleansing.

7. Put on gloves. You must follow standard precautions for your protection.

8. Remove the needle guard. Using your nondominant hand, hold the skin surrounding the injection site in a cushion fashion.

9. With a firm motion, insert the needle into the tissue at a 45-degree angle to the skin surface. Make sure the bevel of the needle is facing upward. Hold the barrel between the thumb and index finger of the dominant hand and insert the needle completely to the hub. A quick, firm motion is less painful to the patient.

Hands On

ADMINISTERING A SUBCUTANEOUS INJECTION (*continued*)

5-6

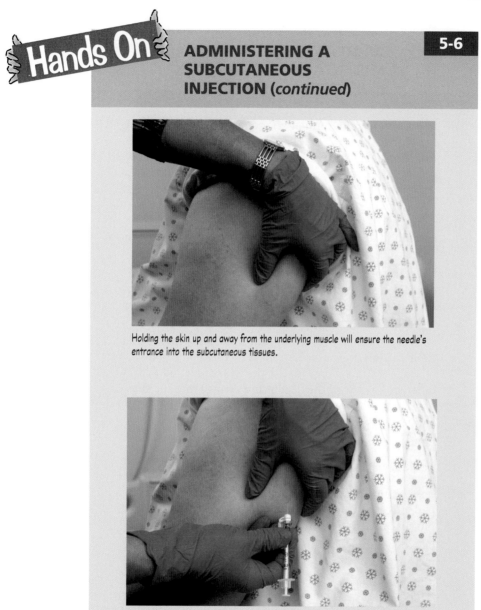

Holding the skin up and away from the underlying muscle will ensure the needle's entrance into the subcutaneous tissues.

Insert the needle at a 45-degree angle. Full insertion of the needle helps to make sure the medication goes into the proper tissue.

(continued)

Hands On

ADMINISTERING A SUBCUTANEOUS INJECTION (continued)

5-6

10. Remove your nondominant hand from the skin. Holding the syringe steady, pull the syringe (aspirate) gently.
    - If blood appears in the hub or the syringe, you've entered a blood vessel. If this happens, don't inject the medication. Injecting the medication into a blood vessel means that the medication may be absorbed too quickly. Remove the needle and prepare a new injection.
    - If blood doesn't appear, you may continue with the procedure.

11. Inject the medication by slowly pressing down on the plunger. If you press down on the plunger too quickly, the pressure will cause discomfort and possibly tissue damage to the patient.

12. Place a gauze pad over the injection site and remove the needle at the angle of insertion. With one hand, gently massage the injection site with the gauze pad and with the other hand, discard the needle and syringe into the sharps container. Don't recap the used needle. Apply an adhesive bandage, if needed.

13. Remove your gloves and wash your hands.

14. An injection for allergy desensitization means the patient must stay in the office for at least 30 minutes so you can observe any reaction the patient might have. Note: If a patient has any unusual reaction after any injection, let the physician know immediately.

15. Document the procedure, site, and results, as well as any instructions to the patient.

Charting Example:
03/04/2007 9:30 A.M. FBS 180. Regular insulin 5 units SQ (R) anterior thigh. _____ P. Collins, RMA

Hands On

ADMINISTERING AN INTRAMUSCULAR INJECTION

This procedure should take ten minutes.

1. Wash your hands and gather supplies, including the physician's order, medication for the injection in an ampule or vial, antiseptic wipes, a needle and syringe of appropriate size, a small gauze pad, a biohazard sharps container, clean examination gloves, an adhesive bandage, and the patient's medical record. Choose the needle and syringe according to the route of administration, type of medication, and size of the patient.

2. Review the medication order and select the correct medication. Check the order carefully against the medication label. Make sure the expiration date hasn't passed. Remember to check the medication label three times—when taking it from the shelf, while drawing it up into the syringe, and when returning it to the shelf.

3. Prepare the injection according to the steps in the Hands On procedure on page 316.

4. Greet and identify the patient. Explain the procedure and ask about any known medication allergies.

5. Select the appropriate site for the injection. Recommended sites include the deltoid, vastus lateralis, dorsogluteal, and ventrogluteal areas. Take into account the patient's age and size, as well as the medication, when choosing a site.

6. Prepare the site by cleansing with an antiseptic wipe. Use a circular motion starting at the injection site and working toward the outside. The circular motion will carry microorganisms away from the site. Don't touch the site after cleansing.

7. Put on gloves. You must follow standard precautions for your protection.

8. Remove the needle guard. Choose one of the following ways to hold the skin surrounding the injection site.
   - Using your nondominant hand, hold the skin surrounding the injection site taut with the thumb and index or middle fingers. This makes the needle easier to insert in an average or overweight individual.

(continued)

Hands On

ADMINISTERING AN INTRAMUSCULAR INJECTION (*continued*)

5-7

- Using your nondominant hand, grasp the muscle. This produces a deeper mass for the injection in a person who is very thin with little body fat.

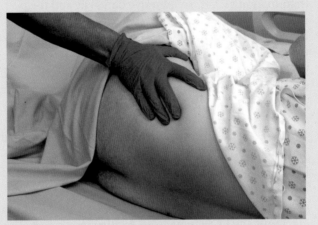

This shows the medical assistant holding the injection site taut with the fingers before administering an intramuscular injection.

9. Hold the syringe like a dart. Use a quick, firm motion to insert the needle into the tissue at a 90-degree angle to the surface. Hold the barrel between the thumb and index finger of your dominant hand and insert the needle completely to the hub. This way, the medication will go into the muscle tissue.

10. Remove your nondominant hand from the skin. Holding the syringe steady, pull back the syringe (aspirate).
    - If blood appears in the hub or the syringe, you've entered a blood vessel. Don't inject the medication! Injecting the medication into a blood vessel means the medication may be absorbed too quickly. Place a gauze pad over the injection site and remove the needle. Prepare a new injection.
    - If blood doesn't appear, you may continue with the procedure.

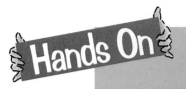

ADMINISTERING AN INTRAMUSCULAR INJECTION (*continued*)

5-7

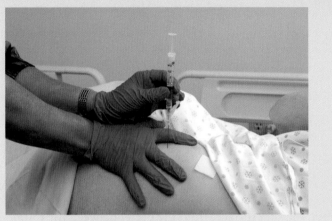

Insert the needle into the tissue at a 90-degree angle.

11. Inject the medication by slowly pressing down on the plunger. If you press down on the plunger too quickly, the pressure will cause discomfort and possibly tissue damage to the patient.

12. Place a gauze pad over the injection site. Remove the needle at the angle of insertion. With one hand, gently massage the injection site with the gauze pad. Massaging helps to distribute the medication. With your other hand, discard the needle and syringe into the biohazard sharps container. Don't recap the needle.

13. Apply an adhesive bandage to the site, if needed. Remove your gloves and wash your hands.

14. Observe the patient for any reactions. If the patient has any unusual reactions, let the physician know immediately.

15. Document the procedure, site, and results, as well as any instructions to the patient.

Charting Example:

07/06/2007 2:40 P.M. Solu-Medrol 20 mg IM (L) DG.

_____O. Campbell, CMA

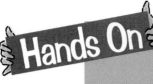

Hands On

ADMINISTERING AN INTRAMUSCULAR INJECTION USING THE Z-TRACK METHOD

5-8

This procedure should take ten minutes.

1. Follow steps 1–7 as described in the Hands On procedure *Administering an Intramuscular Injection* on page 327. Note: The ventrogluteal, vastus lateralis, and dorsogluteal sites work well for the Z-track method, but the deltoid does not.

2. Remove the needle guard. Rather than pulling the skin taut or grasping the muscle tissue, pull the top layer of skin to the side and hold it with the nondominant hand throughout the injection.

3. Hold the syringe like a dart and use a quick, firm motion to insert the needle into the tissue at a 90-degree angle to the skin surface. Hold the barrel between the thumb and index finger and insert the needle completely to the hub.

4. Aspirate by withdrawing the plunger slightly. If no blood appears, push the plunger in slowly and steadily. Count to 10 before withdrawing the needle. This allows time for the tissues to begin absorbing the medication.

5. Place a gauze pad over the injection site. Remove the needle at the same angle at which it was inserted while releasing the skin. Don't massage the area. Discard the needle and syringe into the biohazard sharps container.

6. Apply an adhesive bandage to the site, if needed. Remove your gloves and wash your hands.

7. Observe the patient for any unusual reactions. Note: If a patient has any unusual reaction after any injection, let the physician know immediately.

8. Document the procedure, site, and results, as well as any instructions to the patient.

Charting Example:
07/11/2007 3:30 P.M. Imferon 25 mg IM Z-track (R) DG.

_____ N. Edwards, CMA

Hands On

ADMINISTERING AN INTRAMUSCULAR INJECTION USING THE Z-TRACK METHOD (*continued*)

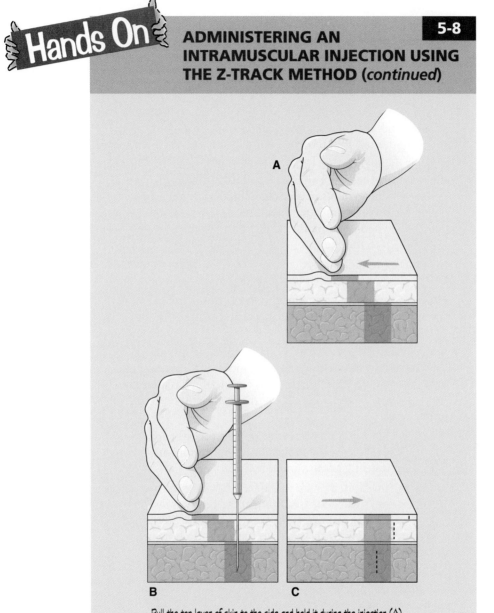

A

B

C

Pull the top layer of skin to the side and hold it during the injection (A). This way, when the needle is withdrawn (B) and the tissue returns to its normal position, the medication doesn't escape from the muscle tissue (C).

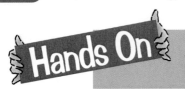

APPLYING TRANSDERMAL MEDICATIONS

5-9

This procedure should take five minutes.

1. Wash your hands and gather supplies, including the physician's order, the medication, clean examination gloves, and the patient's medical record.

2. Review the medication order and select the correct medication. Check the order carefully against the medication label. Make sure the expiration date hasn't passed. Remember to check the medication label three times—when taking it from the shelf, when opening the medication package, and when returning it to the shelf.

3. Greet and identify the patient. Explain the procedure and ask about any known medication allergies.

4. Select the appropriate site for the medication. The usual sites are the upper arm, the chest or back, and behind the ear. These sites should be rotated.

5. Perform any necessary skin preparation. Make sure the skin is clean, dry, and free from any irritation. Trim any hair close with scissors but don't shave areas with hair. Shaving may wear away the skin and cause the medication to be absorbed too quickly.

6. Open the medication package by pulling the two sides apart. Don't touch the area of medication. It may be absorbed into your skin, causing an unwanted reaction.

7. Apply the medicated patch to the patient's skin following the manufacturer's directions. Starting at the center, press the adhesive edges down firmly all the way around. Starting at the center eliminates air spaces. If the edges do not stick, fasten with tape.

8. Wash your hands and document the procedure, including the site of the patch.

Charting Example:
09/14/2007 8:30 A.M. Transdermal nitroglycerine 0.2 mg/hr patch to left anterior chest. _____ R. Evans, RMA

Hands On

INSTILLING EYE MEDICATIONS

5-10

1. Wash your hands and gather your supplies, including the physician's order, the correct medication, sterile gauze, tissues, and gloves. Check the medication label three times. The medication label must specify ophthalmic use. Medications formulated for other uses may be harmful to the eyes.

2. Greet the patient and verify the patient's name. Explain the procedure. Ask the patient about any allergies not recorded in the chart.

3. Position the patient comfortably in a lying or sitting position with the head tilted slightly back. The level of the affected eye should be slightly lower than the unaffected eye. This will keep the medication from running into the unaffected eye.

4. Put on gloves. You may come into contact with fluids from the patient's eye.

5. Using sterile gauze, pull down the lower eyelid to expose the conjunctival sac (the space between the membrane covering the eye and the membrane inside the eyelid). Ask the patient to look up. Looking away from the medication will reduce the blink reflex.

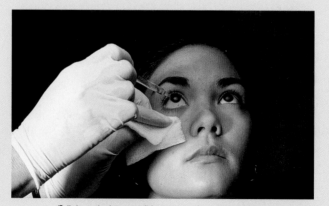

Pull down the lower eyelid to expose the conjunctival sac.

(*continued*)

Hands On

INSTILLING EYE MEDICATIONS (*continued*)

5-10

6. Check the medication label for a second time to be sure it's the right medication. Instill the medication.
   - *Ointment.* Discard the first bead of ointment from the container onto a tissue. It's considered contaminated. Do not touch the tissue because the tissue can contaminate the tip. Moving from the inner canthus (inner corner) outward, place a thin line of ointment across the inside of the eyelid. Placing the ointment in the sac avoids touching the eye with the tip of the ointment tube. Twist the tube slightly to release the ointment.
   - *Drops.* Hold the dropper about half an inch from the conjunctival sac, not touching the patient. Release the proper number of drops into the sac. Discard any medication left in the dropper to prevent contamination of the rest of the container.

7. Release the lower eyelid. Ask the patient to close the eye and gently roll it to disperse the medication.

8. Wipe off any excess medication with the tissue. Instruct the patient to apply light pressure to the puncta lacrimalis (the opening in the eyelid where tears drain) for several minutes. This prevents the medication from running into the nasolacrimal sac and duct (tear duct).

9. Properly care for and dispose of equipment and supplies. When disposing of or putting away the medication, check the label for a third time. Clean the work area and wash your hands.

10. Document the procedure.

Charting Example:
10/14/2007 8:45 A.M. Garamycin ophthalmological ointment applied to left eye. _____ B. Smith, CMA

Hands On

INSTILLING EAR MEDICATIONS

5-11

1. Wash your hands and gather your supplies, including the correct otic medication and cotton balls. Check the medication label to be sure it's the right medication three times. The label should specify otic preparation.

2. Greet the patient and verify the patient's name. Explain the procedure.

3. Ask the patient to sit with the affected ear tilted upward. This position helps the medication flow through the canal to the tympanic membrane.

4. Check the medication label again. Draw up the amount of medication ordered.

5. Straighten the ear canal.
   - *Adults.* Pull the auricle (outer ear) slightly up and back.
   - *Children.* Pull the auricle slightly down and back.

6. Insert the tip of the dropper without touching the patient's skin. This avoids contamination. Let the medication flow along the side of the ear canal. The medication should flow gently to avoid discomfort.

7. Ask the patient to sit or lie with the affected ear up for about five minutes after the instillation. The medication should rest against the tympanic membrane for as long as possible.

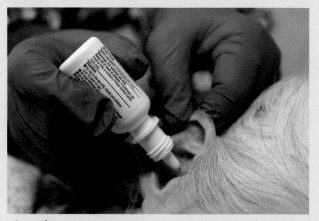

Be careful not to touch the patient's skin when inserting the tip of the dropper.

(continued)

Hands On

INSTILLING EAR MEDICATIONS (*continued*)

5-11

8. If the medication is to be retained in the ear canal, gently insert a moist cotton ball into the external auditory meatus (opening in the ear). The cotton ball keeps the medication in the canal. Because it is moist, it won't wick the medication out.

9. Properly care for and dispose of equipment and supplies. Check the medication label again. Clean the work area and wash your hands.

10. Document the procedure in the patient's chart.

Charting Example:

09/15/2007 12:30 P.M. Neosporin otic solution, 2 gtt instilled into left ear as ordered. _____ D. Barth, CMA

Hands On

INSTILLING NASAL MEDICATIONS

5-12

1. Wash your hands and gather your supplies, including gloves, the correct nasal medication, and tissues. Check the medication label three times to be sure it's the right one. It must be formulated for nasal instillation.

2. Greet the patient and verify the patient's name. Explain the procedure. Tell the patient that the procedure may be uncomfortable, but it shouldn't be painful. Ask about any allergies not recorded in the chart.

3. Position the patient in a comfortable, recumbent (lying down) position. Extend the patient's head beyond the edge of the examination table or place a pillow under the shoulders. Support the patient's neck to avoid strain as the head tilts back. Tilting the head back allows the medication to reach the upper nasal passages.

4. Put on gloves. Administer the medication.
   - *Drops.* Hold the dropper upright just above the nostril. Dispense one drop at a time without touching the patient. Keep the patient recumbent for five minutes to allow the medication to reach the upper nasal passages.
   - *Spray.* Place the tip of the bottle at the naris opening without touching the patient's skin or nasal tissues. Ask the patient to take a deep breath; spray as the patient is inhaling. If the patient breathes out while the medication is being sprayed, it won't reach the nasal passages.

5. For the patient's comfort, wipe away any excess medication from the skin with tissues.

6. Properly care for and dispose of equipment and supplies. Check the medication label as you do so. Clean the work area, remove your gloves, and wash your hands.

7. Record the procedure in the patient's chart.

Charting Example:
06/15/2007 12:00 P.M. Oxymetazoline hydrochloride 0.05% nasal spray, 2 sprays to each nostril as ordered per Dr. Greene.

_____ D. Pratt, CMA

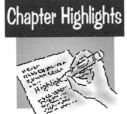

Chapter Highlights

- Medical assistants must be knowledgeable about different medications, their uses, side effects, and potential abuses. The medical assistant may need to administer medications under a physician's supervision and educate patients about using them correctly.

- Most over-the-counter and prescription medications have a chemical name, a generic name, and a trade name. Drugs are manufactured from natural sources and from synthetic materials.

- The Controlled Substances Act of 1970 regulates the manufacture and distribution of dangerous drugs. Physicians who prescribe or administer controlled substances must obtain a registration number from the U.S. Drug Enforcement Agency (DEA).

- Special documentation is required for controlled substances in the medical office. Careful records must be kept of drug purchases, prescriptions, and disposal. Separate dispensing records must be kept for all Schedule II drugs. Federal law requires that an inventory of controlled substances be taken every two years.

- Medical assistants sometimes prepare prescriptions for the physician's signature. They also may phone prescription orders to pharmacies or handle prescription requests from patients. The medical assistant may not sign off on refill requests and it must be seen and initialed by the physician unless there are written standing orders.

- Patients should receive written and verbal instructions regarding their medications. Patients should be encouraged to call the medical office if they have any questions.

- A medication may have a local effect or a systemic effect. The body's reaction depends on the route of administration, the absorption rate, drug metabolism, and excretion. Factors influencing drug effects are age, weight, sex, existing illnesses, and degree of tolerance.

- Drug interactions can occur with other prescribed drugs, over-the-counter medications, herbal supplements, alcohol, and food. In some cases, interactions can produce unwanted effects.

- To calculate dosages, medical assistants may need to convert between different systems of measurement. The most commonly used systems of measurement are the metric system and the household system. The household system is only used by patients at home.

- The ratio method and the formula method can be used to calculate medication dosages for adults. Several formulas are used to calculate children's dosages.

- Medication administration can be divided into two main groups—enteral and parenteral. Enteral routes include medication taken by mouth and medication administered rectally. Parenteral routes include any route other than the enteral ones—for example, injections, intravenous administration, and vaginal application.

- Strict aseptic technique must be followed when administering medication by injection. The three main types of injections are intradermal, subcutaneous, and intramuscular.

- The medical assistant must select the right needle length and gauge for the injection type. Different types of injections have different injection sites and different angles of insertion.

- Intravenous medications are injected through a catheter into the patient's bloodstream. In some cases, medical assistants must set up equipment and fluids for IV and regulate IV fluids. They need to watch for infiltration of the IV fluid into the tissues surrounding the vein.

- Some medications are inhaled using an inhaler or nebulizer. Others are absorbed by the skin through a transdermal patch. Many eye, ear, and nasal medications are instilled drop by drop to produce a local effect.

- Rectal medications are packaged in the form of suppositories or enemas. They are rarely administered in the medical office. They may have local or systemic effects. Vaginal medications usually have local effects.

- Steps for preparing and administering medications must be performed carefully to avoid making errors. Checking the seven "rights" is a good way to reduce the possibility of errors. Any medication errors should be reported to the physician immediately and documented in the patient's chart.

Chapter 6

DIAGNOSTIC TESTING

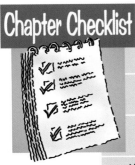

Chapter Checklist

- Explain the difference between radiolucent and radiopaque, using examples

- List ways to protect patients and yourself from radiation hazards

- Describe how to prepare patients for routine x-ray examinations

- List the general steps in a routine radiographic examination

- Discuss how to teach patients about contrast examinations

- Compare and contrast fluoroscopy, MRI, and CT scans

- List three typical uses for sonography

- Describe the medical assistant's role in radiographic procedures

- Explain how to handle and store radiographic film

- Contrast invasive and noninvasive techniques for cardiological diagnosis

- Describe the placement of electrocardiogram electrodes

- Perform electrocardiography

- Identify the main wave forms used for interpretation on an electrocardiogram tracing

- Discuss three types of electrocardiogram artifacts and how to prevent them

- Describe how to apply a Holter monitor

- Define tidal volume and forced expiration

- Perform respiratory testing

- Briefly describe bronchoscopy and arterial blood gas tests

- Explain how to teach a patient to use a peak flowmeter

- Screen and follow up test results

Sometimes, a physician orders specific medical tests to help diagnose a patient's illness. As a medical assistant, it's likely that you'll have to assist with or help educate patients about several different types of diagnostic tests, such as:

- **radiology,** which is a medical specialty that uses different imaging techniques to diagnose and treat diseases

- cardiovascular tests, which are used to diagnose disorders of the heart

- respiratory tests, which are used in the diagnosis and treatment of respiratory conditions

You also may be responsible for screening and following up test results after the procedures have been performed.

Radiology and the Medical Assistant

Among the most common diagnostic tests are those that create a visual image of internal body structures. Because of changing technology, new procedures are continually being developed to help visualize body structures. Physicians who specialize in interpreting these images are called **radiologists.**

Probably the most common radiology technique is the radiograph. **Radiographs** are shadow-like images of internal structures. They're digital or processed on a type of film similar to photography film. The images are created using **x-rays**—invisible, high-energy waves that can penetrate dense objects. The process of making these films is called **radiography.**

The process of radiography and the radiographs themselves are commonly referred to as x-rays. Usually, a patient will ask, "Am I getting an x-ray?" instead of "Am I getting a radiograph?" Medical staff also often refer to *x-rays* instead of *radiographs.* However, it's important to know the technical terms too.

Although you may not perform radiological diagnostic procedures, you have an important role in preparing and educating the patient. Your responsibilities may include:

- preparing patients for radiology procedures
- performing basic x-ray procedures in the medical office
- assisting in educating patients about general radiology processes
- scheduling the procedures

The medical community is making an effort to have as much treatment as possible done on an outpatient basis. Some medical offices have on-site x-ray equipment. Outpatient diagnostic imaging centers also have been created to offer a variety of radiology services. Some companies even specialize in providing basic x-ray services to patients in long-term care facilities or in patients' homes.

> X-rays can't be seen, heard, felt, tasted, or smelled. Patients can hear noises coming from the tube area during an exposure, but it's the equipment that makes these noises–not the x-rays.

X-RAYS AND X-RAY MACHINES

X-rays are produced by electricity of extremely high voltage inside an x-ray tube. The x-rays exit the tube in one direction as a beam and pass though a device designed to control the beam's size. During an x-ray, a beam of light also shines on the patient. This light is not part of the x-ray beam. It's a guide to help the x-ray technician direct and position the x-ray beam.

Many modern x-ray machines are designed to work with computers to produce digital images of the body. Most permanently installed radiography units include a special table. Some tables can be electronically rotated from the horizontal to the vertical to help position the patient.

Before x-ray film is used, it's placed in a special holder called a **cassette** to protect it from light. The cassette slides

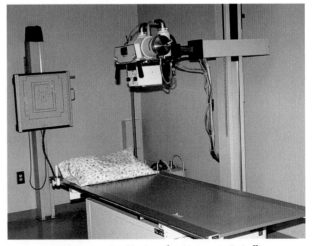

This radiography unit is like those found in many medical offices.

into a slot or opening in the table. Once the film inside the cassette has been exposed to x-rays, the cassette is placed in a special machine that removes the film and processes it. The processed film is the radiograph, or x-ray.

X-RAYS AND THE BODY

Images form as the x-rays either pass through the body and strike the film or are absorbed by body tissues.

- **Radiolucent** substances allow x-rays to pass through them. These structures are not dense, and don't absorb much radiation. They show up as black on the film. An example is the air in the lungs.

- **Radiopaque** substances don't allow x-rays to pass through them. Some tissue is dense and absorbs much of the radiation beam instead. Such tissue appears white on x-ray film. For example, bone is a radiopaque tissue that absorbs radiation. It shows up as white on an x-ray.

- Other body substances vary in density. Examples are muscle, fat, and fluid. They appear as different shades of gray on a radiograph, because of the way each substance absorbs the x-rays.

Patient Positions

A radiograph is a two-dimensional image. However, the human body is a three-dimensional structure. For this reason, x-ray exams usually require at least two exposures taken at 90-degree angles to each other. For example, a chest x-ray generally involves one exposure from the back and another from the side.

Other exams may require three or more x-rays from different angles. The **projection** refers to the body's position in relation to the x-ray beam and the film. Each projection

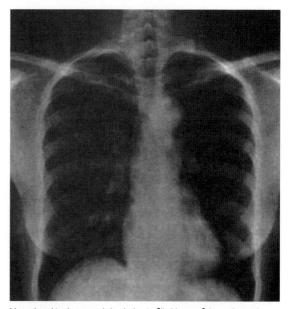

Note the white bones and the dark, air-filled lungs of this radiograph, or x-ray, of a patient's chest.

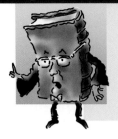

Legal Brief   TAKING X-RAYS

In some states, a medical assistant is allowed to take and process simple images such as chest x-rays or x-rays of bones. The training required to do this varies. In other states, only licensed radiographers may take and process x-rays. You should be familiar with your state's laws and comply with any regulations.

requires the patient to be placed in a specific position. The table on page 345 shows the patient positions for standard projections used in x-ray exams. But first, here are some terms you should be familiar with when positioning patients for x-rays:

- erect—standing
- recumbent—lying down
- supine—lying on the back
- prone—lying face down
- anterior—on the front
- posterior—on the back
- lateral—on the side

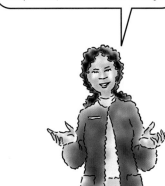

Chest x-rays can help in the diagnosis of pulmonary problems, such as pneumonia, lung cancer, emphysema, tuberculosis, and pulmonary edema, or fluid in the lungs.

Radiation Safety for Patients

Exposure to x-rays can damage the body's cells and genes. The harmful effects are most extreme for cells that reproduce quickly. The results of this damage may not show up for several years, however.

Pregnant women, children, and the reproductive organs of adults are at the highest risk from x-rays. It's important to follow these safety procedures to protect patients.

- Minimize the amount of exposure.
- Avoid unnecessary x-rays.
- Limit the area of the body that's exposed to radiation.
- Shield sensitive body parts, such as the gonads (organs that produce reproductive cells) and the thyroid (a gland in the neck that regulates the body's metabolism).

Standard Projections Used in X-Ray Exams

Projection (medical abbreviation)	Body Position	Illustration (Arrows show the direction of motion of the x-rays.)
Anteroposterior projection (AP)	Patient is erect or supine, with back to the film.	
Posteroanterior projection (PA)	Patient is erect, facing the film.	
Right lateral projection (RL)	Patient is erect, with right side of body nearest to the film.	
Left lateral projection (LL)	Patient is erect, with left side of body nearest to the film.	

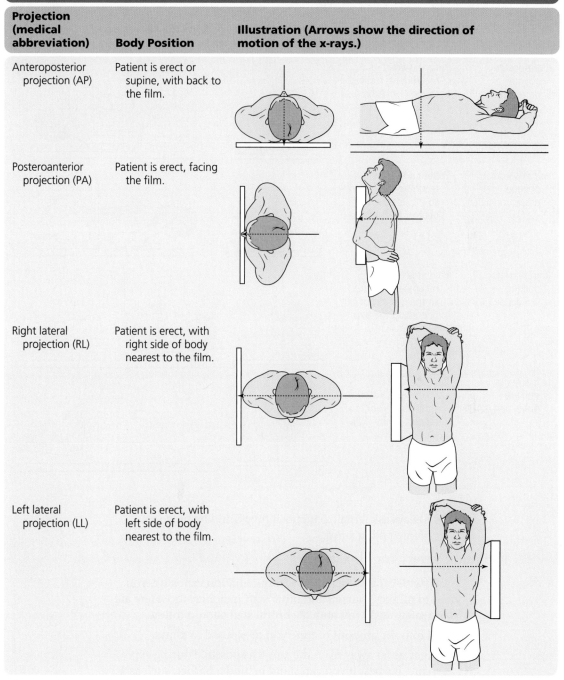

(continued)

Standard Projections Used in X-Ray Exams (*continued*)

Projection (medical abbreviation)	Body Position	Illustration (Arrows show the direction of motion of the x-rays.)
Right posterior oblique projection (RPO)	Patient is erect or recumbent, rotated so the right back is nearest to the film.	
Left posterior oblique projection (LPO)	Patient is erect or recumbent, rotated so the left back is nearest to the film.	
Right anterior oblique projection (RAO)	Patient is erect or recumbent, rotated so the right front is nearest to the film.	
Left anterior oblique projection (LAO)	Patient is erect or recumbent, rotated so the left front is nearest to the film.	

- Always ask female patients if they could be pregnant before taking x-rays.

Radiation Safety for Clinical Staff

Along with protecting patients from radiation exposure, you need to protect yourself and other staff members too. Here are some safety steps you and all clinical staff should follow.

- Limit the amount of time you're exposed to x-rays.
- Stay as far away from the x-rays as possible during exposure. It's best if you can stand behind a barrier, such as a wall lined with lead.

Ask the Professional — CALMING FEARS ABOUT X-RAYS

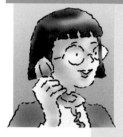

Q: *I have a patient who is concerned about the exposure to radiation from having x-rays taken. What can I tell her to put her mind at ease?*

A: Patients may be worried about the effects of radiation. You can reassure them by letting them know the amount of radiation involved is very small and the body's exposure will be limited. Remind these patients that they will benefit from the procedure because it provides the physician valuable information for diagnosis and treatment.

- Shield yourself using appropriate protective equipment, such as lead aprons and gloves.
- Avoid holding patients during exposures. If necessary, young children may be assisted by a parent wearing a lead apron.
- Wear a **dosimeter.** This is a small device you should clip to the outside of your uniform. It records the amount of radiation to which you're exposed. Your employer should supply dosimeters. They're obtained from companies that specifically monitor radiation exposure for health care workers.
- Ensure x-ray equipment is working properly by scheduling routine maintenance.

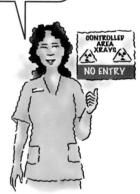

The dangers of radiation have been known for a long time. Pay attention to the warnings posted in the office!

CONTROLLED AREA XRAYS
NO ENTRY

RADIOLOGY AND DIAGNOSIS

The most common diagnostic procedures in radiology are routine x-ray exams. They require little patient preparation, although you may need to explain them and answer patients' questions to reduce anxiety. Here are the preparation procedures that must be followed:

- Typically, patients must remove outer clothing from the area to be x-rayed. A gown should be provided if necessary.
- No metal objects can be worn on any area of the body that will be exposed to x-rays.
- Patients must remove jewelry and clothing with zippers, snaps, or other metal details, including underwire bras.

The table on page 349 describes the preparation needed for routine x-rays of the different body regions.

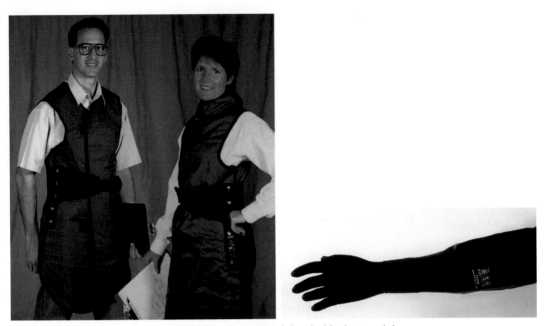

Proper protection when taking x-rays includes a lead-lined apron and gloves.

After patient preparations are finished, the patient is assisted into the proper position for the specific examination. In some cases, the patient may be standing near an upright film holder. In other cases, the patient will be positioned on the x-ray examination table.

After all the x-rays have been taken, the patient may be asked to wait until they're processed. This usually takes less than ten minutes. If the processed x-ray films aren't clear, repeat exposures may be needed. If the x-rays are digital images, there is usually no need for the patient to wait because the images can be checked immediately.

Stay safe by remembering the ALARA principle: Do whatever is necessary to keep radiation exposure As Low As Reasonably Achievable.

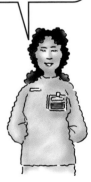

ROUTINE TEST EXAM

Here are the general steps involved in a routine x-ray exam.

1. The film cassette is placed into the table or upright holder. A lead marker may be included to indicate which side of the patient (right or left) is being examined.

2. The patient is placed into the exact position for the specific radiograph.

3. The x-ray tube is moved to a specific distance from the film and body part.

4. Lead shields are positioned to protect the patient from radiation.

5. In the control booth, the radiographer sets the machine for the specific exposure.

6. Final instructions are given to the patient. Patients need to remain perfectly still during the exposure. The patient must hold his breath during certain x-ray positions. Remind the patient that he can breathe again once the x-ray has been taken.

7. The exposure is made.

8. If a different view is needed, a new film is placed in the film holder and the steps are repeated.

Contrast Medium Examinations

Internal organs, like those within the abdomen, don't show up very well on x-ray films. Many structures within the abdomen have similar absorption rates for radiation. In addition, some organs lie behind others in the abdominal cavity. These factors can make it difficult to see the different structures clearly in a two-dimensional x-ray.

In these cases, a **contrast medium** often is used to help differentiate between body structures. A contrast medium is a substance that temporarily changes the absorption rate of a particular structure to highlight a specific organ.

Patient Preparation for Routine X-ray Exams

Region	Areas to Which Preparation Applies	Patient Preparation
Trunk	Chest, ribs, sternum, shoulder, scapula, clavicle, abdomen, hip, pelvis, as well as the sternoclavicular, acromioclavicular, and sacroiliac joints	Disrobing of the area and removing jewelry or clothing that might obscure parts of interest
Extremities	Fingers, thumb, hand, wrist, forearm, elbow, humerus, toes, foot, os calcis, ankle, lower leg, knee, patella, femur	Removing jewelry or clothing that might obscure parts of interest
Spine	Cervical, thoracic, or lumbar spine; sacrum, coccyx	Disrobing of the appropriate area
Head	Skull, sinuses, nasal bones, facial bones and orbits, optic foramen, mandible, temporomandibular joints, mastoid and petrous portion, zygomatic arch	Removing eyewear, false eyes, false teeth, earrings, hairpins, hairpieces

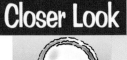

Closer Look MAMMOGRAPHY

Mammography, or x-ray examination of the breast, is used as a screening tool for breast cancer. Each breast is compressed in a special device to even the thickness and allow the best diagnostic image. Using the mammogram as a guide, the physician can do a needle biopsy to withdraw small amounts of cells from suspicious areas for study under a microscope. Mammography thus makes it possible to detect breast cancer in a minimally invasive way.

The American Cancer Society has developed specific guidelines for mammography. By age 40, women should have a screening mammogram. Women who have no symptoms (such as palpable breast masses or masses shown on previous mammograms) should have mammograms on the following schedule:

- for ages 40 to 49, routine screening every 1 to 2 years

- for ages 50 and over, routine screening every year

Contrast media are introduced into the body in several ways. Here are some common ones:

- by mouth

- intravenously

- through a catheter

The method used depends on the type of medium and the area of the body being examined. For example, a patient having an excretory urography will have the contrast medium injected. The anatomical structure of each kidney is evaluated as the medium passes through the urinary tract. The use of the contrast medium allows examination of each structure and its function.

Barium Studies. A patient with gastrointestinal (GI) symptoms may undergo **barium studies** to assist the physician in diagnosis. These are x-ray exams performed after parts of the

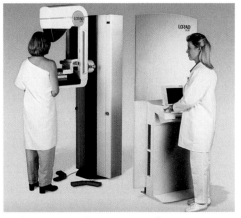

This patient is in the proper position for a mammogram.

patient's GI tract have been highlighted by a contrast medium called barium sulfate. The two most common barium studies are the upper GI examination and the barium enema.

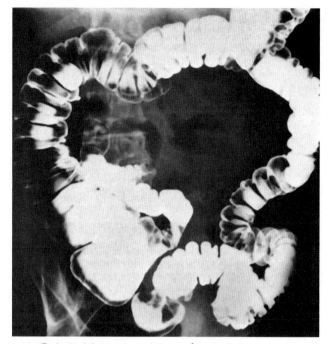

The barium helps to enhance this x-ray of a patient's digestive tract.

- In an upper GI exam, the patient drinks the contrast medium. Then a series of x-rays follows the barium down the patient's esophagus, into the stomach, and into the small intestine. The barium enables the radiologist to examine the x-rays for abnormalities in each organ.

- In a barium enema, the contrast medium is injected through the rectum into the patient's large intestine, or colon. This highlights the organ when the patient's lower abdomen is x-rayed.

Barium studies are becoming less common than in the past. They have been replaced by a technology called endoscopy. Physicians now use scopes to see, biopsy, and even take pictures inside the esophagus, stomach, and large intestine.

CONTRAST MEDIUM: IODINE

Other radiographic examinations require different contrast media. Iodine compounds are used in many areas of the body, including the kidneys and blood vessels. They're also used for some CT scans. (You'll read about computed tomography, or CT, shortly.)

Patients who have an intestinal perforation may be given an iodinated contrast medium instead of barium. That's because barium would be more troublesome to the patient if it leaked into the peritoneum (the lining of the abdominal cavity).

Scheduling X-Rays and Contrast Examinations. Most radiography procedures can be performed in any order, depending on what's convenient. However, some procedures must follow specific sequences. Here are some examples.

> Some patients are allergic to contrast media that contain iodine. Always ask if they have an iodine allergy or if they're allergic to shellfish, which also contain iodine.

- A patient with gallbladder symptoms may go through a series of tests. They begin with a simple, noninvasive oral cholecystogram. This is an x-ray of the gallbladder after the patient drinks a contrast medium. More complex procedures are performed later, such as an operative cholangiogram—an x-ray of the bile ducts after a contrast medium is injected during a surgical procedure.

- If an endoscopic study of the upper gastrointestinal tract is ordered in addition to barium studies, the endoscopy is usually scheduled before any procedure involving barium. That way, the barium will not obstruct or interfere with the visualization of internal structures.

- If an upper GI and a barium enema are ordered, the upper GI is usually scheduled first. But if results are needed quickly, the order is reversed. That's because barium from the small intestine will leave the body through the colon— and the second test can't be done as long as barium from the first test is in the organ to be examined.

Other Diagnostic Procedures

Along with routine x-rays and contrast exams, several other procedures are used to visualize body structures for the purpose of diagnosis. These procedures include:

- fluoroscopy
- computed tomography
- sonography
- magnetic resonance imaging
- nuclear medicine

Fluoroscopy. Fluoroscopy uses a continuous beam of x-rays to observe movement within the body. The image is in "real time" and is displayed on a monitor so the body part and its functioning can be seen in detail. The process may be highlighted by a contrast medium—for example, barium moving through the digestive system. Iodine compounds injected into the blood-

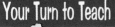

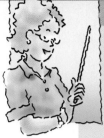

PREPARING PATIENTS FOR CONTRAST EXAMINATIONS

Although most contrast exams are performed outside the medical office, you'll need to tell patients how to prepare for the procedure. You'll also need to tell the patient the time and place where the test has been scheduled. You should make sure patients have both verbal and written instructions on the appointment and preparations.

Patient preparation for a contrast exam of abdominal organs may involve:

- a liquid diet only for the evening meal on the day before the examination

- laxatives the day before the exam to help clean the intestinal tract

- nothing by mouth (NPO) after midnight on the day of the examination. This usually also applies to gum chewing and smoking, because both increase gastric secretions. That could interfere with how the contrast medium coats the walls of the intestine.

- not taking any prescription medicines until after the contrast exam has been completed as prescribed by the physician

Emphasize that patients must follow instructions exactly. Use straightforward language and be sensitive to patient concerns.

Patients are often concerned about contrast exams. You can play a key role in lowering their anxiety. Explaining the importance of the procedure and proper preparation for it is one of the biggest contributions you make to a patient's care in this area.

stream allow the beating of the heart or blood flow through specific blood vessels to be examined.

Fluoroscopy also is used as an aid in treatment. Some ways it can help are in:

- reducing (setting) fractures

- implanting devices such as pacemakers

- inserting feeding tubes and other tubes into a patient's body

Computed Tomography. Computed tomography (CT) is a procedure that feeds x-rays from a tube circling the patient into a computer. All structures in each x-ray are blurred out except those desired. The computer analyzes these x-rays to create a series of cross-sectional "slices" of an organ or the body. Some CT machines can create three-dimensional images, so organs can be viewed from all angles.

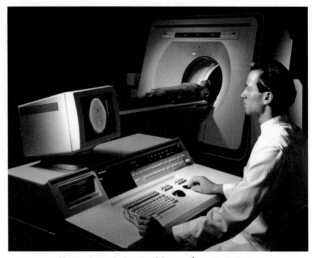

Here a doctor looks at a CT scan of a patient's brain.

CT scans may be done with or without a contrast medium.

Sonography. Sonography, or **ultrasound,** uses high frequency sound waves, instead of x-rays, to create images of the body, usually with the help of a computer. These images may be still or real-time, moving images. Sonography is often used to study heart function, abdominal structures, and pelvic structures. It's also commonly used in prenatal testing to visualize the developing fetus. Many obstetricians schedule at least one sonogram before the fourth month of pregnancy.

Magnetic Resonance Imaging. In **magnetic resonance imaging (MRI),** a combination of high-intensity magnetic fields, radio waves, and computer analysis is used to create cross-section images of the body. Like ultrasound, MRI doesn't use x-rays. The image depends on the chemical makeup of the body. MRI is used commonly for studying the central nervous system, joint structures, and a variety of other studies. Some MRI studies require contrast media.

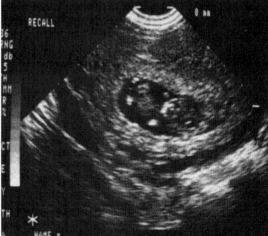

This ultrasound image shows a fetus nine weeks after the patient's last monthly period.

During the MRI, the patient is enclosed for a long period of time in a machine that makes knocking and whirring noises. Some facilities use open MRI, which does not make a patient feel as claustrophobic as a closed MRI.

> Patients with a fear of enclosed places may require a mild sedative before a closed MRI.

Nuclear Medicine. In **nuclear medicine,** the body is injected with small amounts of **radionuclides,** materials that emit radiation. The radionuclides are designed to concentrate in specific areas of the body for short periods of time. Special computer cameras detect the radiation and create an image. This method often is used to examine the thyroid, brain, lungs, liver, spleen, kidney, bone, and breast. These examinations are commonly called scans.

PET scans and SPECT scans are two sophisticated types of nuclear medicine studies.

- *Positron emission tomography* (PET) uses specialized equipment to produce detailed sectional images of physiological processes in the body.
- *Single photon emission computed tomography* (SPECT) produces sectional images of the body as detectors move around the patient.

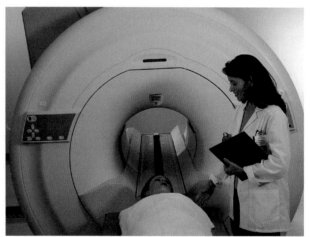

Here's a patient going for an MRI.

Both procedures are useful in the early detection of physiological and cellular abnormalities, such as those associated with cancer.

RADIOLOGY AND TREATMENT

Radiological techniques are used to treat cancer and other conditions. Here are some examples of how radiology helps in treating some specific conditions. For many patients, these tech-

Closer Look TELERADIOLOGY

Teleradiology is the electronic transmission of radiological images, such as x-rays and CTs, from one location to another. Many institutions use a picture archiving and communication system (PACS) in which computers store and transmit images. Images can be transmitted using standard telephone lines, satellite connections, or local area networks (LANs).

Teleradiology has led to improved patient care. Physicians working on difficult cases can send images and information to specialists in other locations. This allows them to obtain expert opinions in a short period of time. For example, rural physicians may use teleradiology to send images taken in their office to a radiologist in a distant location for interpretation and consultation.

niques are so effective, there's no need for surgery. In some cases, they may be lifesaving.

- *Percutaneous transluminal coronary angioplasty* (PTCA) is also known as balloon angioplasty. In this technique, the lumen of a coronary artery is enlarged using a balloon-tipped catheter. Guided by fluoroscopy, the catheter is placed at the point of partial occlusion (blockage) or stenosis (narrowing) of the artery. The balloon is then inflated, compressing the plaque against the sides of the artery. After the balloon is deflated, the catheter is removed. The diameter of the artery remains larger, improving blood flow.

- *Laser angioplasty* uses laser beams to remove deposits in vessels with the aid of fluoroscopy.

- *Vascular stents* are plastic or wire tubes inserted into a constricted or narrowed area of a blood vessel. The stent provides support and keeps the vessel open. Fluoroscopy is used to guide the placement of the stent.

- *Embolization* is a technique for artificially stopping active bleeding from a blood vessel. It also may be used to reduce blood flow to a diseased area or organ.

Radiation Therapy

For many years, radiation therapy has been a major force in the fight against cancer. In radiation therapy, high-energy radiation is used to destroy cancer cells. Because the radiation is so intense, it also may destroy adjacent normal cells. Treatments must be planned carefully and precisely by a radiologist, taking into account:

- the amount of radiation
- the frequency to be used
- the number of exposures during a given period of time

The area of the body to be exposed to radiation must be defined exactly so each treatment is identical. The patient is placed in a position described in the treatment plan, and an exact amount of radiation is directed at the treatment site by a technician. Usually, the patient has little to do but lie still.

The technician may make a small mark on the body to indicate exactly where the radiation should be directed. This helps the technician make sure that the radiation is put in the same spot every time.

Side Effects of Radiation

Most patients have some side effects from radiation therapy. These may include:

- hair loss
- weight loss
- loss of appetite
- skin changes
- digestive system disturbances

Once the treatment plan is completed, most of the side effects disappear.

THE MEDICAL ASSISTANT'S ROLE

As a clinical medical assistant, you're in an ideal position to help reduce patient anxiety over radiology procedures. You can do this by:

- giving patients information about procedures they don't understand
- making patients feel comfortable enough to ask questions
- answering questions using terms patients can understand

You also may have responsibilities that directly involve you with the procedures. These responsibilities may include:

- assisting with examinations
- handling, processing, and storing film

- scheduling appointments
- providing patient education

Educating Patients

Being sensitive to patients' feelings is one of the greatest talents you can possess. It should be an important part of every medical professional's training and personality.

Patients often must undergo procedures they don't understand. The technical aspects of radiology can make understanding its procedures especially difficult. Sometimes, patients feel they don't know enough even to ask the right questions.

Explaining what to do after the procedure is important and can save the patient distress. For example, a barium enema can lead to constipation if a patient does not drink enough fluids after the test.

As a medical assistant, you can affect patients' emotional response to a radiology procedure by explaining what to expect. Use everyday language, not technical medical terms. Keep your explanations simple, and leave the details to the physician. Here are some important topics you should cover:

- what preparations are needed for the procedure
- what to expect during the procedure
- what to do after the procedure

ASSISTING WITH RADIOLOGICAL PROCEDURES

There are several ways you may be required to assist with radiological examinations:

- telling the patient what clothing to remove or assisting with clothing removal as needed
- helping the patient take the position for the procedure. Emphasize the importance of remaining still and following instructions for breathing.
- performing specific procedures, such as bone or chest radiography, as permitted by your state's laws and your education and training
- placing film in an automatic processor and reloading new film into the cassette
- distributing or filing radiographs and reports appropriately

Handling and Storing Film

Automated processing machines are used to develop most x-ray film. This helps eliminate human error and simplifies the process. Processing machines usually can produce a developed image in less than two minutes.

Processors differ, according to their manufacturers. You need to be proficient in the operation of your facility's equipment.

No matter how your office develops x-ray film, here are some general tips for handling and storing it.

- Protect unexposed film from moisture, heat, and light by storing it in a cool, dry place. A lead-lined box is the best storage device.

- Open exposed or unexposed film packets in a darkroom, using only the darkroom light for illumination. The film must be placed in a cassette before using it in any areas outside the darkroom. Intensifying screens in the cassette are used to reduce the amount of exposure required.

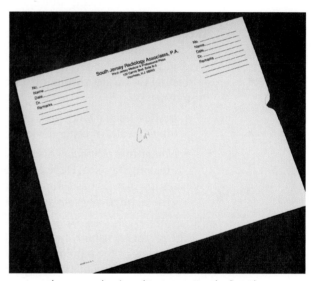

- Store exposed film in special sleeves or envelopes of the right size. Be sure the film has been labeled with the date and the patient's name.

An x-ray envelope is used to store processed radiographs.

Transfer of Study Information

Any radiographic images obtained on site for use by the physician become part of the patient's medical record. Digital images can be saved on a computer diskette or compact disc (CD).

However, in many cases, a physician sends a patient to another office for x-rays or other diagnostic tests. Radiological films belong to the site where the study was performed. The physician or radiologist who examines the films generally writes a summary of the examination. This report is sent to the referring physician. You may need to obtain the patient's permission to have the summary of findings sent to the office physician.

For a short-term referral, the physician who examines the films usually returns the films to the referring physician. Patients who need copies of their reports, often because they changed physicians, may request the information after submitting a written request. The patient also may obtain copies of the actual x-rays. You may be responsible for filling these requests.

Diagnosing Cardiovascular Disorders

Cardiovascular disease is a major cause of illness and death. A **cardiologist** is a physician who specializes in disorders of the heart. Many patients with chronic cardiac conditions are referred to the cardiology office for treatment and follow-up. However, some of these patients are seen in family practice medical offices. You need to understand the common tests and procedures that are ordered for the diagnosis and treatment of cardiac patients.

Testing for cardiovascular disorders may be either invasive or noninvasive.

- *Invasive techniques* require entering the body by using a tube, needle, or other device.

- *Noninvasive techniques* don't involve entering the body or breaking the skin. Depending on the patient's symptoms, testing may be basic and can be done easily during the general physical examination by auscultating the heart and chest.

The physician usually begins the cardiovascular examination with a review of the patient's history and the reason for the visit. She reviews the patient's vital signs and medications, noting any allergies to medications and other substances. The physician also inspects the patient to evaluate:

- the general appearance
- the circulation and any swelling of extremities
- the color of the skin
- any distention of the jugular vein (a large vein on each side of the neck that drains blood to the heart)

Palpation is used to evaluate the efficiency of the circulatory pathways and peripheral pulses. Using a stethoscope, the physician auscultates the sounds made as blood flows through the heart and the valves open and close. This allows the physician to detect abnormal heart sounds such as bruits or **murmurs** (abnormal sounds made as blood moves through the heart valves).

COMMON CARDIOVASCULAR TESTS

After an initial exam, the physician may order additional tests that can be performed in the medical office, including chest radiography and electrocardiogram (ECG). Their results may reveal a need for further testing using more sophisticated procedures.

Some of these tests may take place outside the medical office. For example, invasive procedures are performed at an outpatient surgical center or hospital. The table below shows common invasive and noninvasive cardiovascular tests.

Common Cardiovascular Tests

Cardiac Test	Description	Uses
Chest radiography (noninvasive)	Diagnostic tool using high-energy waves	Detect and follow cardiovascular or other diseases
Electrocardiogram (ECG) (noninvasive)	Graph of electrical activity of the heart from various angles	Obtain a baseline or assess an acute situation
Holter monitor (noninvasive)	Continuous monitor of heart rhythm via portable device worn for an extended period during daily activities	Detect symptoms of rhythm disturbances not shown on ECG or during physical examination
Stress test (noninvasive)	ECG of heart rhythm during exercise on graded treadmill or stationary bicycle	Help diagnose patients with known or suspected heart problems
Echocardiogram (non-invasive)	Ultrasound of heart using sound waves generated by a transducer	Diagnose suspected or known valvular disease, severity of heart failure, or cardiomyopathy (weakness of heart muscle)
Cardiac catheterization (invasive)	Insertion of a catheter into the heart	Diagnose or determine severity of heart disease or atherosclerosis
Coronary arteriography (invasive)	Injection of contrast medium into coronary arteries (after cardiac catheterization) to see, via a monitor, any obstruction of arteries	Assess heart disease and damage after myocardial infarction (MI, death of the heart muscle)

THE ELECTROCARDIOGRAM

One of the most valuable diagnostic tools for evaluating the heart is the electrocardiogram (ECG or EKG). All muscle movements produce electrical impulses. The ECG picks up the electrical signals made by the heart muscle and records them on a graph. This test is often part of a routine physical exam. It's also performed as needed for a patient with chest discomfort or other signs and symptoms of possible cardiac problems.

ECGs help the physician in diagnosing:

- ischemia (insufficient blood flow)
- delays in impulse conduction
- hypertrophy of the cardiac chambers
- arrhythmias (irregular heartbeats)

The table below summarizes the kinds of arrhythmias ECGs can detect. ECGs are not used to detect disorders in the heart's anatomy, such as those that may produce heart murmurs.

Arrhythmias

Type of Arrhythmia	Indications and Symptoms	Possible Causes and Consequences
Sinus tachycardia	Abnormally rapid heartbeat (100–180 bpm) resulting in decreased ventricular filling and low blood pressure	Dehydration, extreme anxiety, heart failure, or hemorrhage; can also result from intense exercise
Sinus bradycardia	Abnormally slow heartbeat (less than 60 bpm), but with a normal rhythm	Can result from myocardial infarction or certain medications (such as digoxin); is also often seen in well-conditioned athletes
Paroxysmal atrial tachycardia (PAT)	Sudden, temporary onset of a heartbeat of 180–250 bpm; often accompanied by patient weakness and the feeling of a pounding or fluttering in the chest	Extreme anxiety or stress, excessive stimulants (such as nicotine or caffeine); also can have no known cause
Premature atrial contraction (PAC)	An electrical impulse starts in the heart before the next expected beat; patient may complain of feeling an "extra" or "skipped" beat	Thyroid disease, heart disease, central nervous system imbalances, stress, or excessive use of stimulants
Premature ventricular contraction (PVC)	Ventricles contract before the next expected beat; patient may complain of feeling an "extra" or "skipped" beat; can be more serious than PAC	Electrolyte imbalances, caffeine or other stimulants, anxiety or stress; may also be a sign of pulmonary disease or an injured or diseased heart
Ventricular tachycardia (V tach)	Heart rate exceeds 100 bpm with 3 or more PVCs per minute; results in decreased cardiac output; patient may complain of pressure and the feeling that the heart is "beating out of my chest"	Similar to causes of PVCS; the longer V tach lasts, the more serious it is because cardiac output drops and the blood supply to organs is decreased; unchecked V tach can lead to V fib
Ventricular fibrillation (V fib)	Ventricles begin twitching, making the heart's pumping action ineffective and stopping the circulation of blood	The most serious of all arrhythmias; death will result if not immediately treated with CPR, a defibrillator, or cardiac drugs

During the ECG, you may be responsible for explaining the procedure to the patient. The patient will lie on her back on the examining table, with her arms, chest, and lower legs exposed. (While patients are waiting, and after the electrodes are placed, you may want to offer female patients a drape to cover the chest area.)

You'll also apply electrodes to the patient's arms, legs, and chest. These electrodes measure the electrical impulses of the heart. There are ten electrodes. Combinations of these electrodes measure the heart's electrical activity in 12 different ways, called **leads.** The ECG machine converts the electrical impulses from each lead into markings on special graph paper.

The ECG tracing is printed on graph paper that is either red or black with a white coating that is sensitive to heat. Graph lines are printed over the white coating and appear as small blocks. Thicker lines outline every five small blocks. On standard ECG paper, each small block is 1 mm square. The large blocks are 5 mm long on each side.

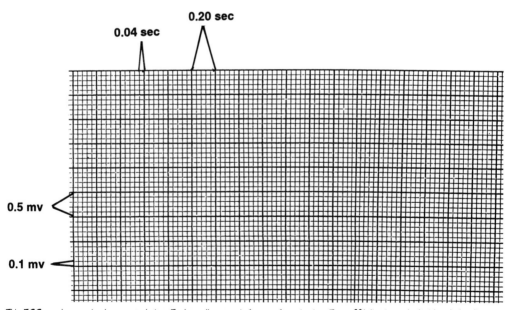

This ECG graph paper is shown actual size. Each small square is 1 mm × 1 mm in size. Every fifth line is marked with a darker line to make a cube of 5 mm × 5 mm.

Some ECG machines contain a stylus that heats and melts the white coating. This exposes the background beneath to record the movement of the stylus as electrical impulses are detected. In newer ECG machines, the stylus uses ink to mark the ECG paper.

Each small horizontal line on the paper represents 0.04 seconds of time. (One large block therefore represents 0.2 seconds and five large blocks measure one second of time.) Each small vertical line represents 0.1 millivolts of electricity. After the heart's electrical activity is traced on the paper, the physician can read the graph to determine the patient's heart rate and the time required for the electrical impulses to spread through the heart.

> ECG paper can be affected by moisture and heat. Handle it carefully to prevent markings that are not related to the test.

Placing the Electrodes

A standard system of electrode placement records the electrical activity of the heart. Each lead records the heart's electrical activity from a different angle. The recordings these leads make on the graph paper give the physician a fairly complete "view" of the entire heart.

Wires from the ECG machine attach to the ten electrodes. Four wires are labeled and color-coded for attachment to electrodes on the limbs. Six electrodes are placed on the anterior chest wall.

- One limb electrode is placed on each arm and leg. You should use muscular areas such as the calves, outer thighs, and the arm above the elbow. The electrodes should not be placed on bony areas. The right leg electrode is the grounding lead. It helps reduce electrical interference and keeps the average voltage for the patient the same as that of the machine. The other limb wires are attached to electrodes on the patient's left leg, right arm, and left arm.

- The chest electrodes must be placed in exact locations for an accurate ECG recording. The diagram on page 365 shows the locations of the chest leads.

> The placement of the limb electrodes may need to be adjusted for patients with amputations, surgery to an extremity, or trauma to the arms and legs.

You'll find the detailed steps for performing the ECG procedure in the Hands On procedure on page 381. The skin to which electrodes are applied must be clean and dry. Body oils, lotions, and sweat must be removed with an alcohol wipe. Body hair generally can be separated by hand to make sure the electrodes make good contact with the skin. However, patients who are extremely hairy may need to have areas on which electrodes are placed shaved or trimmed. Electrodes also cannot be placed on open wounds, bandages, or skin that has recently healed. In such cases, place the electrode as close to the proper site as possible and inform the physician when this occurs.

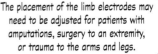

What Electrocardiogram Leads Measure

Different combinations of the electrodes provide 12 different leads to show the electrical activity of the heart. There are three main types of leads:

- *Standard bipolar leads.* These leads measure electrical activity picked up from two limb electrodes. The standard bipolar leads allow a frontal view of the heart's electrical activity from side to side. Roman numerals are used to describe these leads which are known as Leads I, II, and III.

The chest electrodes must be placed in very specific locations for the ECG recording to be accurate.

- *Augmented unipolar leads.* These leads result from a combination of the impulses measured from all three limb electrodes—RA, LA, and LL. (Remember that RL is the ground lead.) They allow visualization of the heart from a frontal view, top to bottom. They're called Leads aVR, aVL, and aVF.

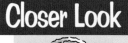

Closer Look SPEAKING ELECTROCARDIOGRAM

Like many other diagnostic tests, there's a special vocabulary associated with the ECG. It's important for you to become familiar with the common abbreviations used in performing ECGs.

- RA—right arm electrode
- LA—left arm electrode
- LL—left leg electrode
- RL—right leg electrode
- V_1–V_6—chest electrodes and leads (each number stands for a different position on the chest)
- aVR—augmented voltage right arm
- aVL—augmented voltage left arm
- aVF—augmented voltage left leg

- *Unipolar precordial leads.* These leads measure electrical impulses picked up from the chest electrodes. Each lead measures the electrical activity from a specific part of the heart. The chest leads are referred to using numbers from 1 to 6—for example, V_1, V_2, and so on.

The table below provides information about each lead and what it measures.

Lead Types and What They Measure

Lead Type	Lead	What's Measured
Standard bipolar leads	Lead I	Electrical activity between LA and RA
	Lead II	Electrical activity between LL and RA
	Lead III	Electrical activity between LL and LA
Augmented unipolar leads	aVR	The electrical activity from LA + LL directed to RA
	aVL	The electrical activity from RA + LL directed to LA
	aVF	The electrical activity from RA + LA directed to LL
Unipolar precordial leads (chest leads)	V_1	The electrical activity from electrode V_1
	V_2	The electrical activity from electrode V_2
	V_3	The electrical activity from electrode V_3
	V_4	The electrical activity from electrode V_4
	V_5	The electrical activity from electrode V_5
	V_6	The electrical activity from electrode V_6

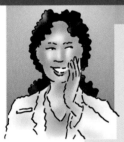

Secrets for Success

ELECTROCARDIOGRAM HOOK-UP HELP FOR CHEST LEADS

If the chest ECG electrodes are not attached in the right places, the ECG leads may not provide an accurate tracing of the heart's electrical activity. The more you practice, the easier it will be to remember where to place the leads. But while you are learning, it might be helpful to take notes to review before working with a patient. Write the abbreviations for the chest leads on the left side of a 3×5 index card. Next to each one, write the location on the body.

V_1 fourth intercostal space at right margin of sternum

V_2 fourth intercostal space at left margin of sternum

V_3 midway between V_2 and V_4

V_4 fifth intercostal space at junction of left midclavicular line

V_5 horizontal level of V_4 at left anterior axillary line

V_6 horizontal level of V_4 and V_5 at midaxillary line

Interpreting the Electrocardiogram

It's not your responsibility to give patients ECG results. But you should still know how to interpret an ECG.

During the ECG procedure, the graph of electrical activity from each lead is printed on the ECG paper. The paper speed on the machine is set at 25 mm per second. This allows the electrical impulses, recorded as waves on the ECG paper, to be measured. The blocks on the paper are used as a reference (each small block is 0.04 seconds). Each lead is marked clearly on the ECG paper as it is printed. In some cases, specific codes are printed on the paper to identify the wave from each lead.

The table below shows the standard codes for ECG leads.

Coding ECG Leads

Lead	Code	Lead	Code
I	.	V_1	-.
II	..	V_2	-..
III	...	V_3	-...
aVR	-	V_4	-....
aVL	–	V_5	-.....
aVF	—	V_6	-......

If the ECG is performed correctly, the physician will be able to examine the wave forms that occur at different parts of the cardiac cycle, the pattern of events in the heart from the beginning of one heart beat to the beginning of the next. Several wave forms are examined. They include the following:

- *P wave.* This impulse measures the contraction of the atria, or upper chambers of the heart, at the beginning of the cardiac cycle, as the heart begins the process of pumping blood.

- *P–R interval.* This part of the wave form shows the electrical activity of the atria as they pump out blood.

- *R wave.* This measures the electrical activity through the left ventricle of the heart.

- *QRS complex.* The QRS segment of the wave form records the electrical activity of the ventricles (the lower, pumping chambers of the heart) as they pump out blood to the body.

- *S–T segment.* This represents the time period between the end of the contraction of the ventricles and the beginning of the period (T wave) when the ventricles are resting.

- *T wave.* This wave shows the resting period of the heart before the next cardiac cycle begins.
- *U wave.* This small "extra" wave is sometimes seen after the T wave in someone whose heart has a slow recovery time because he has a low potassium level or some other metabolic problem.

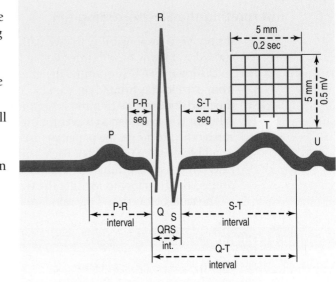

Here is the cardiac cycle with waves, segments, and intervals.

THE ELECTROCARDIOGRAM: WHAT'S THE PHYSICIAN LOOKING FOR?

When interpreting the ECG, the physician takes into consideration:

- heart rate, or how fast the heart is beating
- heart rhythm, the regularity of cardiac cycles and intervals
- axis, or the position of the heart and the direction of electrical movement through the heart
- hypertrophy, the size of the heart
- ischemia, a decrease in blood supply to an area of the heart
- infarction, the death of heart muscle resulting in a loss of function

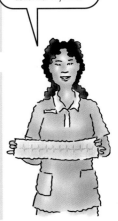

The rhythm strip is useful for identifying cardiac arrhythmias, or abnormal rhythms.

RHYTHM STRIP

Sometimes, the physician requests a **rhythm strip** to provide more information for a particular problem. This is a long strip recording the heart activity for a certain lead or combination of leads. Most ECG machines have a button that automatically records the 12 view in the 12-lead ECG. However, for some machines, you may need to use the manual mode to obtain a rhythm strip.

Getting a Good Electrocardiogram

You are responsible for obtaining good quality ECG tracings and avoiding **artifacts.** An artifact is an abnormal signal that doesn't represent the electrical activity of the heart during the cardiac cycle. Artifacts can result from:

- movement of the patient
- mechanical problems with the ECG machine
- improper technique
- loose electrodes
- broken cables or wires
- 60-cycle (AC) interference

The table below describes three types of artifacts, what they look like, and how to prevent them.

Types of Artifacts

Artifact	Possible Cause	How to Prevent Problems	Example of Appearance
Wandering baseline	Electrodes too tight or too loose; tension on electrodes	Apply electrodes properly; drape wires over patient	
	Electrodes dirty or corroded; gel used when applying electrodes to the patient has dried out	Clean and reapply electrodes or apply new electrodes	
	Machine is picking up patient's breathing movements	Reposition and reapply electrode	
	Poor skin preparation; skin has oil, lotion, or excessive hair	Repeat skin preparation and reapply electrodes	
Somatic muscle tremor	Patient cannot remain still because of tremors	Reassure patient; explain procedure and stress the need to keep still;	

(continued)

Types of Artifacts (*continued*)

Artifact	Possible Cause	How to Prevent Problems	Example of Appearance
Alternating current interference	Improperly grounded ECG machine	patients with tremors or disease may be unable to stay motionless Check cables to ensure machine is grounded properly before beginning test	
	Electrical interference in room	Move patient or unplug appliances in immediate area	
	Dangling lead wires	Arrange wires along contours of patient's body	

ELECTRODE MAINTENANCE

If your ECG machine uses reusable electrodes, here's what you must do to make sure they continue to produce accurate readings.

- Wipe the gel off the electrodes and wash them with a mild detergent solution. Also wash the rubber straps.
- Metal plate electrodes also must be polished. Use a fine grade of scouring powder. Do not use a metal-based powder or steel wool because that kind of cleaning will cause artifacts.
- Rinse and dry the electrodes well before storing them for later use.

HOLTER MONITORS

A Holter monitor is a portable ECG device that can be worn comfortably for long periods of time without interfering with

Ask the Professional

HOW SAFE IS THE ELECTROCARDIOGRAM?

Q: *My patient doesn't want to have the ECG procedure done because she's afraid of having electricity in her body. How can I reassure her?*

A: It's not surprising that some patients feel frightened or worried when they see all the electrodes and leads used in the ECG procedure. Begin by telling the patient it's normal to feel concerned. Explain that the machine is safe and that it's grounded to prevent electrical problems.

Be sure to tell your patient what the ECG machine does in terms she can understand. For example, you might tell your patient the record of the signals provides information that gives the physician a good picture of how her heart is working.

As you talk, make sure your own body language shows you are listening and attentive to your patient's concerns. If the patient still refuses the procedure, tell the physician. The physician may be able to provide a convincing explanation for why it's necessary.

daily activities. In many cases, an ECG that records the electrical activity of the heart for a brief moment in the medical office doesn't reveal cardiac problems. The Holter monitor is especially useful in diagnosing intermittent cardiac arrhythmias and dysfunctions because it records the electrical activity of the heart over periods of 24 hours or more.

The Holter monitor has two different settings:

- *Continuous recording.* The monitor can be set to record throughout the time the patient is wearing the monitor.

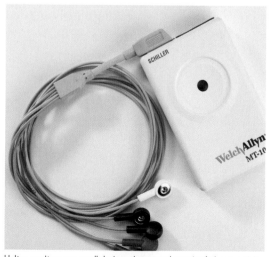

Holter monitors are small devices that record a patient's heart activity over a longer period than a traditional ECG.

- *Incident recording.* The monitor may be set to record only when the patient presses a button called the incident or event button. Patients press the button when they feel symptoms.

> When preparing patients for a Holter monitor, suggest that they wear clothing that buttons down the front. It's more convenient for dressing when the monitor is attached.

You'll find exact steps for applying a Holter monitor in the Hands On procedure on page 385.

When instructing the patient on using a Holter monitor, make sure to explain what to do in case of problems. A flashing light on the monitor indicates a lead is loose, or an electrode has lost contact. If the patient notices right away, the patient can press on the electrodes to try to re-establish contact. You need to remind the patient to call the medical office right away if any problems are noticed.

THE HOLTER DIARIES

When the patient wears a Holter monitor, he or she must keep a diary of daily activities. Patients who press a button when they feel symptoms must record the event or activity that was occurring at the time of the symptoms. All types of activities and the times they took place should be recorded, including:

- working quietly at a desk
- driving a car
- eating a meal
- watching television
- sleeping
- elimination
- sexual intercourse
- laughter
- anger

The physician will interpret the ECG tracing recorded by the Holter monitor and compare these findings to the activities recorded in the diary. This helps to determine what activities, if any, precipitate cardiac arrhythmias.

To ensure an accurate test, tell patients to avoid using electrical devices, such as electric razors or toothbrushes, while wearing the monitor. Emphasize that they also should keep the electrodes dry and in contact with their skin at all times. Patients never should move an electrode or bathe, shower, or swim while wearing the monitor.

OTHER CARDIAC DIAGNOSTIC TESTS

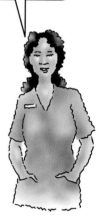

Some Holter monitors have small tape recorders so the patient can keep an audio diary of events instead of a written one.

Physicians often don't rely on one specific test to diagnose problems. They may need to gather information about heart function by looking at the results of several different tests. Many tests for diagnosing cardiovascular conditions typically are performed outside the medical office.

You've already read about x-rays and how they can provide information about the structures of internal body organs. This includes the heart. Other cardiac tests include:

- cardiac stress test
- echocardiography
- cardiac catheterization and coronary arteriography

Cardiac Stress Test

The physician orders a cardiac stress test to measure the response of the cardiac muscle to increased demands for oxy-

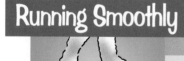

Running Smoothly

USING THE HOLTER MONITOR CORRECTLY

A patient has returned to the office with the Holter monitor and his diary, but one of the leads isn't attached. What should I do?

Check to see if the patient has recorded in his diary when the lead became loose. You may need to check with the physician to see if enough time passed before the lead came loose to obtain sufficient information about the heart function. In some cases, the patient may not be aware the lead became loose. He may need to wear the Holter monitor for another period of time to collect more information.

gen. The patient is attached to an ECG monitor for constant tracing while performing physical activity. The heart is usually tested with the patient walking on a treadmill. The rate or angle of the walk or run is increased periodically during the test. The stress test also may be performed with the patient pedaling a stationary bicycle. The patient's blood pressure is monitored before, during, and after the test.

This procedure typically isn't performed in the medical office. During the procedure, the patient must be monitored carefully for signs of light-headedness. Emergency resuscitation equipment must be available in case of cardiac or respiratory difficulties.

The stress test may be done as part of a routine physical examination. It also may be used as a diagnostic tool for patients who have intermittent periods of angina pectoris (chest pain resulting from lack of oxygen to the heart muscle) or palpitations (irregular heartbeats causing sensations of fluttering or pounding in the chest).

Echocardiography

This procedure uses sound waves to provide an image of the patient's heart. A small device called a transducer generates the sound waves. The waves pass through the cardiac chambers, walls, and valves, and are transmitted back to a monitor for interpretation.

The **echocardiogram,** or image of the heart created by the sound waves, helps the physician diagnose valve disease and

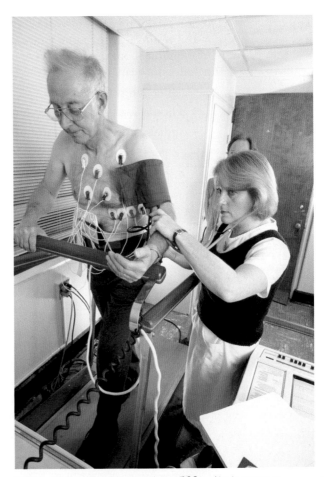

Walking on a treadmill while connected to an ECG machine is one way to determine the heart's ability to tolerate an increased workload.

other defects in the heart. Echocardiograms also help in the diagnosis of:

- the severity of heart disease
- the severity of cardiomyopathy
- injuries to the heart in patients with trauma

Only the most specialized cardiac medical offices have the equipment and personnel (ultrasonographers) to obtain cardiographs. In most instances, your role will be to schedule an outpatient procedure and give the patient any instructions required by the facility. Usually, no patient preparations are needed for the echocardiogram.

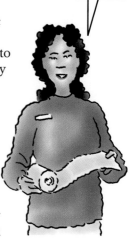

When assisting with an ECG stress test, be sure there is enough paper in the machine or the test might need to be repeated.

Cardiac Catheterization

Cardiac catheterization is a common invasive procedure used to diagnose or treat conditions affecting circulation in the coronary arteries. It involves the insertion of a flexible tube called a catheter into a blood vessel in either the arm or the groin. The physician gently guides the tube toward the heart. It may be performed on patients with various cardiac symptoms, including:

- shortness of breath
- angina
- dizziness
- palpitations
- fluttering in the chest
- rapid heartbeat

This procedure typically is used to determine the severity or cause of the cardiac problem. It is not performed in the medical office. However, you may be responsible for scheduling cardiac catheterizations at a local outpatient facility or hospital. You also will need to give the patient any instructions required by the facility.

If the procedure is for treatment, it must be done at an inpatient facility that has immediate access to open heart surgical equipment and personnel in the event of an emergency.

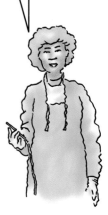

Cardiac catheterization is often used when a cardiac stress test or echocardiogram reveals an abnormality.

Coronary Arteriography

This procedure typically is performed after cardiac catheterization. Once the catheter is in place, a contrast medium is injected to reveal the heart's chambers, valves, great vessels, and coronary arteries on a monitor. If atherosclerotic plaques are found, an angioplasty may be performed or scheduled for later.

RESPIRATORY DISORDERS

The respiratory system works closely with the cardiovascular system to deliver oxygen to every cell in the body. The upper airways, bronchi (two main passages that move air into the lungs), alveoli, and other respiratory structures come into contact with air from the environment. In healthy individuals, body defense mechanisms protect the body from airborne disease and illness. However, disease can occur when the body is overwhelmed by cigarette smoke, air pollution, allergens, infectious organisms, or other irritants.

Respiratory disorders often are grouped according to their location in the body.

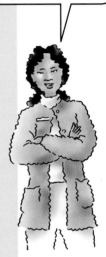

Chronic bronchitis and emphysema are often grouped together as Chronic Obstructive Pulmonary Disease, or COPD, because patients with one disorder usually have symptoms of the other.

- Disorders of the upper respiratory tract involve the structures of the upper respiratory tract, including the nose, throat, and larynx. Common respiratory disorders are caused by infectious microorganisms or allergies. Examples include acute rhinitis, sinusitis, and tonsillitis.

- Lower respiratory tract disorders may be acute or chronic. Acute diseases of the lower respiratory tract include bronchitis and pneumonia. Examples of chronic diseases are asthma, chronic bronchitis, and emphysema.

Respiratory Testing

Many patients with respiratory conditions may be seen in family practice medical offices. You need to understand some of the common tests and procedures required for diagnosing and treating respiratory conditions.

The traditional examination of the chest consists of inspection, palpation, percussion, and auscultation. During this examination, the patient must be sitting up. All clothing should be removed from the waist up. The patient should be given a gown and draped appropriately.

If the examination reveals any abnormalities or suspicious findings, such as crackling or wheezing sounds in the lungs, the physician may order additional respiratory tests. Two common respiratory tests performed in the medical office are:

- pulmonary function tests
- oximetry

PULMONARY FUNCTION TESTS

Pulmonary function tests are procedures for analyzing how well the patient moves air in and out of the lungs. A **spirometer** is a device used to measure the amount of air that is breathed in or out. The patient breathes into a mouthpiece.

During the test, you may ask the patient to perform different breathing maneuvers. The patient's airflow is measured and the results are compared with predicted values for the patient's height, weight, gender, age, and race. With this information, the physician can assess whether the patient has mild, moderate, or severe obstructive or restrictive disease. Two measurements may be obtained during the test.

- *Tidal volume* is the amount of air inhaled or exhaled with each normal breath. Although the human lungs can hold a large capacity of air, only a small amount of the total lung capacity is used during normal breathing.

- *Forced expiration volume* is the amount of air that can be exhaled forcefully after filling the lungs to capacity. The patient is asked to take a deep breath until the lungs are full, and then to exhale as hard and completely as possible.

You'll find the exact steps for performing a pulmonary function test in the Hands On procedure on page 387.

OXIMETRY

Many medical offices may have a pulse oximeter. This is a device that quickly and painlessly determines how much oxygen is in a patient's capillary blood cells. A sensor cable is attached to the nail bed of the patient's finger. The patient's pulse rate and oxygen saturation level are noted on a digital display on the small oximeter unit.

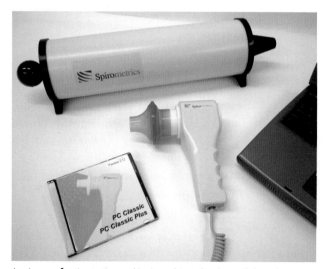

A pulmonary function testing machine is used to analyze how well the patient moves air in and out of the lungs.

A pulse oximeter reading should be obtained as a baseline for patients with chronic respiratory conditions and for those with respiratory signs and symptoms, such as **dyspnea** or wheezing. The results should be recorded as a percentage.

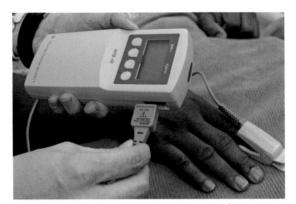

The pulse oximeter is used to measure oxygen saturation of arterial blood.

- Saturation level readings above 95 percent are considered normal.

- Patients with chronic conditions, such as emphysema, may have readings of 90 percent or higher.

- Readings lower than 90 percent should be reported to the physician immediately.

OTHER RESPIRATORY TESTS

The physician may need information from more sophisticated or invasive respiratory tests to make a diagnosis and plan treatment. These tests typically are not performed in a medical office. However, you should be familiar with them in case patients ask questions about tests ordered by the physician.

Bronchoscopy

This endoscopic procedure involves inserting a lighted scope into the trachea and bronchi for direct visualization. This is considered an invasive procedure and requires the patient's written consent. Usually, it's performed in an outpatient surgical setting. You may have to schedule this procedure for patients.

Bronchoscopy is used for many diagnostic purposes, including:

- obtaining sputum specimens
- obtaining tissue for biopsy
- visually assessing airways

It also may be used therapeutically to clear out mucus plugs or remove a foreign body.

Blood Gases

Arterial blood gas (ABG) determination involves drawing a small amount of blood from a patient's artery. The levels of pH and dissolved oxygen and carbon dioxide in the blood are measured. The results can help show whether the lungs are functioning properly to exchange gases.

Drawing blood from an artery requires special training. It isn't done routinely in the medical office. However, you may be required to schedule a patient for an arterial puncture at a laboratory or hospital. You also may need to record the results, which usually are phoned in to the medical office.

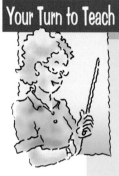

Your Turn to Teach

PEAK FLOW FOR PATIENTS

Patients with asthma may need to use a device called a peak flowmeter, which determines the amount of air moving into and out of the lungs. On days when the patient has no symptoms of asthma, breathing is tested at home using a peak flowmeter and the results are recorded on a chart or diary. This record helps the physician plan treatment for the condition.

You may be responsible for teaching patients how to use a peak flowmeter. You can follow these steps:

1. Wash your hands and gather the equipment. Explain to the patient how to read and reset the gauge after each reading. The peak flowmeter should be held upright.

2. Tell the patient to put the flowmeter's mouthpiece in his mouth. The patient's lips should be closed to form a tight seal around the mouthpiece, without biting down.

3. Ask the patient to take a deep breath and blow hard into the mouthpiece. Be sure to remind the patient not to block the back of the flowmeter, because this will interfere with the movement of the gauge.

4. Show the patient how to measure the airflow by noting the level where the sliding gauge stopped after blowing into the flowmeter.

5. Demonstrate how to set the gauge to zero.

6. Instruct the patient to perform the procedure three times consecutively, in the morning and at night. The highest of the three readings should be recorded on a form. Recording readings on a form also allows the patient to follow his or her progress based on medication therapy or exposure to allergens.

7. Show the patient how to clean the mouthpiece. It must be washed in soapy water and rinsed without immersing the flowmeter in the water.

Following Up Diagnostic Tests

Once diagnostic tests are completed, the testing facility or laboratory will send a report to the medical office. These reports provide important information for patient care and diagnosis. The office may receive reports for many different kinds of diagnostic tests.

- pulmonary tests
- cardiac tests
- radiographic procedures
- blood work
- specimen testing

Reports usually are received through the mail, courier services, or by fax machine. Many medical offices have a specific location to keep reports before they are screened and given to the physician.

As a medical assistant, one of your responsibilities may be to review or screen the reports and decide how the results should be presented to the physician.

- Critical results may need to be reported to the physician right away. Follow the policies in your medical office for notifying the physician of abnormal or urgent results.
- Less urgent results may be placed in a specific location for later review by the physician.

When providing test results for the physician to review, make sure they're accompanied by the patient's medical record. The physician may need to refer to the patient's chart when interpreting the results.

If a patient is coming in for a follow-up appointment based on the testing, it's your responsibility to check to make sure your office has received the results of all the diagnostic tests the physician has ordered. In some cases, you may need to call other medical facilities or hospital record facilities to obtain the test results before the patient's visit. The physician needs to have all the test results to diagnose and treat the patient properly.

After the physician has reviewed the test results, they may be filed in the patient's medical record. Check to see if any additional tests, follow-up procedures, or appointments are required. Depending on office policies, you may be required to notify the patient of test results by phone or through the mail. Always protect patient confidentiality. You'll find exact steps for screening and following up test results in the Hands On procedure on page 389.

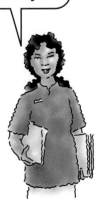

Never file paperwork in a patient's medical record until the physician has reviewed and signed it!

Hands On

PERFORMING A 12-LEAD ELECTROCARDIOGRAM

6-1

1. Wash your hands and assemble the equipment. Greet and identify the patient and explain the procedure. Suggest that the patient use the restroom if necessary.

2. Check that the machine is plugged in and turn on the machine. Make sure all connections and cables are tight. Make sure metal tabs that connect to electrodes are not upside down and that metal is touching metal coating on the electrodes.

3. Enter the appropriate data into the machine, including the patient's name or identification number, age, gender, height, weight, blood pressure, and medications.

4. Ask the patient to disrobe above the waist and provide a gown for privacy. Female patients also should be instructed to remove any nylons or tights. Pants do not have to be removed if they can be pulled up to expose the lower legs for attaching leads.

5. Assist the patient into a comfortable supine position, providing pillows as needed for comfort. Patients in cardiac or respiratory distress may also be placed in a semi-Fowler's or seated position. Drape the patient for privacy. It's important for the patient to feel comfortable. Uncomfortable patients may move during the test, resulting in artifacts on the ECG.

6. You need to prepare the patient's skin by wiping away skin oil and lotions with antiseptic wipes. Shave any hair that will interfere with good contact between the skin and the electrodes.

7. Apply the electrodes against the fleshy, muscular parts of the upper arms and lower legs, following the manufacturer's directions. Make sure the electrodes are snug against the skin, for a proper reading. In case of amputation or an otherwise inaccessible limb, you can place the electrode on the uppermost part of the existing extremity, or on the anterior shoulder (upper extremity) and groin (lower extremity).

8. Connect the lead wires securely according to the color-coded notations on the connectors (RA, LA, RL, LL, V_1–V_6). Untangle the wires before applying them to prevent electri-

(continued)

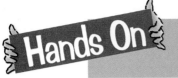

PERFORMING A 12-LEAD ELECTROCARDIOGRAM (*continued*)

6-1

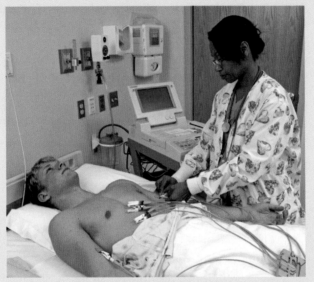

This shows the application of the limb lead.

cal artifacts. Each lead should lie smoothly along the contours of the patient's body. You should double-check the placement of the leads. If the leads are placed improperly, the procedure may have to be repeated.

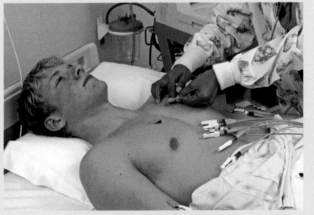

This shows the application of the chest lead.

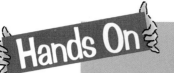

PERFORMING A 12-LEAD ELECTROCARDIOGRAM (continued)

6-1

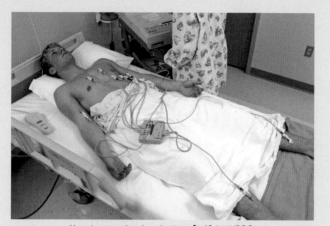

Here is a completed application of a 12-lead ECG.

9. Check the sensitivity, or gain, and paper speed settings on the ECG machine before running the test. Set the sensitivity or gain to 1 and the paper speed to 25 mm/second. These settings are necessary to obtain an accurate ECG and should not be changed without a direct order from the physician. You must note any changes on the final ECG tracing.

10. To start the tracing, press the automatic button on the ECG machine. The machine will move automatically from one lead to the next. If the physician wants a rhythm strip only, use the manual mode of operation and select the lead.

11. When the tracing is printed, you should check for artifacts and a standardization mark. When the sensitivity is set at 1, the standardization mark will be 2 small squares wide and 10 small squares high. It documents the accuracy of the machine and provides a reference point.

12. If the tracing quality is good, turn off the machine. Remove and discard the electrodes. Slowly assist the patient into a sitting position. Some patients become dizzy after lying supine. You can help with dressing if needed.

13. If a single-channel machine was used (each lead is printed on a single roll of paper, one lead at a time), carefully roll the ECG strip. Do not use clips to secure the roll. Folding or

(continued)

Hands On

PERFORMING A 12-LEAD ELECTROCARDIOGRAM (*continued*)

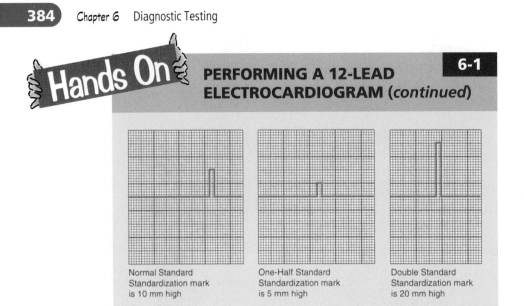

Normal Standard
Standardization mark
is 10 mm high

One-Half Standard
Standardization mark
is 5 mm high

Double Standard
Standardization mark
is 20 mm high

applying clips may make marks on the surface, which can obscure the reading. This ECG must be mounted on a special form or 8 × 11-inch paper before going into the patient's medical record. Follow the policies in your medical office.

14. Record the procedure in the patient's medical record.

15. Place the ECG tracing and the patient's medical record on the physician's desk, or give it directly to the physician, as instructed.

Charting Example:
02/02/2007 9:45 A.M. Preop 12-lead ECG obtained and placed in chart, given to Dr. Bruno for evaluation. Pt. discharged, no follow-up required at this time._____ A. Perez, CMA

Hands On

APPLYING A HOLTER MONITOR

6-2

1. Wash your hands and gather the equipment. Greet and identify the patient.

2. Explain the procedure, including how to use and care for the Holter monitor. You'll need to remind the patient of the need to carry out all normal activities for the duration of the test. A normal routine is necessary to allow the physician to identify areas of concern.

3. Explain the purpose of the incident diary. Emphasize the need to carry it at all times during the test. Ask the patient to remove all clothing from the waist up and to put on the gown. The patient must be exposed for placement of the electrodes. Drape patient appropriately for privacy.

4. With the patient seated, prepare the skin for electrode attachment. Be sensitive to patient privacy! Shave the skin only if necessary, and cleanse with antiseptic wipes. Clean skin will help the electrodes adhere properly.

5. Expose the adhesive backing of the electrodes. Follow the manufacturer's directions to attach each one firmly. Apply the electrodes at the specified sites:
   A. right manubrium border
   B. left manubrium border
   C. right sternal border at fifth rib
   D. fifth rib space at the left anterior axillary line
   E. fifth rib space at the right anterior axillary line as a ground lead

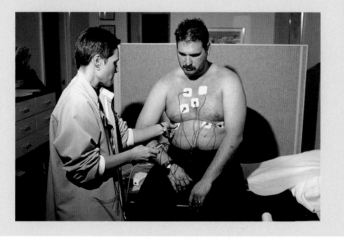

(continued)

Hands On

APPLYING A HOLTER MONITOR (*continued*)

6. Check the security of the attachments.

7. Position electrode connectors down toward the patient's feet. Attach the lead wires and secure them with adhesive tape. Putting tape over the connections helps to make sure the leads don't work loose.

8. Connect the cable and run a baseline ECG by hooking the Holter monitor to the ECG machine with the proper cable hookup. You need to make sure the Holter monitor is working properly.

9. Assist the patient in dressing carefully, with the cable extending through the garment opening. You want to prevent any pulling or straining on the connectors or wires.

10. Plug the cable into the recorder and mark the diary. If needed, explain the purpose of the diary to the patient again. Give instructions for a return appointment to evaluate the recording and the diary.

11. Record the procedure in the patient's medical record.

Charting Example:

11/28/2007 1:00 P.M. Holter monitor ordered and applied; baseline ECG done. Oral and written instructions given regarding care and use of monitor. Instruction for completion of diary also given. Pt. verbalized understanding of use of monitor and completion of diary. To RTO tomorrow P.M. for removal of monitor._____ R. Steele, CMA

Hands On

PERFORMING A PULMONARY FUNCTION TEST
6-3

1. Wash your hands and assemble the equipment. Greet and identify the patient and explain the procedure.

2. Turn the pulmonary function test machine on. If necessary, calibrate the spirometer using the calibration syringe, according to the manufacturer's directions. The spirometer must be calibrated daily to ensure accurate results. Record the calibration in the appropriate log book, following office policy.

3. With the machine on and calibrated, attach the appropriate cable, tubing, and mouthpiece according to the type of machine being used. One cable is plugged into an electrical outlet and another is connected to the spirometer and the patient's mouthpiece.

4. Using the keyboard on the machine, enter the patient's name or identification number, age, weight, height, sex, race, and smoking history. The spirometer automatically takes these parameters into consideration when providing results.

5. Ask the patient to remove any clothing that may restrict the chest from expanding. Show the patient how to apply the nose clip to stop air from being expelled through the nose during the test.

6. Ask the patient to stand, breathe in deeply, and blow into the mouthpiece as hard as possible. The machine will indicate when the patient should stop blowing. The indicator may be a buzz, beep, or visual signal you can use to instruct the patient. Make sure a chair is available, and watch the patient carefully for signs of dizziness or imbalance.

7. During the procedure, coach the patient as necessary to obtain each reading. Many patients feel they have exhaled all air from the lungs when the machine is instructing them to continue. The machine will indicate whether the reading is adequate. Three repetitions usually are required to obtain the patient's best result. Allow the patient to rest between them if necessary.

8. After printing the results, properly care for the equipment. Dispose of the mouthpiece in the biohazard container.

(continued)

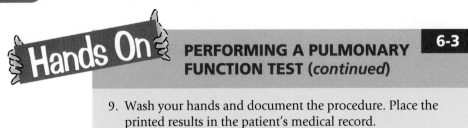

**PERFORMING A PULMONARY
FUNCTION TEST** (*continued*)   6-3

9. Wash your hands and document the procedure. Place the
   printed results in the patient's medical record.

Charting Example:
06/12/2007 3:00 P.M. PFT performed for employment physical
as ordered by Dr. John. 3 maneuvers obtained with no difficulty. Dr. John notified for results in chart. _____
_____P. Hill, CMA

Hands On

FOLLOWING UP TEST RESULTS

6-4

1. Gather supplies, including patient diagnostic test results, a pen, a telephone, etc.

2. Review diagnostic reports to determine whether results are urgent or can be set aside for physician's later review.

3. Get the patient's medical record.

4. Double-check the patient's name or identifying numbers on the chart to be sure they match those on the results. Review the results and initial and date the results. Attach the results to the front of the patient's chart for the physician to review.

5. If the results are urgent, follow the procedures in your medical office for notifying the physician. If not, place the chart in the appropriate location for review by the physician at a later time. In many medical offices, received reports and results are placed in a specific location in the physician's office.

6. After the physician has reviewed the results, check to see if the physician has written any orders in response to the results. Often, physicians write comments or information on the results. Also check that the physician has dated and initialed the report.

7. Results that state "Within Normal Limits" may require follow-up after a specified interval of time has passed. Follow the policies in your medical office for creating a reminder for following up. In some offices, a tickler card is made and placed in a tickler file for patient reminders.

8. If requested by the physician, inform the patient of the results following standard office policies. When telephoning patients, be sure not to leave confidential information on answering machines unless the patient has asked you to do so specifically.

9. Document the procedure in the patient's medical record.

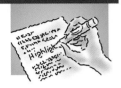

Chapter Highlights

- Radiology is a medical specialty that involves different imaging techniques to diagnose and treat diseases. These techniques include radiographs (x-rays), fluoroscopy, sonography (ultrasound), computed tomography (CT scans), magnetic resonance imaging (MRI), and nuclear medicine techniques. Radiologists interpret the images and send a report to the medical office.

- To produce a radiograph (commonly referred to as an x-ray), a beam of x-rays passes through the patient to record an image on radiographic film. Radiolucent tissues allow the x-rays to pass through and appear as black on the film. Radiopaque tissues are dense and absorb the x-rays, showing up as white on an x-ray.

- In some states, medical assistants are permitted to take and process simple x-ray images of the bones or chest. In other states, only licensed radiographers may take and process x-rays.

- Medical assistants who work in facilities where radiographs are performed may need to help prepare patients. Preparation includes removing any metal objects, including jewelry and clothing with metal fasteners.

- For some radiological procedures, contrast media are used to make it easier to differentiate body structures. A contrast medium may be introduced into the body by mouth, intravenously, or through a catheter.

- The medical assistant has a key role in educating patients about radiological examinations. Patients need information about what to expect during the procedure, what preparations they need to make, and what to do after the procedure.

- Diagnostic tests for cardiac disorders may be invasive or noninvasive. Some noninvasive tests are performed in the medical office, such as the electrocardiogram (ECG).

- The 12-lead electrocardiogram machine picks up electrical signals from the heart and records them on a graph. Sometimes, it is performed as part of a routine physician examination. It also can be used in the diagnosis of heart problems such as arrhythmias and ischemia. Placement of the electrodes is important for providing an accurate ECG tracing.

- Medical assistants are responsible for obtaining an accurate ECG. It's important to avoid artifacts that do not represent the electrical activity of the heart. Common factors that can produce artifacts are movement of the patient, mechanical problems with the ECG machine, and improper technique.

- The Holter monitor is a small, portable ECG worn by patients for a long period of time. It is useful in diagnosing intermittent cardiac arrhythmias and dysfunctions. While wearing the Holter monitor, the patient must keep a diary of all activities.

- Many cardiac procedures are not performed in the medical office. Some of these procedures are the stress test, echocardiography, cardiac catheterization, and coronary arteriography.

- The basic examination for respiratory disorders includes inspection, palpation, percussion, and auscultation. If the examination reveals abnormalities, the physician may order additional tests, such as pulmonary function tests, oximetry, bronchoscopy, or an arterial blood gas.

- When the results of diagnostic tests are received in the medical office, the medical assistant screens them to determine if they require immediate attention. The medical assistant attaches the test results to the patient's medical record for review by the physician.

- After the physician has reviewed the test results, the medical assistant places them in the patient's medical record. The medical assistant may be required to inform patients of test results.

Chapter 7

PATIENT EDUCATION

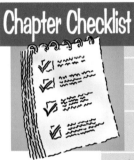

Chapter Checklist

- List the five main steps in a teaching plan

- Describe four different teaching strategies

- List five conditions necessary for learning

- Summarize Maslow's hierarchy of needs and explain how to use it

- Identify three factors that can promote learning

- Provide instruction for health maintenance and disease prevention

- Discuss four obstacles that can interfere with patient learning

- Identify some considerations for adapting teaching materials to meet the needs of specific patients

- Instruct individuals according to their needs

- Identify community resources

- List the recommended annual screenings for maintaining good health

- List and describe the main food groups in the food groups system

- Explain how to modify a basic diet to treat a medical condition

- Define range-of-motion exercises and explain why they're used

- Explain what to teach patients about herbal supplements

- Identify different stressors associated with illness or disease

- Describe three relaxation techniques for managing stress

- Explain the role of the medical assistant in educating patients about substance abuse

As you've noticed from reading previous chapters, patient education is an important part of a clinical medical assistant's job. Educating patients involves more than telling them what medications to take or which behaviors they need to change. To educate patients effectively, you need to:

- help them adjust to and accept their illness or condition
- involve them in gaining knowledge that will change their attitudes or behaviors
- provide them with positive reinforcement, or encouragement

The Process of Patient Education

Effective patient education involves five basic steps:

- assessment
- planning
- implementation
- evaluation
- documentation

Together, these five steps form a teaching plan. The plan may be written as the process is occurring, or it may be documented after the teaching has taken place.

ASSESSMENT

Assessment is a process that involves gathering information about a patient's abilities and needs. Before you begin this first step, you need to review your own attitudes. This means being aware of your personal feelings about:

- the patient
- the material to be taught

At times, you may be uncomfortable with the situation, the material, or the patient. However, as an educator, you must set aside your feelings, beliefs, and experiences. For example, you may be asked to instruct a patient about something you personally oppose. Your job is to teach objectively—that is, without making judgments or opinions—and to the best of your ability.

Always consider how your actions and responses will affect the patient. Treat each patient fairly and without prejudice.

GETTING A GOOD ASSESSMENT

In doing a good assessment, here are some of the things you should consider:

- the patient's current health care needs
- the patient's past medical and surgical conditions
- the patient's current understanding and acceptance of her health problems and status
- the patient's need for additional information
- factors that may hinder the patient's learning

> If you talk to family or friends when doing a teaching assessment, be extra careful not to violate the patient's privacy. Don't share any medical information.

You can get this information from a variety of sources. The best source is the patient's medical record. It includes all the information about current diagnoses, treatments, medications, past medical history, and other documentation. Most medical records have a problem list on the inside cover. This can give you a snapshot of the patient and may save you time. Other sources of information might be:

- the physician
- the patient's family members
- the patient's significant other, if any
- other members of the health care team

PLANNING

In **planning**, you use the information gathered during the assessment phase to decide how to approach the patient's instruction. Try to involve the patient in this part of the process if you can. Work with the patient to establish goals and objectives.

- The **learning goal** is what the patient should achieve at

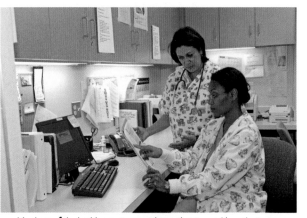

Members of the health care team work together to provide patient care.

the end of the program. This might be knowledge, an action or behavior, or even an attitude toward something. Whatever it is, the learning goal is the desired outcome of your teaching.

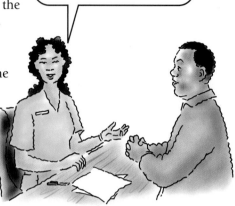

Learning goals and objectives that you establish in cooperation with the patient are the most meaningful to the patient.

- **Learning objectives** are tasks to help reach the goal that will be performed at different points in the program. The learning objectives must be specific to each patient. They also must be measurable. That way, you will be able to determine whether the patient has successfully completed them.

Consider this example: A patient must learn to limit his fluid intake. Which of these two objectives would better allow you to measure the patient's progress in reaching the learning goal?

1. The patient understands why he should limit his fluid intake.

2. The patient is able to prepare a schedule for daily fluid intake and explain why it's important that he limits his fluids.

The second objective is better because it requires the patient to demonstrate that he understands.

Having patients prepare their own schedules also gets them involved in their own health care. It lets them create schedules to fit their lifestyles. This will be likely to increase a patient's **compliance,** or how well the patient follows the physician's recommendations.

IMPLEMENTATION

After you and the patient agree on goals and objectives, you begin to put them into practice. **Implementation** is the process used to perform the actual teaching. You'll find general steps to help guide your teaching in the Hands On procedure on page 437.

The implementing stage may occur once or several times over a longer period. The length of the teaching process depends on:

- the patient's disease process

- the patient's ability to understand

- the patient's access to resources

For example, teaching a patient about diabetes probably will require several sessions. The first session may focus on what diabetes is. Later teachings might include topics such as diet, foot care, glucose monitoring, and insulin injection.

Teaching Methods

You'll probably use one or more of these methods in the teaching process. Choose teaching methods that will best help that particular patient understand and remember the learning. The subject to be taught also will influence which of these methods you choose. Each teaching session is usually carried out in several steps. You should use more than one method.

Lecture and Demonstration. Lecture and demonstration are both good ways to present basic information to the patient. However, no patient participation is involved. Participation helps patients remember the information.

Role Playing and Demonstration. During role playing and demonstration, the patient watches you perform a medical procedure. Then the patient performs it in a return demonstration. Active participation will help the patient remember the information.

First explain to the patient how to use the crutches, and then demonstrate how to do it. Next, ask the patient to try it out.

Discussion. A discussion is a two-way exchange of information. It works well when teaching patients about lifestyle changes. This method isn't as useful for teaching about medical procedures.

Audiovisual Material. DVDs, videos, and CDs often can be taken home. Patients and family members can then review the material as needed. This provides reinforcement of your teaching. This type of material also provides auditory and visual stimulation.

Printed Material and Programmed Instructions. When you give a patient printed instructions or other material, you need to make sure he understands it. Discuss the information with the patient to clarify points. Encourage the patient to ask questions.

Teaching Aids

Patients also can benefit from the use of teaching aids. Here are some aids you might find useful:

- drawings
- charts and posters

- graphs

- pamphlets and booklets

- videos and DVDs

- audiocassettes and CDs

- mannequins or models

Booklets, DVDs, and CDs provide handy references for patients to use at home.

EVALUATION

After you've taught a patient, you need to determine if your teaching was effective. The process of finding this out is called **evaluation.** It begins by asking some basic open-ended questions.

- How is the patient progressing?

- How well did the teaching plan work?

- What kind of changes does the plan need, if any?

Contact with patients in the medical office is limited. So part of the evaluation process might have to be done by patients at home. If you can't schedule office visits for direct observation of patients, they'll be responsible for phoning in and reporting their status. When you speak to these patients on the phone, you need to find out:

- if the patient can do the task you taught

- if the patient is having trouble with the task

If the patient mentions any concerns, or seems unclear about the instructions, try to resolve the problems over the phone. However, you may need to schedule an office appointment.

During the evaluation, you may discover **noncompliance.** This is the patient's inability or refusal to follow a prescribed order. When you discover noncompliance, your first step is to find out why. The patient may have misunderstood the instructions. In some cases, the noncompliance is because the patient simply refuses to follow them. In either case, you need to notify the physician.

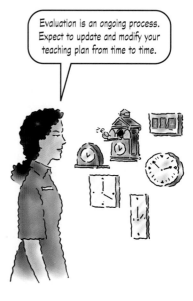

Evaluation is an ongoing process. Expect to update and modify your teaching plan from time to time.

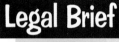

THE RIGHT TO REFUSE

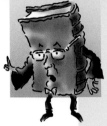

A patient has a legal right to refuse medical treatment if she is determined to be mentally competent. The right to refuse also includes patient education. If the patient refuses to participate in the teaching you have planned, you should notify the physician. Patients who refuse medical treatment or teaching need to be informed of the consequences of their actions. The physician will decide what to do next.

DOCUMENTATION

All teachings must be documented in the patient's chart. The table below shows what kinds of information a teaching note should contain.

Documenting Patient Education

Things to Be Documented	Example
Date and time of teaching	06/03/2007 4:15 P.M.
What information was taught	Diabetes foot care was discussed. It consisted of the proper method for toenail cutting and the need for regular examination by a podiatrist.
How the information was taught	ADA (American Diabetes Association) foot care video was shown to the patient.
Evaluation of the teaching	Patient verbalized the need to make an appointment with a podiatrist.
Any additional teaching planned	Patient will return on 6/10/2007 to the office with his wife for glucose monitoring instructions.

Your signature implies that you did the teaching. If another staff member helped, make sure you clearly note that in the patient's chart. Also include the names of any interpreters who were involved.

Documenting patient education is important for phone conversations too. You might write, "Spoke with patient by phone today; he said he is testing his blood sugar every morning without problem."

CHARTING SAMPLE FOR PATIENT EDUCATION

It's important to document patient education. Here's an example of how to do it.

11/27/2007 11:15 A.M. Patient arrived in the office for teaching on the glucose meter; brought meter from home. Following steps were demonstrated by me: calibration of meter strips, battery change, finger sticks, strip insertion into machine, use of the patient logbook. Normal BGM ranges were reviewed along with treatment of high and low blood sugar. Pt returned demonstration without problem and verbalized understanding of the teaching. Reviewed glucose meter instruction manual with pt. Pt. instructed to bring logbook to each MD appointment.

_____ Bea Zame, CMA

Conditions Needed for Patient Education

Patients will have a hard time learning new information and skills if the conditions aren't right. Here are some of the things that are necessary.

- a patient's perceived need to learn and readiness to learn
- an appropriate environment
- the right equipment
- a knowledgeable teacher
- different ways to teach the information

THE NEED TO LEARN

Learning isn't likely to occur unless a patient perceives, or sees, a need to learn. Suppose you're planning to teach a patient with hypertension about low-sodium diets to help manage high blood pressure. However, the patient doesn't feel his hypertension is a problem. Because he hasn't accepted the need for teaching, he isn't motivated to learn the diet. Before you begin teaching this patient, three things must occur.

1. The patient must accept that hypertension needs to be managed.
2. The patient has to accept that there's a relationship between high sodium intake and hypertension.
3. The patient needs to be willing to make a dietary change.

MASLOW'S HIERARCHY OF NEEDS

Basic human needs must be met before people can focus on higher needs, such as taking personal responsibility for their health. A psychiatrist named Abraham Maslow viewed human needs as being like a pyramid. Basic needs are at the bottom or foundation of the pyramid, while higher needs are at the top. The patient makes upward progress as different levels of needs are met. If the patient reaches the highest level, she has reached a state of health and well-being. A patient can move up and down the pyramid depending on her situation.

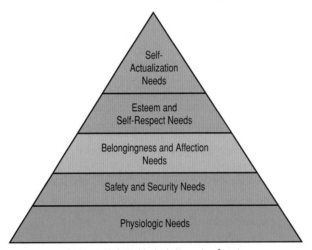

This pyramid shows Maslow's hierarchy of needs.

Physiological Needs

At the base of Maslow's pyramid are basic needs like water, food, rest, and comfort. Until these needs are met, the patient can't begin the process of meeting higher needs. Everyone has a different level of tolerance and expectation for basic needs. For example, one person might expect to have his food in three meals with drinks and dessert. Another may skip lunch regularly to attend work meetings.

> If the patient believes that her basic needs are met, you should accept that. Don't judge the situation.

Safety and Security

These needs include a safe environment and freedom from fear and anxiety. Patients can be affected by fear and anxiety because of their medical conditions. Some people who are diagnosed with cancer may be so frightened that they're unable to think of anything but dying. Patients who have experienced trauma or disaster may place the need to feel safe above all other needs.

Belonging and Affection

The need for love and belonging is essential for feeling connected and important to others. A sense of love and belonging can be an important motivation for patients to try to regain good health.

Esteem and Self-Respect

These needs involve our need to feel self-worth. We can develop esteem ourselves, or it can come from those who admire us. If others value us, or we value ourselves, we are more likely to strive to maintain good health. Patients who lack self-esteem are less likely to accept education that targets improving their health. They aren't likely to have much motivation to learn.

Self-Actualization

A person at the top of the pyramid has satisfied all the lower level needs. This person feels responsible and in control of his own life. Self-actualized patients will work eagerly to control their state of wellness by following medical teaching and orders. They even may help others achieve wellness. Not all patients will reach this level. But patients who have reached it will be ready to learn health care skills. They will work to regain good health and maintain it. They also will follow guidelines to prevent possible medical problems in the future.

THE TEACHING ENVIRONMENT

You need to teach in an environment that will promote learning. For example, it's not appropriate to teach patients in a hallway, a waiting room, or any other high-traffic area. The room where you teach should meet the following criteria.

- well lighted
- quiet
- private
- free of distractions

Patients learn best when they feel relaxed. For example, it wouldn't be worthwhile to teach a patient who's still on the examination table with her feet in the stirrups. Little learning will take place until she's more comfortable. First, remove her from the stirrups and have the patient get dressed. Then invite her to sit in a chair. If the patient had a procedure done in the

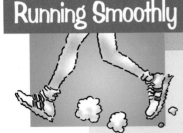

Running Smoothly

USING MASLOW'S HIERARCHY OF NEEDS

How can I use Maslow's hierarchy of needs to help in teaching patients?

You need to be aware that patients must have their basic needs met before they'll be willing or able to learn to take care of their health. Of course, not everyone starts at the bottom of the pyramid. At the same time, some patients will never reach the top. Others may be at the top and slide backward as a result of unfortunate circumstances. Figuring out where a patient is on the pyramid will help you decide what type of education is appropriate, if any.

- If a patient isn't meeting basic needs, you should help in arranging for him to get those needs met before beginning teaching.

- Patients who are in the middle levels may be able to focus and learn certain skills, but they may not be ready for complex teachings. In this case, you should involve family or significant others in the teaching process, if possible.

room and bloody dressings or suture equipment are still present, clean the area and then return for teaching. Try to make the patient as comfortable as possible.

TEACHING WITH EQUIPMENT

Often, you'll need to teach patients to perform a **psychomotor skill.** A psychomotor skill requires the patient to perform a physical task. Some examples of psychomotor skills are:

- crutch walking
- glucose monitoring
- eye drop instillation
- dressing changes

In order to teach the skill, you need to have the equipment on hand and ready to use. If possible, the equipment should be from the patient's home or be an exact copy of what the patient will use.

TEACHING A PSYCHOMOTOR SKILL

Here are the steps you need to follow when teaching a psychomotor skill.

1. Demonstrate the entire skill.

2. Then, demonstrate the skill again, step by step. Explain each step as you complete it.

3. Have the patient demonstrate the skill with your help.

4. Have the patient demonstrate the skill without your help.

Give the patient positive reinforcement as she completes the steps. Complete the teaching by giving the patient written instructions for the skill she has just demonstrated. If the patient is taking the equipment home, include written instructions about proper care of it as well.

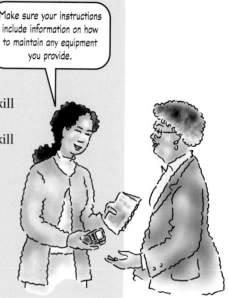

Make sure your instructions include information on how to maintain any equipment you provide.

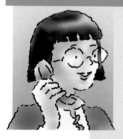

Ask the Professional   WHEN YOU DON'T KNOW

Q: *Yesterday, when I was teaching a patient, she asked me a question and I wasn't sure how to answer. So I guessed at it. Was that the right thing to do?*

A: Never guess or imply that you know something you don't know. Instead, tell the patient that you aren't sure about that specific piece of information and that you'll find out. Then research the answer or ask for help from another health care professional.

Whenever you're teaching, you need to have a solid knowledge of the material. If you're not comfortable or don't feel knowledgeable about the topic, ask for help before you begin teaching the patient. You don't need to be an expert on the topic, but you need to feel comfortable with the information.

USING DIFFERENT STRATEGIES

For patient education to be effective, you should use several techniques or approaches. The more techniques you use, the more the patient will learn and remember. People learn in three different ways:

- by seeing
- by hearing
- by touching

Your teaching should involve at least two of these three senses. When there are different ways to learn the material, patients are more motivated to learn. They also will learn more information.

Here's an example. Suppose you were teaching a patient about the dangers of smoking. Which method would be the most effective?

1. Giving the patient a pamphlet that explains the dangers of smoking, along with statistical data.

2. Showing a patient photos comparing a smoker's and a nonsmoker's lung, explaining what happens to the lungs when the patient smokes, and giving the patient pamphlets about smoking cessation programs.

The teaching in the second approach will be more effective. The patient sees the photos and hears your explanations about the dangers of smoking. He also receives a brochure with practical hands-on information he can refer to later.

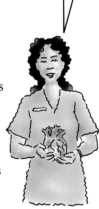

In addition to traditional teaching aids like pamphlets, diagrams, and DVDs, you can use tools such as mannequins and models of body parts to make points. Food, food labels, and websites are other tools.

AIDING LEARNING IN SPECIAL SITUATIONS

Along with the main conditions that must be present for patient learning, other factors can be important. Here are some additional aids that can help depending on the situation.

- Family or significant others may need to be present if the information is complex, or if it requires their help. Family members are essential if the patient is confused or unreliable.

- Patients should be wearing any sensory devices they need (for example, glasses, hearing aids, etc.).

- Some patients may require a qualified interpreter.

Obstacles to Patient Education

Even when you have the right conditions for learning, some factors can get in the way of the process. You need to recognize these factors and be able to intervene, if appropriate. In some cases, your teaching may be delayed. Also, you may need to adjust your teaching plan. Some of the factors that can interfere with patient learning are:

- illness and pain
- the patient's age
- the patient' educational background
- any physical impairments

EXISTING ILLNESS AND PAIN

The type of illness patients have will play a key role in their ability and willingness to learn. In general, patients with acute, short-term illnesses will be motivated to learn a skill that will speed up healing. Some examples of such illnesses are:

- colds and viruses
- some orthopedic injuries, such as uncomplicated fractures and sprains

However, many illnesses have symptoms and complications that may make learning more difficult. Untreated or persistent pain can affect the healing process and affect the patient's quality of life. The table below shows several kinds of illness or conditions that will negatively affect learning.

Medical Conditions That Affect Patient Education

Condition	Examples
Illness that results in moderate to severe pain	Neuropathies, bone cancer, kidney stones, recent surgical procedures
Illness with poor prognosis or limited rehabilitation potential	Progressive neurological disorders, certain cancers, traumatic events
Illness with weakness or general malaise as a primary symptom	Gastrointestinal disorders that cause vomiting or diarrhea, anemia, Lyme disease, recent blood transfusions
Illness that impairs the patient's mental health or cognitive abilities	Brain tumors, Alzheimer's disease, substance abuse, psychiatric disorders
More than one chronic illness	Diabetes with cardiac, renal, or integumentary (relating to skin, hair, and nails) complications
Illness that results in respiratory distress or difficulty breathing	Chronic obstructive pulmonary disease, pneumonias, lung cancer, asthma

AGE

You need to consider the age of the patient when deciding on the amount and type of education you can do. Children need to be educated at an age-appropriate level. For example, it wouldn't be appropriate to teach a two-year-old how to assemble an asthma nebulizer. You would need to teach that to the parent or caregiver. However, it would be appropriate to explain to the child that the nebulizer is not a toy and that it contains medication.

It's important to focus on safety issues when teaching small children and their parents.

Children

Children mature at different rates. You need to assess what information a specific child can handle, and what information should not be shared with the child. To do this, talk to the child's parents first, to gather information about the child's developmental stage.

Here's an example. A seven-year-old child has just been diagnosed with diabetes. He needs to know the signs and symptoms of low blood sugar and how to treat it. But the child may not be ready to learn about the long-term complications of the disease, such as blindness or renal failure. You need only to teach the child that the disease must be well controlled to prevent future problems. You don't want to provide so much information that the child becomes fearful.

Adults

The challenge in teaching adults is that they often have many responsibilities and obligations. These may relate to children, spouses, or aging parents. Social or work obligations also limit their free time. As a result, adults may be less willing to learn or have little time to learn something new. Your teaching may have to occur in short sessions over long periods of time.

Older Patients

Elderly patients may be challenging to teach for several reasons, including:

- confusion
- lack of interest
- overall poor health
- sensory deficits

But remember never to stereotype any of your patients. Some older patients can be the most attentive and curious learners.

EDUCATIONAL BACKGROUND

On most assessment forms, patients are asked to fill out the level of education they've obtained. This information can help you determine their ability to understand written information. You need to be careful in making this assessment, however. Education level may not guarantee how well the patient can read. You'll need to use tact and diplomacy to evaluate the situation.

Also keep in mind that patients who have an educational background in health care may need the same attention and teaching as other patients.

> Don't assume you can skip teaching a skill just because your patient is a nurse or a physician. Her specialty may be in an unrelated area.

PHYSICAL IMPAIRMENTS AND OTHER FACTORS

For patients with physical impairments, some types of learning may be difficult. For example, patients with severe arthritis in their hands may have difficulty performing certain psychomotor skills, such as giving themselves insulin. For patients with physical impairments, an occupational therapist is the best resource to assist you. Speak to the physician to obtain the proper referrals.

Along with physical impairments, other factors may hinder your efforts to teach patients.

- A patient's culture may guide which teaching methods you use.

- Patients with financial troubles may feel distracted and have a difficult time focusing on your instruction. This applies to any patients under a good deal of stress.

It's important for you to assess the patient's readiness to learn, and to try to remove any obstacles that may be present. You can learn more about instructing a patient according to his individual needs in the Hands On procedure on page 437.

USING COMMUNITY RESOURCES

Sometimes, patients will need help with problems that are beyond what your office or even the health care system can provide. Resources in the community may be able to meet these needs. Being aware of these resources is part of being an effective teacher. You should be able to provide patients with information about community resources that can help meet their needs. The Hands On procedure on page 438 shows you how to develop and use lists of community resources.

Patient Teaching Plans

Medical assistants usually are given only a small amount of time for patient teaching. Often, you may find yourself needing to teach without a written plan. To make sure the teaching process follows a logical order, develop a general plan in your mind. Following the steps you learned earlier in the chapter—assessing, planning, implementing, evaluating, and documenting—will help you do this.

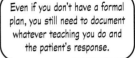

Even if you don't have a formal plan, you still need to document whatever teaching you do and the patient's response.

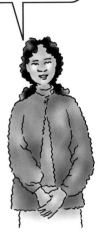

TEACHING DURING CRUNCH

Here are some other suggestions for teaching when you don't have much time to plan.

- *Preprinted plans.* Many facilities have preprinted teaching plans for common problem areas, such as "Controlling Diabetes," "Living with Multiple Sclerosis," and "Coping with Hearing Loss." Although these save time, they're not tailored to the individual patient. If you use teaching plans prepared by others, be sure to adapt them to suit the learning needs and abilities of each patient.

- *Teaching plan resource books.* If there are no preprinted plans, consult teaching plan resource books. These may contain the information you need in an outline form. You can take material from these sources and transfer it to the format that's used in your office. Then, you can add your own comments to fit the patient's needs.

Using commercially prepared materials to start a teaching library will give you much of the information you need right at your fingertips.

ELEMENTS OF A TEACHING PLAN

No matter what the design, all teaching plans need these elements:

- *Learning goal.* This is a description of what the patient should learn from your teaching.

- *Material to be covered.* This should include all the major topics you will teach.

- *Learning objectives.* These are the steps or procedures the patient needs to understand or demonstrate to meet the learning goal.

- *Evaluation.* You need to describe how you will measure the patient's progress.

- *Comments.* The plan should include a place for remarks about circumstances that may be preventing the patient from reaching the learning objectives. It also includes how the patient is meeting the objectives and revisions to the teaching plan.

ADAPTING TEACHING MATERIAL

A huge amount of material is available for patient education. Although the physician or office may provide much of the material you use, you may be responsible for selecting some teaching aids. Here are several things to consider when choosing this material:

Teaching Plan: 32-year-old female with Iron Deficiency Anemia
Patient Learning Goal: Increase patient's knowledge of Iron Deficiency Anemia, its complications, and treatments
Material to be Covered: Description of disorder, complications, diet, medications, procedures

Learning Objectives Comments	Teaching Methods/Tools	Procedure Explained/Demonstrated Date/Initial	PT Demonstrated/ Objectives Met Date/Initial
1. Patient describes what happens when body's demand for oxygen is not met. a. oxygen and hgb concentration decrease b. signs/symptoms of anemia c. anemia occurs only after body stores of iron are depleted	Instruction		
2. Patient describes complications caused by decrease of oxygen concentration a. chronic fatigue b. dyspnea c. inability to concentrate, think d. decrease in tissue repair e. increase of infection f. increase in heart rate	Instruction		
3. Patient discusses importance of diet in prevention of iron deficiency anemia a. including iron-rich foods in diet (beef, poultry, green vegetables) b. including foods that contain ascorbic acid to assist in absorbing iron in body (fruits) c. importance of limiting large meals if fatigued; stress importance of several small meals	Instruction/Video: "Your Diet: Why It Is Important"		
4. Patient describes prescribed medication, its purpose, dosage, route, and side effects	Instruction/Pamphlet: *Taking Your Iron Supplements*		
5. Patient aware of importance of follow-up appointments for evaluation of prescribed plan of treatment	Instruction/Appointment slip with next scheduled appointment		

Here's an example of a teaching plan. Note that it contains all the elements of a good plan. Also note that it provides a place to document the teaching and evaluation of each learning objective.

- The material should be clear and easy to read. Look at its format (physical appearance on the page), headings, illustrations, vocabulary, and writing style.
- Make sure the information in commercial materials is accurate and truthful.
- Be sure the information in any outside source you use agrees with your office's policies and procedures.

A good rule of thumb is to use commercial material only from nationally recognized organizations or government agencies.

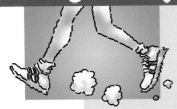

Running Smoothly

CREATING A TEACHING PLAN

There's no teaching plan or outline available on a topic I need to teach. How can I meet my patient's needs?

Sometimes, you may need to create your own teaching materials. Review available resources and teaching aids. Then, adapt the information to benefit your patient. Here are some important things to remember when developing teaching material.

- Include the objective of the information.
- Personalize the information so the patient will want to learn.
- Make sure the information is clear and well-organized.
- Use lists and outlines, which are easier to read and remember than paragraphs.
- Avoid medical jargon as much as possible.
- Focus on the key points.
- Select appropriate printing type or font.
- Use diagrams that are simple, clear, and well-labeled.
- Include names and telephone numbers of people or organizations whom patients can call with further questions.
- Suggest websites or books that have appropriate information.

After patients have been using the material for a while, you should review it to evaluate its effectiveness. If necessary, adjust the material to make it more useful for patients.

Teaching Specific Health Care Topics

Medical assistants' roles in patient education vary greatly. The topics you will teach can depend not only on the patient, but also on your medical office and the physician's wishes. Some of the topics medical assistants teach about include:

- preventive medicine
- medications
- nutrition
- exercise
- alternative medicine
- stress management
- smoking cessation
- substance abuse
- diseases, such as hypertension and diabetes

You'll find general steps for instructing patients about health maintenance and disease prevention in the Hands On procedure on page 439.

PREVENTIVE MEDICINE

Preventive medicine is the branch of medicine that's concerned with promoting health and avoiding disease. Preventing health problems is the key to living a long, healthy life. As a medical assistant, you have two important roles in preventive medicine:

- promoting preventive screenings
- teaching safety tips to prevent injury

Many hospitals and clinics offer free preventive screenings for patients. Public health departments also may have this service available. Your office should keep a list of which free screenings are available.

In addition to free screenings, you should recommend:

- regular physical examinations for all age groups
- annual flu and regular pneumonia vaccinations
- adult immunizations for tetanus, influenza, and hepatitis A and B
- childhood immunizations
- regular dental checkups
- regular blood pressure checkups
- monthly breast self-examinations for women

- mammograms on a regular basis for certain groups of women
- annual Papanicolaou (Pap) tests for women
- bone density tests for women
- monthly testicular self-examinations for men
- prostate-specific antigen (PSA) blood tests for all men, along with the need for regular digital rectal examinations

TEACHING SAFETY TIPS

Another large part of preventive medicine is teaching safety tips. Preventable injury is the leading cause of death in people between the ages of 1 and 21. In addition, about 25 percent of children will require at least one emergency room visit for treatment of a preventable accident during childhood. Preventable injuries and deaths can arise from:

Toys can cause injury when they are broken or used by a child who's too young for them.

- bicycle and car accidents
- poisoning
- fires
- choking
- falls
- drowning
- firearms
- lawn mowers

The American Academy of Pediatrics (AAP) offers injury prevention tips for parents and health care providers. You'll find valuable teaching tips to give to parents from their website. The AAP also provides educational materials that can be mailed to physicians' offices for distribution to patients.

PREVENTING FALLS

One in three adults over age 65 will fall. These falls account for most of the 340,000 patients who are admitted to hospitals each year for hip fractures. Hip fractures require long hospitalizations and often rehabilitation in a nursing home.

Most falls occur at home and are preventable. Fall prevention tips should be taught to all older patients. You also should teach these tips to any patient who has a problem maintaining balance or who uses a device such as a cane or walker.

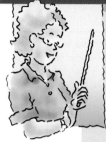

Your Turn to Teach

TEACHING FALL PREVENTION

Offer these tips to older patients and others who are at high risk for falls.

- Encourage patients to remove all scatter rugs in their home. Use double-sided rug tape to keep area rugs in place.
- Remind patients to keep hallways clutter-free.
- Advise patients to ensure adequate lighting in all rooms and hallways.
- Advise patients to avoid steps. Encourage one-floor living.
- Encourage patients to store frequently used items in low shelves and cabinets so they don't need a step stool to get to these items.
- Ensure that patients have well-soled shoes or sneakers. Advise patients to avoid slippers with soft soles. Advise female patients to avoid wearing shoes with heels.
- Instruct patients to place nonskid surfaces in bathtubs and to purchase a shower chair.
- Encourage patients to install handrails or grab bars in bathtubs, hallways, and stairwells.
- Encourage patients to have smoke detectors installed and remind them to change the batteries twice a year.
- Advise patients taking medications that lower their blood pressure to stand up slowly and get their balance before they begin to walk.
- Advise patients to have regular eye examinations and have their glasses adjusted as needed.
- Encourage patients to have a plan for power outages and severe storms.

MEDICATIONS

With new medications available all the time, patient education becomes even more essential. Some medication information comes in package inserts. If this isn't available, the patient may not understand the importance of the medication therapy. This could lead to noncompliance, drug interactions, or other serious side effects. You may be responsible for gathering the information needed and preparing teaching materials for patients. Your teaching will help prevent complications.

When preparing a teaching tool about medication therapy, you need to consider factors such as the patient's financial abilities, social or cultural demands, physical disabilities, and age. Be sure to include the following information in any teaching:

- medication name (generic or brand)
- dosage to be taken
- route of administration
- what the medication is for
- why the medication must be taken as prescribed
- possible changes in bodily functions (for example, colored urine)
- possible side effects
- other medications (including over-the-counter ones and natural supplements) that might interfere with the action of this medication
- foods, liquids, and any medications to be avoided
- activities to be avoided
- a phone number to call for any questions or concerns

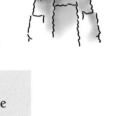

Make sure you cover all the information when teaching about over-the-counter medications, too. Many patients mistakenly think these medications are 100 percent safe, but they can pose dangers.

TEACHING ABOUT SCHEDULING

For patients taking many medications, scheduling can be a prime concern. For example, the patient may be taking several types of medications at different times of the day or week. Evaluate the patient's daily routine to see how a medication schedule will affect his lifestyle. Some questions you might ask the patient are:

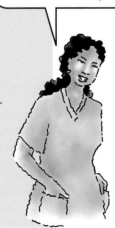

You might need to instruct patients how to administer their medication. You learned about different methods of administration in Chapter 5.

- How late do you sleep each morning?
- What time do you go to bed?
- When do you usually eat?

Once you've collected information about the patient's lifestyle, you can create a scheduling tool. This will help remind your patient what medications to take when.

Pillboxes also can help remind patients to take their medications. Pillboxes are plastic containers prelabeled with the days of the week and times. They're sold in most pharmacies. You may need to instruct the patient on how to fill the pillbox.

NUTRITION

Nutrition is the study of what people eat and how the body uses food to maintain and repair itself. Proper nutrition is important for everyone, not just people who are ill. Here is some basic information you can teach all patients.

- There are no "quick fixes" for losing weight.
- Moderation is key. It's not necessary to totally eliminate favorites like ice cream, candy, or chips.
- A good dinner or meal consists of a rainbow of colors.
- Limit salt and sodium intake.
- Eat three balanced meals a day.
- Avoid eating at least two hours before going to bed.
- Drink plenty of water. Avoid ingesting large amounts of soda or caffeine.

The Food Guide

Materials are available to help you instruct patients about healthy eating. The U.S. Department of Agriculture (USDA) has developed a basic food group system and a Food Guide Pyramid. The USDA system organizes foods into five main groups, plus an extra category for oils.

Grains. *Grains* include any foods made from wheat, rice, oats, cornmeal, barley or other grains (cereals, pasta, bread, tortillas).

Vegetables. *Vegetables* are any raw or cooked vegetable, or 100 percent vegetable juice.

Fruits. *Fruits* include any fruit or 100 percent fruit juice.

Milk and Milk Products. *Milk and milk products* consist of all milk fluids (including flavored milks) and different products made from milk, such as cheese or yogurt.

Meats and Beans. *Meats and beans*, often called proteins, include different kinds of meats as well as poultry, fish, eggs, nuts, seeds, and legumes.

Oils. *Oils* are fats that are liquid at room temperature. This group includes oils that are used for cooking, such as canola oil or corn oil, as well as oils used for flavorings (for example, sesame oil). The group also includes foods that are naturally high in oils, such as olives, nuts, avocados, and some fish.

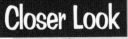

GETTING GOOD GRAINS

Although there are many kinds of grains, not all have the same nutritional benefits. Patients need to be aware that there are two main types of grains.

- *Whole grains* refers to the entire grain kernel. These include brown rice, products made with whole wheat flour, oatmeal, and bulgur.

- *Refined grains* have been processed. Processing gives the grains a longer shelf life and a finer texture. But products made with refined grains contain fewer nutrients than products made with whole grains. Examples of refined-grain products include most cornmeal products, pita, couscous, and products made with white flour.

Some products are made with a mixture of whole and refined grains. Many refined grain products have vitamins added to them. These are referred to as **enriched.** Teach patients to check the ingredient list for the word *enriched* on products made with refined grains.

Teaching with a Personal Food Pyramid

The amounts of food needed from each food group vary depending on a person's age, gender, and activity level. The USDA website allows you to create an individual food guide pyramid for anyone more than two years old. The website also includes a general food pyramid and learning information designed specifically for teaching nutrition to children ages 6 to 11. The table on page 418 gives some specific tips for teaching adult patients about different food categories.

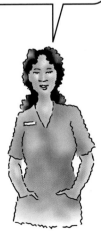

When you're teaching nutrition, you can provide patients with their own personal food pyramid. Visit the USDA's website at www.mypyramid.gov.

General Dietary Guidelines

In addition to the food guide and food pyramid, the USDA and the U.S. Department of Health and Human Services have general guidelines for improving diet. Here are some of the key recommendations.

- Choose a variety of foods from the five basic food groups.
- Maintain a healthy weight by balancing the food you eat with physical activity.

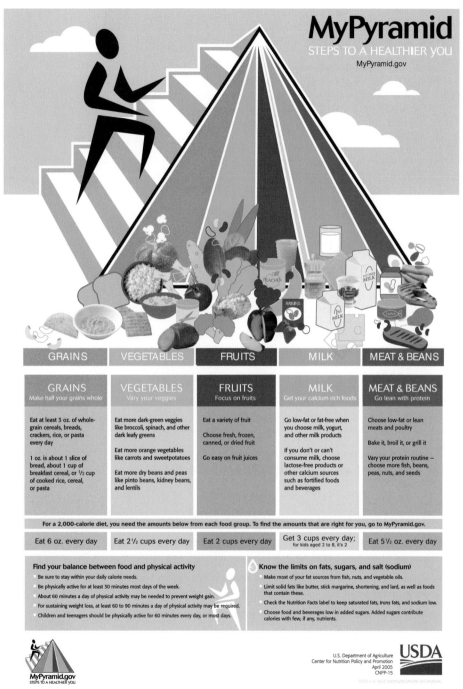

The Food Pyramid consists of six main food groups. The widths of the colored food group bands show the proportion of food that should be chosen from each group.

Teaching Tips for Food Group Categories

Food Group	What to Teach Patients
Grains	• At least half of the grains eaten each day should be whole grains. • Eat three or more ounces of whole grain products per day. Look for *whole* before the word *grain* on the ingredient list. • Avoid croissants, biscuits, sweet rolls, and pastries. • The best cereals are oat, bran, and whole grain cereal. Avoid frosted or sweet cereals.
Milk	• Use skim or 1% milk. Avoid creams and buttermilks. • Eat low-fat cheeses, such as 1% cottage cheese. • Choose low-fat or nonfat yogurt.
Fruits	• Eat a variety of fruits each day. Canned, frozen, and dried fruits are all acceptable. • When choosing canned fruits, look for fruits canned in water or fruit juice instead of syrup. • Avoid drinking too many fruit juices. Fruit juices should be less than half of the total fruit intake.
Vegetables	• Choose a variety of vegetables each day. Try to eat vegetables from different groups (dark green, orange, starchy vegetables, legumes, other vegetables) several times a week. • Fresh, frozen, or canned vegetables all count. Low-salt or no-salt versions of canned vegetables are best.
Meats and Beans	• Choose low-fat or lean meats and poultry. Use USDA-select grade beef, and avoid beef with large amounts of marbling (fat). • Limit bacon to small serving sizes and limit its frequency. • Use preparation methods that don't add fat, such as roasting, broiling, or grilling. • Fish should be fresh. Cook unbreaded and avoid sauces. Good fish choices are salmon, trout, and herring.
Oils	• Limit solid fats like butter, shortening, stick margarine, and lard. • Choose low-fat snacks such as air-popped popcorn, pretzels, and rice cakes to avoid saturated or trans fats. • Use low-fat versions of salad dressings and mayonnaise.

- Keep your diet low in saturated fats and keep trans fats as low as possible.
- Choose a diet with plenty of vegetables, fruits, and whole grain products.
- Prepare and choose foods with little salt or added sugar.
- Drink alcoholic beverages in moderation.

Food Labels

When teaching patients about nutrition, you need to encourage them to read the labels on food containers. These labels provide several important pieces of information:

- the nutritional value of the product
- the specific ingredients that were used
- what additives are in the food

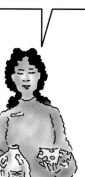

Calcium is an essential mineral for preventing osteoporosis, or loss of bone density. Be sure patients are taking in enough calcium when you assess their diets.

All information on food labels is based on the portion or serving size. Remind patients that if they eat double the portion, they need to double the nutritional facts. The serving size is at the top of the label. Below the serving size is the number of servings per container. For certain foods, it's easy to determine the serving size. The label may say two cookies or one slice of bread. In other cases, it may be more difficult. Generally, serving sizes are listed in grams.

When teaching about the nutritional facts on a label, you should point out the key information on the label that patients should look for. You'll find exact steps for teaching patients how to read food labels in the Hands On procedure on page 440.

SIZING UP PORTIONS

Teach your patients these simple rules for measuring.

- 50 grams of cheese is about the size of 2 thumbs.
- 50 to 100 grams of meat is about the size of the palm of an adult's hand.
- One cup of raw greens or salad is about the size of a fist.

Fats. Total fat is the first nutritional fact on the food label. It lists the total grams of fat in one serving.

The average diet consists of 2,000 calories per day. Each gram of fat contains 9 calories. On a 2,000-calorie diet, the maximum grams of fat per day should be less than 65, with less then 20 grams of saturated fat. Teach patients to add their total grams of fat per day.

The label also will list a percentage number. The percentage refers to what percent of allowed fat is contained in one serving. However, most patients will find it easier to add up the total grams of fat they eat instead. Different kinds of fat also are listed under the total fat heading on the label. Remind patients to look for foods that are low in saturated and trans fats.

Carbohydrates. Carbohydrates are the sugars and starches found in many foods. They are converted to simple sugars in the body to provide energy for body cells. Any portion of sugar the body doesn't use is stored as fat.

The nutrition label tells how many carbohydrates are in each serving. Each gram of carbohydrates contains 4 calories. Based on a 2,000-calorie diet, the total carbohydrates per day should not exceed 300 grams. Patients should add their total carbohydrate intake for 24 hours. It's essential that patients learn to count carbohydrates if they have diabetes.

Carbohydrates also include **fiber** (also called roughage). Fiber is the parts of fruits and vegetables that can't be digested. It helps digestion by stimulating peristalsis—muscle contractions that push food through the digestive tract. It also helps lower blood cholesterol levels (LDL).

Sodium, Cholesterol, and Protein. Amounts for these nutrients are also listed on food labels. Patients with special diets can use this information to determine how much of a particular nutrient they're eating. Amounts are listed in grams per serving, as well as by the percentage of the nutrient in an average 2,000-calorie diet. Each gram of protein contains 4 calories.

Large fast food chains will have this information available at each of their stores. You should encourage your patients to ask for and read this information.

Vitamins and Minerals. Food labels also list percentages for vitamins and minerals. These percentages show how much of the daily recommended amount of a vitamin or mineral is contained in a serving. Recommended amounts are different for each vitamin and mineral. Food labels are not required to show all the vitamins and minerals in the food.

Nutrition Facts

Serving Size ¹/₁₂ package
(44g, about 1/4 cup dry mix)
Servings Per Container 12

Amount Per Serving	Mix	Baked
Calories	190	280
Calories from Fat	45	140

	% Daily Value**	
Total Fat 5g*	8%	24%
Saturated Fat 2g	10%	13%
Cholesterol 0mg	0%	23%
Sodium 300mg	13%	13%
Total Carbohydrate 34g	11%	11%
Dietary Fiber 0g	0%	0%
Sugars 18g		
Protein 2g		

Vitamin A	0%	0%
Vitamin C	0%	0%
Calcium	6%	8%
Iron	2%	4%

* Amount in Mix
** Percent Daily Values are based on a 2,000 calorie diet. Your daily values may be higher or lower depending on your calorie needs:

		Calories:	2,000	2,500
Total Fat	Less than		65g	80g
Sat Fat	Less than		20g	25g
Cholesterol	Less than		300mg	300mg
Sodium	Less than		2,400mg	2,400mg
Total Carbohydrate			300g	375g
Dietary Fiber			25g	30g

Calories per gram:
Fat 9 • Carbohydrate 4 • Protein 4

This food label shows all of the important nutrition facts.

Closer Look

THE FACTS ON FATS

Small amounts of some fats and oils are necessary for good health. Fats store fuel and supply energy to the body. They also contain essential **fatty acids**, substances that are necessary to repair and maintain body cells. Fatty acids help the body absorb some vitamins, such as vitamin A and vitamin D.

However, some fats are associated with heart disease, stroke, or other illnesses. Fats in the diet can affect the levels of **cholesterol** in the blood. Cholesterol is a fatty substance that is used by the body to produce hormones. It's carried by substances called lipoproteins. High-density lipoproteins (HDL), also called "good cholesterol," protect against cardiovascular diseases. But low-density lipoproteins (LDL), also known as "bad cholesterol," may form deposits called plaque on artery walls. By choosing the right fats in the diet, you can lower the risk of cardiovascular diseases.

- *Unsaturated fats* are the best choices for healthy eating. They are found in products made from plant sources, including vegetable oils, seeds, and nuts, and some fish. Unsaturated fats may be called *monounsaturated* (canola, olive, and peanut oils) or *polyunsaturated* (sunflower, corn, soybean oil) on food labels. Both types of unsaturated fats can reduce the risk of heart disease.

- *Saturated fats* typically are found in products that are solid at room temperature. They are found in meat, seafood, egg yolks, and dairy products made with whole milk. They are also found in products made with coconut, coconut oil, or palm oil. Saturated fats raise the levels of LDL ("bad" cholesterol) in the blood.

- *Trans fats* are created when hydrogen is added to vegetable oil during a food-manufacturing process. The ingredient lists on food products list them as hydrogenated or partially hydrogenated fats and oils. Trans fats are found in baked goods like crackers, cookies, and other snack foods, as well as in shortening and some margarine. Like saturated fats, diets with high levels of trans fats increase the risk of cardiovascular disease.

Patients who have a balanced diet will take in enough vitamins and minerals in the foods they eat. It's important to emphasize that patients eat a variety of foods from the basic food groups. Sometimes processing, storing, or cooking can reduce the vitamin content of foods. The physician may recommend a daily multivitamin to be sure the patient is getting the proper amounts of vitamins and minerals.

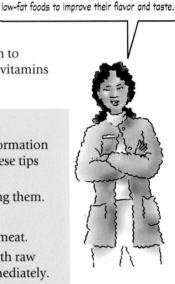

Explain to patients that "fat-free" or "low fat" on the label doesn't guarantee that a food is healthy. Manufacturers often add extra carbohydrates to low-fat foods to improve their flavor and taste.

HEALTHY FOOD PREPARATION

After discussing healthy foods, provide some information about healthy food preparation. Give patients these tips for preparing healthy foods:

- Broil, bake, roast, or grill meats instead of frying them.
- Trim the fat from beef.
- Use a cooking rack so fat drips away from the meat.
- Remove the skin from chicken. Use caution with raw chicken. Wash hands and cutting surfaces immediately.
- Homemade soups or gravies should be chilled after they're cooked. Then, skim the fat off the top and reheat to use.
- Use unsaturated oils (canola, corn, sunflower). Use non-stick spray when possible. Avoid saturated oils (butter, lard).

Other Dietary Considerations

As with any patient teaching, you need to consider several factors before sending a patient home with a preprinted diet form. Some factors that influence how well a patient complies with dietary changes are:

- age
- culture
- religion
- geographic background
- social and financial circumstances

Some patients may have questions about vegetarian diets. Vegetarian diets typically have low levels of saturated fat and high levels of fiber and vitamins. There are three types of vegetarian diets.

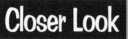

MODIFYING DIETS FOR MEDICAL CONDITIONS

Diets that limit or balance the intake of specific nutrients are used to treat some diseases. Some examples are listed in the table below.

Special Diets for Medical Conditions

Type of Diet	Description	Disease
Bland diet	Foods that contain irritating chemicals (peppers, spices, caffeine) or bulky fiber are eliminated.	gastrointestinal disorders
Diabetic diet	Food intake is controlled to keep blood glucose levels under control. Foods are grouped according to protein, carbohydrates, and fats.	diabetes mellitus types 1 and 2
Elimination diet	Specific foods are limited (for example, milk, eggs, wheat).	food allergies
Low sodium diet	Foods that are high in sodium are eliminated (for example, avoid processed foods and canned vegetables with added salt).	hypertension (high blood pressure)

- **Lacto-ovovegetarian** means that a diet of vegetables is supplemented with milk, eggs, and cheese.
- **Lactovegetarian** means the diet is supplemented only with milk and cheese.
- Pure **vegetarian** means that the diet is only vegetables and excludes all foods of animal origin.

Other patients may require special diets to help treat an illness or disease. The patient's normal diet is assessed and then modified. A specific nutrient may need to be limited through careful diet planning.

EXERCISE

Exercise can be any activity that uses muscles to help maintain fitness. If done in moderation, there are several reasons why it benefits the body:

- maintains healthy body weight
- increases circulation

- strengthens the heart and lungs
- increases muscle tone
- keeps bones strong
- decreases stress and helps patients manage depression
- helps patients sleep better

All patients should get some form of exercise on a regular basis. Patients who are under age 35 and in good health usually don't need medical clearance before starting a routine exercise program. However, a physician consultation is recommended for patients aged 35 or older who have not been active in several years. Patients with known medical disorders also should check with the physician before exercising. These disorders include:

- hypertension
- cardiovascular problems
- family history of strokes

Pregnant patients should consult their obstetrician before beginning an exercise program.

RANGE-OF-MOTION EXERCISES

If patients are unable to perform exercises without assistance, it may be necessary to instruct them or their family members on **range-of-motion** (ROM) exercises. In these exercises, the patient moves the affected limb or joint through all of the movements that the joint is capable of making, until resistance is met.

In most cases, ROM exercises are ordered by the physician to prevent further loss of motion or disfigurement after a musculoskeletal injury, surgery, or neurological damage. ROM exercises are performed several times a day on each involved joint.

Some patients are unable to perform any exercise on the affected area. In that case, passive ROM is performed. This requires someone else to exercise the limb or joint for the patient. ROM exercises help promote blood circulation and improve muscle tone. If they're not performed as ordered, the patient may not be able to regain use of the affected area.

Some of the motions that you are likely to see in practice include:

- abduction—the movement of a body part or limb away from the body or axis of limb; for example, lifting the leg laterally away from the body
- adduction—the movement of a body part or limb toward the body or axis of the limb; for example, returning one leg toward the other leg and lifting beyond it if possible
- flexion—the movement that brings two parts of the body closer together or closes joints; for example, bending fingers to make a fist
- extension—the movement that spreads apart two parts of the body or opens joints; for example, straightening fingers out
- rotation—the movement of a body part or limb around its axis; for example, moving the head from side to side bringing chin toward shoulder

Patients with a major loss of motor skills often will be referred to physical therapy or occupational therapy for intense ROM teachings. In these cases, your role will be to assess their compliance in going to their therapy appointments and to provide positive reinforcement.

ALTERNATIVE MEDICINE

Alternative medicine is health care practices that are used instead of standard medical treatments. Some ancient remedies that were once dismissed by Western medicine have proven to be beneficial in some circumstances. There are many kinds of alternative medicine. Let's look at four of the most common therapies.

Acupuncture

Acupuncture is one of the oldest forms of Chinese medicine. It's based on the principle that there are 2,000 acupuncture points in the human body. These points are connected throughout the body by 12 pathways called meridians. When the meridians are triggered, they conduct energy, or qi (pronounced "chee"), in the body. The trigger comes in the form of very thin needles that are inserted at certain acupuncture points. When a meridian is stimulated, it prompts the brain to release certain chemicals and hormones.

Acupuncture is used to treat many conditions. Here are some of the more common ones:

- addictions, such as smoking
- fibromyalgia
- osteoarthritis
- asthma
- chronic back pain

Acupuncture is also sometimes used to treat children with attention deficit/hyperactivity disorder (ADHD). About 40 states require that acupuncturists be licensed to practice. Training and licensing requirements vary by state.

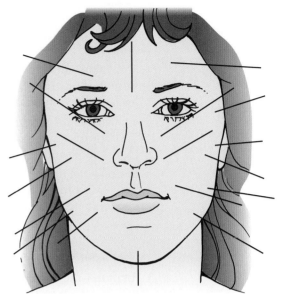

Here's an example of acupuncture needles placed in a patient's face.

Acupressure

Acupressure is similar to acupuncture, but it does not use needles. The practitioner applies pressure to the meridians through direct touch. Acupressure has several uses:

- to treat nausea and vomiting associated with chemotherapy
- to ease chronic pain
- to boost the immune system

Training and requirements vary among states.

Hypnosis

On television, hypnosis is portrayed as a magical method for reaching the inner workings of the brain. However, when conducted properly, there are some health care benefits. Here are some of its most common uses:

- in weight loss programs
- treating obsessive-compulsive disorder (OCD)
- for smoking cessation

In most areas, licensure is not required. Training varies greatly from state to state.

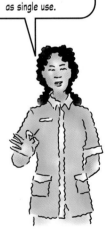

In 1996, the Food and Drug Administration required that all acupuncture needles be labeled as single use.

Yoga

Yoga is useful for relieving stress and improving flexibility. It involves a mix of physical exercises, posture, breathing exercises, and meditation. There are many types or forms of yoga.

HERBAL SUPPLEMENTS

Many people think of herbal supplements as "natural" and therefore, safe. However, the Food and Drug Administration (FDA) does not regulate herbal supplements and similar substances. Patients need to understand that there's been no formal government testing or approval of these substances. Without testing, many aspects of herbal supplement use are unclear, including:

- What are appropriate dosages?
- What side effects may exist?
- What potential interactions with other substances may exist?
- What are the possible benefits of these supplements?

There's also no guarantee that what the label claims is in the bottle is actually there.

The quality and purity of herbal supplements can vary greatly, depending on the manufacturer. Advise patients who wish to use them to buy only supplements that are stamped with a U.S. Pharmacopeia bar code. This bar code means that the manufacturing site has met certain standards. However, it does not mean that the supplement has been tested for health care benefits.

The use of some herbal supplements has evolved through folklore, various cultures, or clinical research. In some cases, the supplement may involve an element of the **placebo effect.** The placebo effect is the power of believing that something will make you better when there's no chemical action from the substance that creates a medical benefit.

Some supplements may have scientific studies to document their effects, however. The table below lists some common herbal supplements and their reported benefits.

As a medical assistant, you need to assess whether patients are using any alternative therapies. Your assessment should include the length of time they have used these treatments and

Commonly Used Herbal Supplements

Supplement	Reported Benefit
Echinacea	Treatment of colds; stimulates immune system, attacks viruses
Garlic	Treatment of colds; diuretic; prevention of cardiac diseases
Ginkgo	Increased blood flow to the brain; treatment of Alzheimer's disease
Ginseng	Mood elevator; antihypertensive
Glucosamine	Treats arthritis symptoms; improves joint mobility

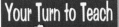

TEACHING ABOUT HERBAL SUPPLEMENTS

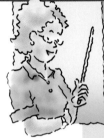

Here are a few general teaching tips on herbal supplements:

- Emphasize that it's important for patients to always tell the physician or other health care provider about any herbal supplements they're taking.

- Caution patients that *natural* products are not necessarily safe. A good example is mushrooms. All mushrooms are natural, but some are very poisonous.

- Teach patients to look for the USP (United States Pharmacopeia) label. Patients also should look for expiration dates on all supplements.

- Advise patients not to depend on health store clerks for information about supplements. They should speak to physicians or pharmacists.

- Caution patients not to trust advertisements that use words like *magical* or *breakthrough* or that claim to *detoxify the whole body.*

- Teach patients to check in with the physician about taking herbal supplements at least two weeks prior to surgery. Tell them they also must advise the surgeon what supplements they've been taking, how much, and for how long. Some supplements can increase bleeding time.

- Warn diabetic patients that many supplements will interfere with blood sugar levels.

- Advise patients to avoid giving herbal supplements to their children unless approved by a physician.

- Advise pregnant or breast-feeding patients to consult with a pharmacist or physician before taking any supplements.

> Patients should seek a physician's approval before taking herbal supplements and other alternative medicine therapies.

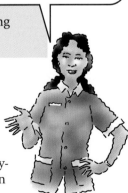

any side effects or benefits the patient has noted. You should report this information to the physician.

STRESS MANAGEMENT

When people are affected by illness or injury, they often experience stress. **Stress** is a state of physiological and/or psychological strain that may disturb normal functioning. It can result from forces such as fear, anger, anxiety, crisis, or joy.

When the body is healthy, it can handle stress more easily. But when dealing with an illness or injury, a patient may face:

- physical pain
- the inability to perform self-care
- treatments, procedures, and possible hospitalization
- changes in self-image and in roles in life
- loss of control and independence
- changes in relationships with friends and family

If patients are able to deal with stress factors, they're more likely to adjust to lifestyle changes. Patients with chronic conditions may need more time to adjust than those with acute illnesses. Also, some patients may not be capable of coping with stress on their own, even with the help of teaching by medical office staff. These patients may need professional counseling.

Positive and Negative Stress

Two types of stress affect all of us—positive stress and negative stress. Positive stress motivates us to work efficiently and to perform to the best of our abilities. Examples of positive stress include:

- working on a challenging new job or project
- getting married
- giving a speech or performance

Many people work best under positive stress. When faced with this kind of stress, our brain releases chemicals that increase our heart rate and breathing capacity. Our body releases stored glucose that gives us an energy boost.

Once a stressful situation is over, we must take time to relax, to prepare for the next one. Positive stress can become negative stress if relaxation techniques aren't part of our daily routine. Negative stress is the inability to relax after a stressful encounter. Left unchecked, it can lead to physical responses such as:

- headache
- nausea and diarrhea
- sweating palms
- insomnia
- malaise
- rapid heart rate

If stress is not relieved, patients will progress to higher anxiety levels. It will require all their energy and attention to focus on the problem at hand. Most mental and physical activity will be directed at relief of the stress. Patients try to avoid the ultimate anxiety level known as **panic**— a sudden, overwhelming state of anxiety or terror.

Long-term physical effects of unrelieved stress include increases in:

- blood pressure
- glucose levels
- metabolism
- intraocular pressure

Stress also can lead to exhaustion.

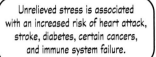

Unrelieved stress is associated with an increased risk of heart attack, stroke, diabetes, certain cancers, and immune system failure.

Dealing with Stress

Most people have developed methods for reducing the effects of intense stress. These methods are referred to as **coping skills.** Usually, we have no conscious control of them. They're a psychological defense against unpleasant situations. Here are some common coping skills.

- *Repression* means the mind blocks uncomfortable or distressing ideas from conscious awareness.
- *Denial* is when a person rejects a fact that's painful or difficult to accept.
- *Rationalization* is the process of finding excuses for thoughts or feelings that would otherwise be hard to accept.

STRESS COPING SKILLS

There are several coping skills you can teach to patients suffering from psychological effects of negative stress. Applying these skills may help them manage their stress.

- Encourage patients to try to reduce stressors (things that cause stress), but make it clear that it's not possible to remove all stressors. Caution them that trying to make everything perfect adds its own stress.
- Encourage patients to organize and limit their activities as needed.
- Try to lessen patients' fear of failure so they just do the best they can.
- Encourage patients to talk to someone when they're feeling anxious or stressed. Talking about their problems allows them to "let off steam."
- Teach patients relaxation techniques to help them regain control over their stressors.

Relaxation Techniques

There are several relaxation techniques that patients might use. To find what works best for them, they must first consider how much time they have and what type of relaxation they need. Three different types of relaxation techniques are:

- breathing techniques
- visualization
- physical exercise

Breathing Techniques. Breathing exercises can be done anywhere. Most people are shallow breathers and need to be instructed on deep-breathing techniques. Deep breathing can get the oxygen flowing through the body at a faster rate. It sometimes can relieve boredom, tension, and stress.

Follow these steps for instructing patients to use deep breathing exercises:

1. Tell the patient to sit up straight and place the hands on the stomach.
2. Instruct the patient to take a deep breath through the nose. The patient should keep breathing in as the hands are pushed away by the stomach. This may feel awkward, because most people try to pull their stomach in when they breathe deeply.
3. Tell the patient to hold the breath for a few seconds.
4. Instruct the patient to exhale through pursed lips. The hands will be pulled in.

This exercise allows for good control of the rate of exhalation.

Visualization. This relaxation technique involves allowing the imagination to run free and focus on positive and relaxing situations. It's similar to "daydreaming." It can help the patient feel removed from a stressful situation and help the mind to relax.

Instruct the patient to find a quiet place, close the eyes, and visualize a soothing scene. Remind the patient that it's important to choose appropriate times for this daydreaming technique.

Physical Exercise. As you read earlier in the chapter, exercise has many health benefits. Another important benefit of exercise is that it relieves tension and anxiety. Most people who exercise regularly say that it helps them relax and rest better at night.

The key to using exercise to manage stress is to find the type of exercise that is right for the individual. Here are some tips to teach your patients.

- The vigorous activity in recreational sports such as squash or tennis can help the body cope with stress.

- Even a brisk 20-minute walk every day can help relieve tension and stress.
- If possible, break up the workday by exercising for a short period of time every 90 minutes. Exercises at work can include stretching, walking up and down stairs, or a short walk outside. A 10-minute break can help relax a person's mind and reduce tension.

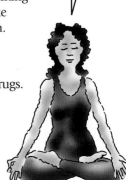

> Don't forget to practice stress reduction and relaxation techniques yourself! A heavy workload can lead to stress or burnout.

SUBSTANCE ABUSE

Substance abuse is the excessive use of and dependency on drugs. Some abused substances are legal (for example, alcohol and nicotine), whereas others are illegal (for example, marijuana and cocaine). Patients affected by commonly abused substances usually work with trained specialists or counselors.

Substance abuse can have serious effects on patients' health. It's important that you give them information about substance abuse if they ask for it. This information may come from various national organizations. You also should have information available about any local organizations or groups that may help these patients.

A patient with a substance abuse problem may need **detoxification** before counseling. Detoxification is the process of clearing drugs out of the patient's body. Factors that affect the detoxification process include:

- the type of substance that's been abused
- the length of time the patient has abused the substance
- the patient's overall level of health
- any physical or mental effects that result from the body's withdrawal from the substance

In some cases, detoxification may require hospitalization.

The most important role of the medical assistant in educating patients about any type of substance abuse is to be supportive.

- Provide positive reinforcements as appropriate.
- Offer services to patients for cessation programs.
- Never condemn a patient for not seeking help. Always be non-judgmental.

Smoking Cessation

Nicotine is highly addictive, whether it's ingested by smoking or chewing. This drug reaches the brain in six seconds. It damages blood vessels, decreases heart strength, and is associated with many cancers. Patients who try to stop smoking experience withdrawal symptoms, such as:

- anxiety
- progressive restlessness
- irritability
- sleep disturbances

Many different methods are used to try to stop smoking. Some programs have the patient stop gradually. Others try a total, abrupt stoppage. There is research data to support both methods.

Here are some suggestions to help patients stop smoking:

- Find local smoking cessation support groups. Provide phone numbers and contact names of these groups to your patients.
- If you don't have a local group, the American Heart Association, American Lung Association, or American Cancer Society may help.
- Discuss with the physician the options of prescribing various patches, gums, or other interventions for the patient. Some products have side effects and the physician may choose not to order them. The decision may be based on the patient's age or other medical illnesses.

Alcohol

Alcohol is chemically classified as a mind-altering substance because it contains ethanol. Ethanol depresses the action of the central nervous system and affects motor coordination, speech, and vision.

Many people use alcohol in moderation. However, in large amounts, alcohol can affect respiration and heart rate. There are also several long-term effects of alcohol use or abuse:

- liver failure
- various types of cancer
- strokes
- nutritional deficiencies

The leading organization for treating alcoholism is Alcoholics Anonymous (AA). Patients complete a 12-step program during recovery. Recovering alcoholics provide many of its support services. AA has many chapters and support services for patients and patient families. There are also special services for teenage alcoholics.

Recovering alcoholics should avoid over-the-counter and prescription medications that contain alcohol. This is a common ingredient in many cough and cold medicines.

Illegal Drugs

Many people assume that users of illegal drugs have criminal tendencies or come from a certain type of background. However, drug abuse affects a wide range of people from different cultures and with different social experiences. The abuse of prescription drugs or the use of illegal drugs can have long-term effects on brain function. It's important to understand drug abuse so you can work to help prevent it.

Drug abuse can affect several areas of an individual's life.

- *Personality changes* might include mood swings, depression, or frequent lying. Some individuals may become verbally or physically abusive.
- *Changes in physical appearance* may be noticeable. Some examples are neglecting personal hygiene, changes in sleeping behavior or activity level, and changes in weight.
- *Changes in social activity* may include withdrawal from family and friends, dropping social connections, or a loss of interest in school and work.

There are also other effects related to the type of drug being abused.

Marijuana. Marijuana and hashish have many effects on the brain and body. Here are just a few:

- impaired short-term memory
- impaired comprehension
- reduced ability to perform tasks requiring concentration or coordination
- increased heart rate
- increased appetite

Long-term users may develop psychological dependence. Because these drugs are inhaled as unfiltered smoke, users take in more cancer-causing agents and do more damage to the respiratory system than with regular filtered tobacco smoke.

Cocaine and Crack. These drugs stimulate the central nervous system and are extremely addictive. Crack cocaine is particularly dangerous. This pure form of cocaine is usually smoked and absorbed rapidly into the bloodstream. It can cause sudden death. The use of cocaine can cause psychological and physical dependency. There are many side effects, such as:

- dilated pupils
- increased pulse rate
- elevated blood pressure
- insomnia

- loss of appetite
- paranoia
- seizures

Cocaine also can cause death by disrupting the brain's control of the heart and respiration.

Amphetamines. Amphetamines and other stimulants boost the central nervous system and have similar effects as cocaine. Some stimulants are legally prescribed to treat medical conditions, such as depression or ADHD. However, when they are abused or used illegally, these drugs can be addictive and dangerous. They cause increased heart rate and blood pressure. Symptoms of stimulant use include dizziness, sleeplessness, and anxiety. Amphetamine use causes:

- psychosis
- hallucinations
- paranoia
- physical collapse (in extreme cases)

The long-term effects of these substances are hypertension, heart disease, stroke, and renal and liver failure.

Depressants. Depressants and barbiturates are sometimes referred to as "downers." That's because they may calm nerves, relax muscles, and have a tranquilizing effect. Chemically, they depress the action of the central nervous system. Use of these substances can cause physical and psychological dependence.

Some depressants are prescribed to treat medical conditions. However, illegal use or abuse of these drugs can have serious effects, such as respiratory depression, coma, and even death. Withdrawal from them can lead to:

Depressants are especially dangerous when taken with alcohol.

- restlessness
- insomnia
- convulsions
- death

Hallucinogens. There are many different types of hallucinogens. These substances interrupt the brain's messages that control thinking and the processing of sensory experiences. They affect individuals by causing them to hallucinate—to hear, see, or feel things that aren't really there. Here are some examples of hallucinogens:

- lysergic acid diethylamide (LSD)
- phencyclidine (PCP or "angel dust")

- mescaline
- peyote

Large doses of hallucinogens can produce seizures, coma, and heart and lung failure. Chronic users complain of memory problems and speech difficulties for up to a year after they stop using the drugs.

One effect of hallucinogens is that they stop the brain's pain sensors. Users can hurt themselves and not even know it.

Narcotics. Narcotics are addictive drugs that relieve pain by preventing pain messages from being sent to the brain. They include natural substances derived from the opium poppy as well as synthetic substances designed to have similar effects. Narcotics may be prescribed to ease pain, to suppress coughing, or to produce anesthesia. Some examples are codeine and morphine.

You read about the regulations for prescribing narcotics (controlled substances) in Chapter 5. Because they are addictive, narcotics are highly susceptible to abuse. Some narcotics are illegal substances, such as heroin. Others are commonly prescribed drugs.

Narcotics have many effects on the body. Here are some of the common ones:

- feelings of euphoria
- drowsiness
- fluctuations in blood pressure
- fluctuations in pulse

An overdose of narcotics can lead to seizures, coma, cardiac arrest, and death.

Many substances of abuse can harm a fetus; some examples include fetal alcohol syndrome and cocaine dependency in babies. Teach all pregnant women about the dangers of these substances to their unborn children.

Secrets for Success

USING INTERNET RESOURCES FOR PATIENT EDUCATION

When you're teaching patients, you'll need to find reliable information to use. Also, patients may want to use the Internet to search for information on their own. It's important to be knowledgeable about websites that will provide solid information based on facts and research. Look for websites with extensions such as *.org*, *.gov*, or *.edu*. Avoid personal or commercial websites (for example, *.com*). The table on the next page shows some websites you can use to search for more information.

Internet Resources for Patient Education

Organization	Website
Alcoholics Anonymous	www.alcoholics-anonymous.org
American Academy of Pediatrics	www.aap.org
American Cancer Society	www.cancer.org
American Heart Association	www.americanheart.org
American Lung Association	www.lungusa.org
Food and Drug Administration	www.fda.gov
Food and Nutrition Information Center	www.nal.usda.gov/fnic
National Center for Complementary and Alternative Medicine	nccam.nih.gov
National Institute of Drug Abuse	www.nida.nih.gov

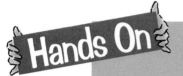

IMPLEMENTING INDIVIDUALIZED TEACHING

7-1

1. Gather your supplies, including the patient's medical record and physician's orders. Read the physician's orders. Clarify any questions you have before you begin.
2. Identify factors that may get in the way of the teaching or learning process.
3. Consult resources for the specific topic you are teaching the patient.
4. Create a set of instructions you can give to the patient. This may involve adapting existing instructions from resources in your medical office. If your teaching involves equipment, include instructions on how to maintain it.
5. After you have prepared your materials, greet and identify the patient. If necessary, involve the patient's parent or legal guardian.
6. Explain the procedure to the patient in a logical, step by step manner.
7. Show the patient how to perform the procedure.
8. Ask the patient to return the demonstration. Provide feedback and positive reinforcement to the patient.
9. Ask questions to check whether the patient has understood the information. You also can use questions to determine whether the patient is compliant.
10. Provide the patient with the prepared instructions and any other materials such as pamphlets, DVDs, or CDs.
11. Document your teaching in the patient's medical record.

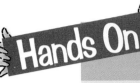

IDENTIFYING AND USING COMMUNITY RESOURCES

7-2

1. Determine what types of resources will be most useful for the patients in your medical office. These may include support groups and/or services for:
   - patients with serious and fatal diseases (for example, cancer, multiple sclerosis)
   - patients suffering from abuse
   - patients who are ill or elderly and need assistance
   - patients with limited financial resources
   - patients who are hearing-impaired or sight-impaired
   - patients with mental disabilities
   - patients with chronic diseases

2. Compile a contact list of resources you can use to find out about community services. Your list may include:
   - social service departments at hospitals
   - local public health departments
   - nursing home associations
   - local charities and church organizations
   - community services in the phone book
   - websites

3. Contact the resources to determine what services they offer. Create a list of services available. Include addresses, e-mail addresses, websites (if available), and phone numbers. Store this master list on your office computer.

4. When needed, use this master list to create a list of services specific to your patient's needs. Answer any questions your patient may have about the services available.

5. Offer to make contact with the service for your patient. However, some patients may prefer to do this for themselves. Be sensitive to your patient's wishes.

6. Document in your patient's chart that you provided the information.

Charting Example:
03/04/2007 2:30 P.M. Provided pt. with list of support groups for alcohol abuse. Pt. verbalized understanding. Pt. states he will contact one of the support groups within 7 days. Pt. will contact the office if he has any questions or concerns.

_____ C. Perez, CMA

Hands On

TEACHING PATIENTS ABOUT HEALTH CARE AND DISEASE PREVENTION

7-3

1. Gather your supplies, including the patient's medical record and physician's orders.
2. Identify topics for educating the patient about health and disease.
3. Identify factors that may hinder the teaching or learning process.
4. Consult resources and gather materials for teaching the patient about the specific topic. Collect any printed materials or pamphlets that you can give to the patient.
5. Create an oral presentation that will cover the key points of the topic.
6. After you have prepared your teaching, greet and identify the patient.
7. Present the information to the patient. Follow a logical order and speak in a clear, sincere tone of voice. It's important not to "talk down" to the patient.
8. Ask open-ended questions to check whether the patient has understood the information. You also can use questions to determine whether the patient is compliant.
9. Provide the patient with supplemental materials such as pamphlets, DVDs, or CDs.
10. Document your teaching in the patient's medical record.

Charting Example:
02/08/2007 10:40 A.M. Discussed nutrition and food preparation with pt. Pt. verbalized understanding. Provided pt. with copies of food group guidelines and cooking tips.

_____ B. Schultz, RMA

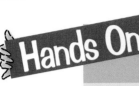

USING FOOD LABELS TO TEACH NUTRITION INFORMATION

7-4

1. Gather your supplies, including examples of low-fat foods and snack foods, the patient's medical record, paper, printed information such as cooking or shopping tips, and a pencil.

2. Greet the patient by name. Explain that you are going to show the patient how to use the nutritional information on food labels for shopping and meal planning.

3. Ask the patient what label information they usually notice when shopping for foods. This helps you assess what the patient knows about food labels.

4. Using one of the foods as an example, explain the different nutrients listed on the food label. Be sure to discuss the importance of looking at the serving size.

5. Ask the patient to choose two foods. Have the patient compare the two foods by looking at the food labels and writing down nutritional facts such as:
   - serving size
   - total number of calories
   - sugar content (carbohydrates)
   - total fats
   - amount of fiber

   Writing down the information will involve the patient in the learning process.

6. Discuss the significance of the different types of fats in the diet. Ask the patient to look at the sample foods and find an example of a food that is low in saturated fats and a food that is high in saturated and trans fats. Remind the patient about the importance of a low-fat diet.

7. Have the patient tell you how to use label information when shopping for foods. This allows you to evaluate the patient's level of understanding. Provide feedback and discussion as necessary.

8. Provide the patient with printed materials to take home for reference.

9. Document the teaching in the patient's medical record.

Charting Example:
01/09/2007 1:50 P.M. Discussed nutrition and food labeling. Pt. demonstrated knowledge of nutritional facts and verbalized understanding. Gave pt. printed materials on low-fat diets.

_____ M. Jones, CMA

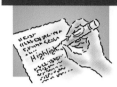
Chapter Highlights

- Medical assistants have an important role in patient education. They teach patients information about health care and disease prevention. They also help patients to accept their illnesses and provide support and encouragement.
- Effective patient education requires a teaching plan. Five main steps in the teaching plan are assessment, planning, implementation, evaluation, and documentation.
- Medical assistants use different strategies to implement the teaching plan. Some of these are lectures, demonstrations, role playing, discussion, audiovisual presentations, and printed materials. Teaching aids such as diagrams, charts, or audiocassettes are useful.
- All teaching must be documented in the patient's medical record. Documentation must include the date and time of teaching, how the information was taught, and an evaluation of the teaching.
- Before they can learn new information, patients need to be motivated or realize they need to learn. Basic needs must be met before patients will be ready to learn health care skills.
- Factors that may be obstacles to learning are existing illness and/or pain, age, educational background, and physical impairments. The medical assistant should try to remove any obstacles to learning.
- Medical assistants often teach preventative medicine. They focus on promoting preventive screenings and teaching safety tips to prevent injury. Teaching patients about medications helps to prevent non-compliance and to avoid drug interactions or other serious side effects.
- Food labels can provide patients with nutritional information. Medical assistants may teach patients to look for the serving size when assessing the nutrients in a food product. Patients with specific medical conditions may need special diets.
- All patients should participate in some form of exercise on a regular basis. If patients are not able to exercise without assistance, range-of-motion exercises may be necessary.
- Alternative medicines may be useful for treating some medical conditions. Four therapies that have proven effective are acupuncture, acupressure, hypnosis, and yoga.
- Herbal supplements are not regulated by the Food and Drug Administration. Medical assistants need to assess whether

patients are using herbal supplements, how long they have been using them, and any reported benefits. This information should be reported to the physician.

- Illness or disease often can lead to stress as patients experience changes in lifestyle, relationships, and anxiety associated with medical procedures. Medical assistants may teach patients about relaxation techniques to cope with stress. Three main relaxation techniques are controlled breathing, visualization, and physical exercise.

- Substance abuse can have serious health effects. Medical assistants provide patients with information from national organizations and may help patients find community resources if they ask for them. The most important role of the medical assistant is to be supportive.

Chapter 8

MEDICAL OFFICE EMERGENCIES

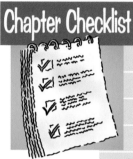

Chapter Checklist

- Identify five duties that may be required of a medical assistant during an emergency

- List the key elements for a medical office emergency action plan

- List seven signs that may indicate an emergency

- Describe the general steps to take after identifying an emergency

- Discuss the steps involved in the primary assessment of a patient in an emergency

- Compare the two methods for opening an airway and explain when each is used

- Describe the steps involved in cardiopulmonary resuscitation (CPR)

- Describe the purpose and use of the automatic external defibrillator (AED)

- Describe the signs, symptoms, and treatment of shock

- Explain how to control severe bleeding from a wound

- Explain how to classify burn injuries and how to assess the extent of a burn using the rule of nines

- Describe the differences between sprains, strains, fractures, and dislocations and explain the emergency treatment for each

- Identify the early symptoms of heart attack

- Explain the signs of seizure and how to manage a seizure patient

- Identify the signs and symptoms of an anaphylactic reaction

- List the information needed before calling a poison control center

- Contrast hyperthermia and hypothermia and list the dangers of each condition

- Discuss the difference between a psychiatric emergency and an emotional crisis

- Describe the steps in managing a patient who has fainted

- Explain the key elements in managing patients with severe diarrhea and severe vomiting

- Explain how to control a nosebleed

- Identify unusual patterns of illness or patient behavior that could suggest bioterrorism

- Explain how and why heat and cold are used in emergency treatments and identify adverse reactions to watch for

A medical emergency can happen anytime, anywhere, and to anyone. Consider the following scenarios.

- A patient getting a routine exam could have a heart attack.
- A patient might have a seizure in the waiting area.
- A staff member could fall and hit her head on something.
- A passer-by might come into the office with a recently sprained ankle.

In this chapter, you'll learn about different types of emergencies that may come up in the medical office. You'll also learn how to handle them effectively.

Emergency Care in the Medical Office

Emergency medical care is immediate care given to persons who are sick or injured. Proper emergency care can sometimes mean the difference between:

- temporary disability and permanent disability
- rapid recovery and a long recovery
- life and death

You're likely to encounter two types of medical emergencies during your medical assisting career.

- medical emergencies suffered by patients or staff while in the medical office
- situations that arise when a patient arrives seeking emergency medical treatment

In general, a medical office should respond to both types of emergencies in one of two ways. For major emergencies, treat the patient until help arrives to handle the situation and transport the patient to a hospital emergency room. For minor emergencies, treat the patient and send him home with instructions for follow-up care.

STEPS FOR HANDLING MEDICAL EMERGENCIES

Providing proper care and treatment in medical emergencies requires medical office workers to take these steps.

1. Correctly identify the emergency.
2. Deliver basic first aid.
3. If needed, provide temporary help or basic life support until an emergency response team arrives.

As a medical assistant, you'll be a valuable member of the team when medical emergencies occur. Here are some of the duties that may be required of you.

- providing basic life support or assisting in life support procedures
- providing or assisting in basic first aid and other treatments
- contacting emergency rescue help and providing information about the situation when they arrive
- documenting emergency treatment delivered by medical office personnel
- calming the patient's relatives, other patients in the office, and any other bystanders during the emergency

The Emergency Action Plan

Every medical office should have an emergency action plan. Here's what the plan should include.

- the local emergency rescue service phone number
- the location of the nearest hospital emergency department

Closer Look

OUTSIDE EMERGENCY TRAINING

This chapter provides an overview of medical office emergencies and how they are handled. It's not a substitute for comprehensive training in emergency care. Your office may provide you with such training, as well as training in its own policies and procedures for handling emergencies. Other training may be available from the following organizations.

- the American Red Cross
- the American Heart Association
- the American Health and Safety Institute
- the National Safety Council

- the phone number of the local or regional poison control center
- the location and list of contents of the emergency medical kit or crash cart
- procedures for various emergencies
- a list of office personnel who are trained in CPR

You should be able to find the emergency action plan in the procedure manual for your medical office. Read it carefully so you know your office's protocol.

As a medical assistant, you should be certified in **cardiopulmonary resuscitation** (CPR). This is a technique to temporarily circulate blood through the body when the heart has stopped. You also should know how to clear a person's airway when it's blocked by an object.

Providing emergency care requires you to coordinate many different events. Emergency situations often can be complicated by added factors. Here are just a few examples.

- panicky family members
- arrival of emergency personnel
- language barriers

You need to stay calm, no matter what happens. You also need to perform your work competently, professionally, and within your scope of practice and state guidelines.

> The American Association of Medical Assistants has required that certified medical assistants show proof of current CPR certification in order to renew their CMA credential.

THE EMERGENCY MEDICAL KIT

Proper equipment and supplies always must be ready in case of a medical emergency. The equipment and supplies in a medical office may vary with the medical specialty. However, emergency equipment and supplies are fairly standard. They should be kept in a place where all staff members can get to them.

Items used during an emergency must be replaced as soon as possible. In addition, a staff member should check the emergency kit or crash cart regularly to make sure:

- all necessary items are present
- items have not passed their expiration dates

WHAT'S IN AN EMERGENCY MEDICAL KIT?

Standard supplies for an emergency medical kit include:

- activated charcoal
- adhesive strip bandages, assorted sizes
- adhesive tape, one- and two-inch rolls
- alcohol (70 percent)
- alcohol wipes
- antimicrobial skin ointment
- chemical ice pack
- cotton balls
- cotton swabs
- disposable gloves, latex
- elastic bandages, two- and three-inch widths
- gauze pads, two-by-two and four-by-four-inch widths
- rolls of self-adhesive gauze, two- and four-inch widths
- safety pins, various sizes
- scissors
- syrup of ipecac
- thermometer
- triangular bandage
- tweezers

In addition to these supplies, the following equipment should be available:

- blood pressure cuff (pediatric and adult)
- stethoscope

- bag-valve mask device with assorted size masks
- flashlight or penlight
- portable oxygen tank with regulator
- suction unit and catheters

If possible, the following additional equipment also could be included:

- various sizes of endotracheal tubes
- laryngoscope handle and various sizes of blades
- automatic external defibrillator
- intravenous supplies (catheters, administration set tubing, assorted solutions)
- emergency drugs (atropine, epinephrine, sodium bicarbonate)

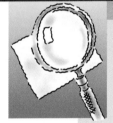

Closer Look

THE EMERGENCY MEDICAL SERVICES SYSTEM

All citizens need access to fast emergency care by specially trained medical staff. Emergency medical services are designed to provide this service.

- *Communities with a 911 system.* Most communities have a 911 system. This allows citizens to report emergencies and call for help by phone. The communications operator at the local EMS station answers these calls. The operator takes information and alerts the EMS, fire, or police department as needed.

- *Communities without a 911 system.* When there is no 911 system, emergency calls usually are made directly to the local ambulance, fire, or police department.

Most major U.S. cities have an enhanced 911 system that automatically identifies the caller's phone number and location. If the telephone is disconnected, or the caller loses consciousness, the communications operator can still send emergency personnel to the scene. You should know what emergency system is used in your community.

RECOGNIZING AN EMERGENCY

You may rarely see some kinds of emergencies in your medical office. However, you still should be aware of the signs. Here are some signs that can indicate an emergency situation.

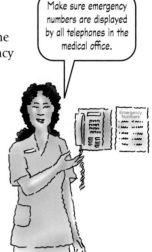

Make sure emergency numbers are displayed by all telephones in the medical office.

- fainting or loss of consciousness
- difficulty breathing or shortness of breath
- chest pain
- choking
- coughing up or vomiting blood
- persistent vomiting
- continuous bleeding or large wound
- change in mental status (confusion, unusual behavior)
- ingestion of a poisonous substance
- head or spine injury
- sudden injury, such as burns, smoke inhalation, a motor vehicle accident, or near drowning

You should be able to recognize when an emergency situation exists and notify emergency medical services (EMS) if it's life threatening or could become life threatening.

WHAT TO DO IN A MEDICAL EMERGENCY

In an emergency, the victim is always your first priority. Once you've identified the emergency, here are the general steps to follow.

1. Provide immediate care to the patient, including CPR if necessary.
2. While you're providing emergency care, direct another staff member to notify the physician.
3. Continue to provide first aid, or assist the physician in providing first aid, as the physician assesses the patient. Direct another staff member to notify EMS unless the physician tells you to do so.
4. When EMS arrives, assist EMS workers as necessary. Let them examine the patient and take over emergency care.

The staff member who calls EMS must be able to describe the emergency to the communications operator. This will tell the operator what level of emergency personnel and rescue equipment to send.

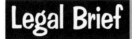

GOOD SAMARITAN LAWS

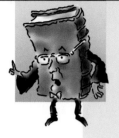

Emergencies can happen anywhere. You may encounter an emergency outside the medical office. Good Samaritan laws protect off-duty health care professionals when they give emergency aid only if they provide care within their scope of practice. These prevent a victim from suing a health care professional for injuries resulting from a genuine attempt to help.

Good Samaritan laws vary from state to state. Most require that you perform as you would for a patient in your office. That is, you must perform only the procedures you've been trained to do. You should know the details of the Good Samaritan laws in your state.

After EMS arrives and takes over patient care, you still have some tasks. First, clear any objects that might get in the way of removing the patient on a stretcher. You also can support any family members who may be present. Family members should be moved to a private room away from the emergency area.

Good communication and cooperation between staff members is critical during an emergency!

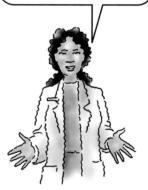

DOCUMENTING THE EMERGENCY

Once other medical staff members have taken over the emergency, you should turn to documenting the events. For example, EMS personnel will need several pieces of information when they arrive:

- the patient's symptoms
- the nature of the emergency
- any treatment already provided
- age
- medications the patient is currently taking
- allergies

Place this information in the patient's medical record. Record events in chronological order as they occurred or as treatments were performed. In some cases, the emergency may involve visitors or staff. Treatment of these persons also must be documented. You can use a blank paper or progress note page to record the details of the emergency and the care provided.

HOW TO DOCUMENT AN EMERGENCY

Whether the victim is a patient, a visitor, or a staff member, the information you record should include:

- basic identification, including the person's name, age, address, and an emergency contact if known
- the chief complaint, if known
- times of events, beginning with recognition of the emergency, management techniques, and changes in the person's condition
- the person's vital signs
- specific emergency management performed in the office. Some examples might be CPR, bandaging, splinting, or any medications given by the office before, during, and after the emergency
- observations of the patient's condition, such as slurred speech, lethargy, or confusion
- any medical history, allergies, or current medications, if known

Taking Emergency Action: The First Steps

In any emergency situation, you have two immediate goals.

- to identify and correct any life-threatening problems
- to provide necessary care

Meeting these goals requires an emergency assessment of the patient. There are three main steps to an emergency assessment. Each step must be managed effectively before proceeding to the next one.

- primary assessment
- secondary assessment
- physical examination

You'll need to survey the scene quickly to identify any hazards to the patient and any clues to the patient's condition.

- Don't assume the obvious injuries are the only ones. Less noticeable or internal injuries also may have occurred.
- Look for the causes of the injury. They may provide a clue to the extent of the physical damage.

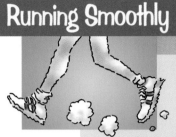

Running Smoothly

WHEN A PATIENT CALLS WITH AN EMERGENCY

What should I do if a patient phones in with an emergency?

Your office should have a policy for evaluating emergency calls. Being familiar with the office policy will help you know what to do. But here are some general guidelines.

Usually, you will put the call through to the physician or office nurse if the caller reports symptoms such as:

- chest pain
- shortness of breath
- loss of consciousness
- severe bleeding
- severe vomiting or diarrhea
- temperature greater than 102 degrees
- severe headache with neck stiffness
- abdominal pain with symptoms of appendicitis

A patient with any of these symptoms most likely will need to go to a hospital emergency room.

Some emergency callers may need to be seen in the office the same day. This can happen when a caller reports:

- a fever for more than two days
- a headache
- a sore throat

Whatever the case, the doctor or nurse will decide what to tell the caller. Your job is to know which calls are emergencies and which are not. Be sure to follow the policies in your office.

For example, a patient who fell down stairs may have a noticeable bump on his forehead. He also may have an injury to the spine that is not as easily noticed.

THE PRIMARY ASSESSMENT

When you reach the patient, do a quick check to assess the situation. The primary assessment is usually done in less than 45 seconds. The purpose is to identify and correct any life-threatening problems. Here's what you must immediately assess:

- *Responsiveness.* Is the patient conscious or unconscious? In some emergencies, the patient may be conscious and able to respond to your voice. If the patient is unconscious, try to wake him or her. Speak and touch the patient's shoulder. If there's no response, assess the patient's airway.

> In any injury involving the head or back, a spinal fracture may be possible. Be careful not to move the patient any more than necessary.

- *Airway.* Is the airway clear? You need to check the patient's airway to be sure it's not blocked. As you'll learn later in this chapter, the method you'll use to open the airway depends on the patient's condition.

- *Breathing.* Once you've determined that the airway is open, evaluate the patient's breathing. For an unconscious patient, look at the patient's chest to see if it's rising and falling. Listen for breathing sounds and feel for air moving out of the patient's mouth or nose. If the patient isn't breathing, start artificial respiration or **rescue breathing** immediately.

- *Circulation.* In adults and children, you evaluate circulation by checking the carotid pulse. For infants, you need to use the brachial pulse. If no pulse is found, you must begin cardiopulmonary resuscitation (CPR) immediately. If a pulse is present, or becomes palpable during CPR, note the rate and quality.

Check the patient's pulse frequently. Evaluate **perfusion,** or blood flow through the tissues, by checking the temperature and moisture of the skin. While assessing circulation, you also should check for any hemorrhage. Control any bleeding quickly.

Once you're sure the patient's heart is beating, you should recheck the patient's breathing. Respirations that are too fast, too slow, or irregular will require medical intervention. Immediate intervention for these conditions may include:

- breathing into a mask or paper bag to treat **hyperventilation** (respirations that are too fast)

- administering oxygen as directed by the physician

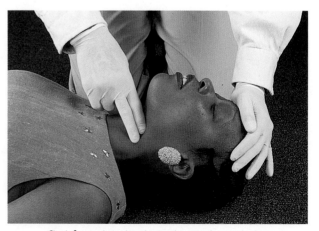

Check for circulation by palpating the patient's carotid pulse.

Any obvious noises, such as stridor (a harsh, high-pitched sound heard when breathing in) or wheezes (continuous high-pitched sounds heard when breathing in and out), are noted and reported to the physician.

Assessing and Opening the Airway

There are two ways to assess the airway. The patient's condition will determine which one you'll use.

- For an unconscious patient, you normally assess the airway using the head tilt-chin lift technique.
- Unconscious patients who may have neck injuries should have the airway opened using the jaw thrust technique.

An unconscious patient who is supine may have a partial or total airway obstruction, if the tongue has fallen back into the oropharynx. This would produce either snoring respirations or a total airway obstruction. In either case, you will need to open the patient's airway to allow for adequate respirations. The table below explains how to do this.

Opening a Patient's Airway

Patient's Situation	Airway-Opening Technique	Description of Technique
Patient is unconscious and unresponsive.	Head Tilt-Chin Lift	Tilt the head backward with one hand on the forehead. Lift the chin forward with the fingers of the other hand.

(continued)

Opening a Patient's Airway (*continued*)

Patient's Situation	Airway-Opening Technique	Description of Technique
Patient is unconscious and may have neck injuries.	Jaw Thrust Technique 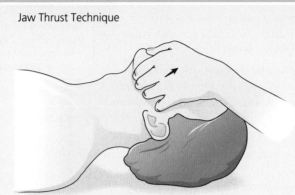	Place your hands on either side of the patient's head. Grasp behind the angle of the jaw with your fingers on both sides, and gently bring the jaw up.

Closer Look DEALING WITH A BLOCKED AIRWAY

The way to help a patient with a blocked airway will depend on the patient's condition. For a conscious patient, first ask, "Are you choking?" If the patient can speak or cough, the obstruction isn't complete. The patient can breathe. Observe the patient closely, and assist as needed. The patient may be able to remove the obstruction without help. Don't perform abdominal thrusts, as this may cause injury to the patient.

For a conscious patient who can't speak or cough:

1. Have a coworker notify the physician and EMS according to office policy.

2. Ask for permission to help the patient.

3. Stand behind the patient. Wrap your arms around the patient's waist.

4. Make a fist with your nondominant hand. Place the thumb side against the patient's abdomen between the navel and the xiphoid process.

5. Grasp your fist with your dominant hand. Give quick upward thrusts. Completely relax your arms

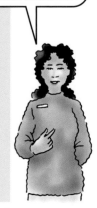

The xiphoid process is a small extension to the lower part of the sternum. It's located at the meeting of the ribs under the sternum.

(continued)

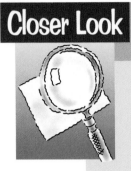

Closer Look

DEALING WITH A BLOCKED AIRWAY (*continued*)

between each thrust. Each thrust should be forceful enough to dislodge the obstruction.

6. Repeat the thrusts until the object is expelled. Several thrusts may be necessary to expel the object. Continue thrusts until the patient can breathe or becomes unconscious.

> Don't perform abdominal thrusts on obese or pregnant patients. They'll require chest thrusts. Also, you shouldn't perform abdominal thrusts on children younger than eight.

If the patient is unconscious or becomes unconscious:

1. Put on clean examination gloves, if available. Perform a tongue-jaw lift. Then perform a finger sweep to clear the mouth area.

2. Open the airway and try to perform rescue breathing. (You can review the rescue breathing procedure later in the chapter.)

3. If rescue breaths are obstructed, begin abdominal thrusts:
   - Straddle the patient's hips.
   - Place the palm of one hand between the patient's navel and xiphoid process.
   - Lace your fingers with the other hand against the back of the properly positioned hand.
   - Give five abdominal thrusts.

> If you can't breathe air into the patient's lungs, keep repeating steps 3 and 4 until you can or until EMS arrives.

4. After performing five abdominal thrusts, repeat the tongue-jaw lift and finger sweep. Attempt rescue breathing again. If rescue breaths ventilate the lungs, continue rescue breathing until the patient resumes breathing or EMS arrives.

Rescue Breathing

In your primary assessment, you'll determine whether the patient is breathing or not. If the patient isn't breathing, here's what to do.

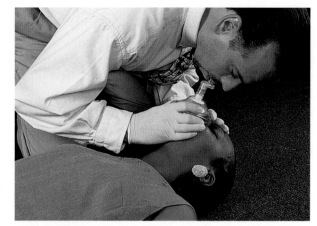

This rescuer is using a bag-mask valve to do rescue breathing on an unconscious patient.

1. Open the patient's airway.

2. With the airway open, use one hand to pinch the patient's nostrils shut. This stops air from escaping through the patient's nose. Rest the heel of the hand on the patient's forehead to help keep the head tilted back.

3. If available, place a one-way CPR valve or bag-mask valve over the patient's mouth. This prevents transmission of disease. If not using a breathing mask, be sure to seal your mouth over the patient's mouth while blowing to prevent the air from escaping.

4. Turn your head to the side. Listen and watch for signs of breathing. If there are no signs of breathing, deliver two long, slow breaths.

5. If the patient's lungs don't inflate, the airway may be obstructed. Reposition th patient's head and give two long, slow breaths again.

6. Check for signs of breathing and check the patient's pulse.
   - If the patient is still not breathing but has a pulse, give one slow breath every five seconds for 12 breaths. Repeat until the patient begins breathing or until EMS arrives. Stop if you are too exhausted or when the patient begins breathing.
   - If the patient has no pulse, you'll need to perform CPR.

Cardiopulmonary Resuscitation

Cardiopulmonary resuscitation is used to keep the patient's blood circulating until the patient can receive appropriate medical care. There are two main components of CPR.

- rescue breathing
- chest compressions

STEPS FOR CARDIOPULMONARY RESUSCITATION

During rescue breathing, you should periodically palpate the patient's carotid artery for a pulse. If there's no pulse, you must continue chest compressions.

1. Before starting CPR, you should tilt the patient's head back and listen for breathing. If the patient is not breathing, pinch his nose and, if available, place a one-way CPR valve or bag-mask valve over the patient's mouth. Give two long, slow breaths. If the patient is not breathing, begin chest compressions.

2. Place hands in the center of the chest, between the nipples.

3. Place the palm of the other hand on top of the hand. Lace your fingers together.

4. Position yourself so your upper body is perpendicular to the patient's chest. Lock your elbows. Press straight down, compressing the chest about 1.5 to 2 inches.

5. Keep your hands in position as you release the compression. You need to allow the patient's chest to completely expand before starting the next compression.

6. Alternate compressions and rescue breathing. After every 30 compressions, give 2 rescue breaths.

7. Continue CPR until EMS arrives or a pulse is palpated. Stop if you are too exhausted or the patient is breathing and has a heartbeat.

Be sure to document the procedure as soon as you can.

Charting Example:
10/14/2007 10:30 A.M. Pt. arrived complaining of chest pain. Skin diaphoretic, color pale. Pulse 125 and regular, BP 88/54 (L.). Collapsed in exam room, Dr. Barton notified. Pulse and respirations absent, CPR started. EMS notified. _____ S. Pencil, CMA
10/14/2007 10:40 A.M. CPR continued per EMS. Pt. transported to General Hospital. _____
_____ S. Pencil, CMA

> If the patient's pulse returns but breathing doesn't, you need to continue with rescue breathing until EMS arrives.

Defibrillation

Some medical offices may have an automatic external defibrillator (AED) as part of the emergency medical kit. **Defibrillation** is the process of using electric shock to restore normal heart rhythm. The AED device shouldn't be used on infants. However, adults and children with life-threatening heart rhythms will have increased changes of survival if defibrillated quickly and appropriately.

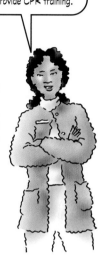

Training to use the AED is offered by many organizations that provide CPR training.

STEPS FOR USING AN AUTOMATIC EXTERNAL DEFIBRILLATOR

The AED is normally used after CPR has been started. Here's a brief summary of the steps involved in using an AED device.

1. While another rescuer performs CPR, remove the patient's shirt. Prepare the chest for electrodes.
   - Remove any medication patches that interfere with placement of the electrodes. Wipe away medication.
   - Make sure the chest is dry so the electrodes will have good contact.
   - Make sure the patient is not in water or is dried off
   - Make sure the patient is not on any metal

2. Stop chest compressions. Remove sticky paper backing and press electrodes onto chest.
   - Place the first electrode on the upper right chest.
   - Place the second electrode on the lower left chest.

3. Connect the wire from the electrodes to the AED. Turn on the AED.

4. The AED will analyze the heart rhythm. Don't touch the patient or perform CPR. Make sure the patient is not moving or in a moving vehicle. Follow instructions on the device.
   - If no shock is indicated, the AED will instruct you to restart CPR. Before you resume, check the patient for respirations and a carotid pulse.
   - If the AED indicates that electrical shock is needed, make sure no one is touching the patient or the examination table. Deliver the electrical shock by pressing the button on the AED.

5. After delivering a shock, begin CPR immediately, starting with chest compressions. Check the victim's rhythm after giving about five cycles of CPR (about 2 minutes).

6. Continue the process until the EMS team arrives.

As with any procedure, defibrillation must be documented.

Charting Example:
11/15/2007 3:15 P.M. Pt. became unresponsive while waiting in reception area; no pulse or respiratory effort. Dr. Barton and EMS notified. CPR started. _____ J. Crete, CMA
11/15/2007 3:20 P.M. AED applied, 2 electrical shocks delivered, pulse returned, no respiratory effort. Rescue breathing resumed. _____ J. Crete, CMA
11/15/2007 3:25 P.M. EMS here. Patient's pulse and respiration returned. R12 P68. Pt. transported to General Hospital. _____ J. Crete, CMA

AEDs can be used for children over the age of one after five cycles of CPR. Ideally, you should use a child-friendly AED with smaller child pads, but if one is not available just use the adult machine.

THE SECONDARY ASSESSMENT

By the end of the primary assessment, you will have checked and corrected the patient's airway, breathing, and circulation. Once this is done, and if EMS or other help has not yet arrived, you need to perform the secondary assessment. Here's what a secondary assessment involves:

- asking the patient questions to get more information
- a more thorough physical evaluation to find less obvious problems

When you evaluate the patient, you'll be assessing four things.

- general appearance
- level of consciousness
- vital signs
- skin

General Appearance

The patient's skin color and moisture, facial expression, posture, motor activity, speech, and state of alertness are all clues to the patient's mental and physical condition. Check for a medical bracelet or necklace. Medicine bottles in a pocket or purse also can give you useful information.

Level of Consciousness

After examining the patient's general appearance, you may have a good indication of his level of consciousness. Many conditions can alter a patient's level of consciousness, such as:

- a decrease in oxygen to the cells of the brain
- neurological damage from a cerebrovascular accident (CVA or "stroke")
- intracranial swelling

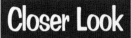

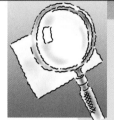

CARDIOPULMONARY RESUSCITATION FOR INFANTS AND CHILDREN

The CPR procedure for infants and children is slightly different from the procedure for adults. Here are the steps to follow.

1. Check for responsiveness. For children, gently shake and call to the child. For infants, flick the bottom of the foot.

2. If the patient is unresponsive, have another person notify EMS.

3. Place the infant or child on her back on a flat surface.

4. Open the airway as described earlier. Don't tilt the head too far back. Doing that could cause airway obstructions in infants.

5. Check for breathing signs. If the patient isn't breathing, begin rescue breathing.
   - For children, pinch the nostrils and breathe into the mouth. If available, use a one-way CPR valve or bag-mask valve.
   - For infants, use your mouth to cover the mouth and nose. If available, use a one-way CPR valve or bag-mask valve.

6. Check for a pulse.
   - For children, check the carotid pulse as you would for an adult.
   - For infants, check the brachial pulse.
   - As you palpate for a pulse, assess the patient's circulation.

7. If you feel a pulse and there are no signs of breathing, continue rescue breathing.
   - For children, give one breath every three to five seconds.
   - For infants, give one breath every three to five seconds.

8. If there's no pulse, begin chest compressions.
   - For children, place your hand in the same position as for adults. Use only one hand. Compress to approximately one-third the depth of the chest. Give compressions at a rate of at least 100 per minute.
   - For infants, use two fingers to compress the middle of the chest just below the nipples. Compress to approximately one-third the depth of the chest. The rate of compressions should be about 100 per minute.

(continued)

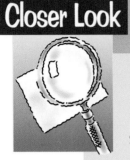

Closer Look

CARDIOPULMONARY RESUSCITATION FOR INFANTS AND CHILDREN (*continued*)

- Give 2 breaths for every 30 compressions if you're delivering CPR on you own. If there are two rescuers attempting CPR on a child, give 2 breaths for every 15 compressions.

9. Every few minutes, check for pulse and signs of circulation. If there's still no pulse, continue CPR until EMS arrives.

> When it comes to CPR, a child is any person between one year of age and the onset of puberty.

Changes in the level of consciousness can be an indication of how well the patient's brain is working.

Vital Signs

The third part of the secondary assessment is taking vital signs, including pulse, respiratory rates, and blood pressure. It's also important to remember to check the patient's temperature. Temperature assessment is essential for:

- patients who have altered skin temperature
- patients who have been exposed to extreme environment conditions
- patients with a history of infection, chill, or fever
- children with seizures

Skin

You'll have already noted the temperature and moisture of the skin during the primary assessment. A more thorough look is performed in the secondary assessment. Skin is normally dry and somewhat warm. Moist, cool skin may indicate poor blood flow to the tissues and likely, shock. The color of the skin provides information about:

- circulation near the surface of the body
- oxygenation of tissues

The table on page 463 summarizes what various skin colors can mean.

PHYSICAL EXAMINATION

After the primary and secondary assessments are done, the patient should be examined from head to toe. The physician

Abnormal Skin Colors and Their Causes

Skin Color	Possible Causes	Possible Conditions
pink	vasodilation increased blood flow	heat illness hot environment exertion fever alcohol consumption
white, pale	decreased blood flow decreased red blood cells vasoconstriction	shock fainting anemia cold exposure
blue	inadequate oxygenation	airway obstruction congestive heart failure chronic bronchitis

yellow	increased bilirubin (a waste product formed
	   by the liver when breaking down red
	   blood cells)
	retention of urinary elements
		liver disease
		
		renal disease

usually performs this examination, but you should be prepared to assist. It's important for you to keep providing reassurance to the patient.

Head and Neck

If a cervical spine injury is suspected, the patient's spine must be immobilized immediately. Also avoid moving the neck when the head is examined. The head examination should include:

- inspecting the face for edema, bruising, bleeding, and drainage from the nose and ears
- examining the mouth for loose teeth and dentures
- inspecting the eyes with a flashlight or penlight

Checking the pupils of the eyes can show the condition and severity of a neurological injury. This can help to assess patients with altered consciousness. The pupils should be checked for several characteristics.

- equality in size
- dilation bilaterally in darkness or in dim light
- rapid constriction to light in both eyes
- equal reaction to light

To evaluate the pupils, you or the physician must shade the eyes from the light. A small flashlight or penlight is held six to eight inches from each eye. A conscious patient should not look

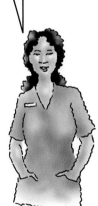

To _immobilize_ something means to prevent it from moving.

Closer Look · CERVICAL FRACTURES

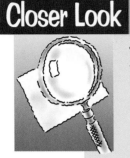

The degree of injury to the patient depends on which cervical vertebrae have been fractured. There are seven cervical vertebrae in the neck.

- *C-1.* Fractures to the first cervical vertebra are often fatal. They must be treated immediately and aggressively by EMS before the patient is transported to the hospital.

- *C-2 and C-3.* Fractures to the second and third cervical vertebrae often result in permanent or long-term respiratory dependency.

- *C-4 to C-7.* Fractures of the fourth to seventh cervical vertebrae usually result in different levels of paralysis and motor impairment.

If you think a patient has a cervical or spinal fracture, keep the patient still and call for EMS. Don't move the patient unless the patient is in immediate danger.

directly into the light. If you perform the examination, you should report the findings to the physician.

Chest, Back, and Abdomen

You may have examined the chest somewhat when you checked for respirations. You may need to remove clothing from the chest for a more thorough examination. Patients who should have a more thorough examination include:

- patients with trauma
- patients with abnormal vital signs
- patients with cardiac or respiratory complaints

Palpation of the chest and back also may reveal possible fractures.

The abdomen of all patients is examined. This examination is particularly important for these types of patients:

- patients with GI symptoms
- patients with vaginal bleeding
- patients with vomiting
- patients with melena (blood in the stool)

The abdomen is inspected for scars, bruises, and masses.

> A distended abdomen may indicate hemorrhage in the abdominal cavity.

Arms and Legs

Examination of the arms and legs is the last step in the head-to-toe survey. Arms and legs should be inspected for:

- swelling
- deformity
- tenderness

Also, any tremors in the hands should be noted.

The neurological status of the arms and legs is checked by assessing four things.

- strength
- movement
- range of motion
- sensation

Each side of the body is compared to the other side.

- Muscle strength in the upper extremities is checked by having the patient squeeze both the examiner's hands at the same time. Leg strength is assessed by having the patient push each foot against the examiner's hand, again at the same time.
- Sensation is assessed by using a safety pin or other tool on the arms and legs to determine the patient's response to pain.
- The examiner must compare both sides and note any weakness or decreased sensation in one side compared to the other.

While the physician normally performs these tests, you should be prepared to assist as needed.

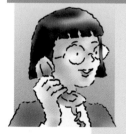

Ask the Professional   STAYING CALM

Q: *A patient in the office had an emergency situation. I tried to help, but she was so upset I couldn't understand what she was saying. Finally, I started getting upset too. What could I have done to make things better?*

A: To help the patient, you need to stay calm too. Do this by focusing on the information you need from her. Explain that some information is necessary in order to help her. Then give her your full attention, if possible. If you think family members are contributing to the patient's agitation, ask a staff member to take them to another room.

Types of Emergencies

Many different kinds of emergencies could need handling in a medical office. Although the physician or EMS probably will provide most of the emergency treatment, you may need to assist or care for the patient until help arrives. Knowing about the different types of emergencies you could encounter will prepare you for what to expect.

SHOCK

Shock is a lack of oxygen to individual cells of the body, including the brain. It results from a decrease in blood pressure. The reasons for this decrease can vary. But the body reacts to any type of shock in much the same way.

- The strength of heart contractions increases.
- The heart rate increases.
- Blood vessels constrict (narrow in diameter) throughout the body.

As shock progresses, the body has more difficulty trying to adjust. Eventually, tissues and organs have such severe damage that the shock becomes irreversible, causing death.

Signs and symptoms of shock are:

- low blood pressure
- restlessness or signs of fear
- thirst
- nausea
- cool, clammy skin
- pale skin with cyanosis (bluish color) at the lips and earlobes
- rapid and weak pulse

Types of Shock

There are several types of shock. Each has a different set of causes.

Hypovolemic Shock. **Hypovolemic shock** is caused by loss of blood or other body fluids. If the cause is blood loss, it's hemorrhagic shock. Dehydration caused by diarrhea, vomiting, or heavy sweating also can lead to hypovolemic shock.

Cardiogenic Shock. **Cardiogenic shock** is an extreme form of heart failure. It occurs when the heart's left ventricle is so impaired it can't pump adequate blood to body tissues. This type of shock may follow the death of cardiac tissue during a myocardial infarction (heart attack).

Neurogenic Shock. **Neurogenic shock** is caused by a dysfunction of the nervous system following an injury to the spinal cord. After a spinal cord injury, the nervous system loses control of the diameter of the blood vessels. This results in vasodilation. Once the blood vessels are dilated, there is not enough blood in the general circulation. Blood pressure falls and shock occurs.

Anaphylactic Shock. **Anaphylactic shock** is an acute general allergic reaction. It occurs within minutes or hours after the body has been exposed to an offending foreign substance. You must observe patients carefully for this type of shock after giving medications and during allergy testing.

Septic Shock. **Septic shock** is caused by a general infection of the bloodstream. It may be associated with an infection such as pneumonia or meningitis. It also may occur without any apparent source of infection, especially in infants and children. The patient appears seriously ill. Initially, a fever is present, but the body temperature falls. This fall in temperature is a clinical sign suggesting sepsis.

Managing Patients in Shock

Shock can occur following many types of medical crisis or trauma. After doing primary and secondary assessments, you'll need to care for the patient. Here's a list of guidelines for managing a patient in shock.

1. Maintain an open airway and adequate breathing.
2. Control any bleeding.
3. Administer oxygen as directed by the physician.
4. Immobilize the patient if spinal injuries may be present.
5. Splint any fractures. (Techniques will be reviewed later in the chapter.)
6. Prevent loss of body heat by covering the patient with a blanket, especially if the patient is cold.
7. Assist the physician with starting an intravenous line, as directed.
8. If the patient's blood pressure is low, elevate his or her feet and legs.
9. Do not let the patient move unnecessarily.
10. Do not let the patient eat, drink, or smoke.

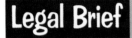

WHEN PATIENTS CAN'T GIVE INFORMED CONSENT

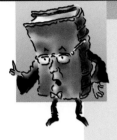

In some emergency situations, patients aren't able to give informed consent. For example, if the patient is unconscious, it's not possible to obtain her consent.

If treatment can be delayed without putting the patient in danger, the physician should obtain consent first. Conscious patients have the right to make choices about their emergency care.

If the patient is not competent or is unable to give consent, a surrogate may be asked to give it. A surrogate is a person authorized to make decisions on the patient's behalf. However, if no surrogate can be found and the patient's life is at stake, the physician can provide emergency treatment without informed consent.

11. Be sure that someone stays with the patient at all times. The patient should not be unattended.

12. Call EMS to transport the patient to the hospital as soon as possible.

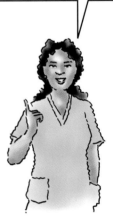

If you need to leave a patient in shock for any reason, be sure to find someone to stay with the patient while you're away. Patients in shock should never be left alone.

SOFT TISSUE INJURIES AND BLEEDING

Soft tissue injuries involve the skin and/or the muscles underlying the skin. An open injury to these tissues is referred to as an **open wound.**

When a blunt object strikes the body, it may crush the tissue beneath the skin. Although the skin doesn't always break, severe damage to the tissues and blood vessels may cause bleeding within a confined area. This is called a **closed wound.**

Closed Wounds

There are three main types of closed wounds.

- A **contusion** is a collection of blood under the skin or in damaged tissue. The site may swell immediately, or 24 to 48 hours later. As blood gathers in the area, a characteristic black and blue mark called **ecchymosis,** or a bruise, can be seen.

- A **hematoma** is a blood clot that forms at the injury site. This often occurs when large areas of tissue are damaged. When a large bone is fractured, as much as a liter of blood can be lost in the soft tissue.

- Crush injuries are usually caused by extreme external forces that crush both tissue and bone. Even though the skin remains intact, the organs underneath may be severely damaged.

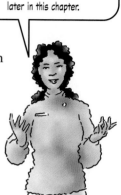

Many emergency treatments involve the application of cold or heat. You'll read more about these procedures later in this chapter.

No matter what type of swelling occurs in a closed wound, the treatment is the same. You need to apply ice to the area to reduce and prevent more swelling.

Open Wounds

In an open wound, the skin is broken. This exposes the patient to external hemorrhage and wound contamination. You need to follow standard precautions to:

- protect yourself against disease transmission
- protect the patient from further contamination

There are several kinds of open wounds. Some are more serious than others and each presents its own set of problems. The table on page 470 describes the common types of open wounds.

Managing Soft Tissue Injuries and Bleeding

Open wounds often involve bleeding. Here are some essential steps for controlling bleeding.

- Have the patient lie down to reduce the risk of fainting.
- Raise the body part above the level of the heart, if possible.
- Apply direct pressure to the wound by using a clean gauze pad and holding it firmly on the wound.
- If blood soaks through the gauze pad, place another pad on top. Keep applying pressure.
- Don't remove a pad that is soaked with blood. You could disrupt the process of blood clotting.
- If bleeding stops, secure the gauze pads with a bandage.

Remember that you learned about bandaging in Chapter 4.

Amputations. Some types of open wounds require special treatment. For amputations, you need to control the bleeding. However, you also need to preserve the severed part for possible reattachment later. Here are the steps for preserving a severed body part.

Types of Open Wounds

Type of Wound	Description	Examples/Causes
Abrasion	The least serious open wound; it's basically a scratch on the skin's surface. All abrasions are painful because they affect nerve endings.	Scrapes
Laceration	Results from snagging or tearing of tissue, leaving jagged edges; skin may be partly or completely torn away.	Wound caused by broken bottle or piece of jagged metal
Major arterial laceration	Sharp or jagged instrument cuts the wall of a blood vessel; it may result in shock or death if bleeding is not controlled.	Same causes as lacerations
Puncture wound	Results from penetration of skin by sharp, narrow object; it also can be caused by high-speed penetrating objects, such as bullets.	Wound caused by knife, nail, or ice pick
Impaled object wound	Like a puncture wound; however, the object that caused the injury remains in the wound.	Wound with steel rod, stick, or glass
Avulsion	A wound with a flap of skin torn loose; the flap may remain hanging or tear off altogether. This wound usually bleeds profusely.	Wounds caused by machinery, lawn mowers or power tools
Amputation	This is a wound caused by a force that is strong enough to rip away or crush limbs from the body.	Wounds caused in industrial or automobile accidents

- Place the severed part in a plastic bag.
- Place this bag in a second plastic bag. This will provide added protection against moisture loss from the severed part.
- Place both sealed bags in a container of ice or ice water. Don't use dry ice.

Impaled Objects. Wounds with impaled objects also require special attention.

- The object should not be removed.
- The patient and injured area of the body should be immobilized.

Movement of the impaled object might cause more damage to the wound and underlying tissue. Place gauze pads around the object and stabilize. The immobilized, impaled object can be removed carefully after the patient is transported to the hospital.

Closer Look ## CONTROLLING SEVERE BLEEDING

Elevation and pressure to the wound alone may not stop severe bleeding. You also may need to apply direct pressure to an artery. **Pressure points** are specific places where you can press an artery against a bone. This will slow the flow of blood.

Here are some tips for using pressure points:

- Apply pressure to the artery at a point between the wound and the heart. Continue to apply direct pressure to the wound.

- Check if bleeding has stopped by slowly removing your fingers from the pressure point. However, keep direct pressure on the wound.

- Once the bleeding has stopped, don't continue to apply pressure to the artery.

- Only use pressure points if direct pressure doesn't stop the bleeding. Body tissues can be damaged without sufficient blood flow.

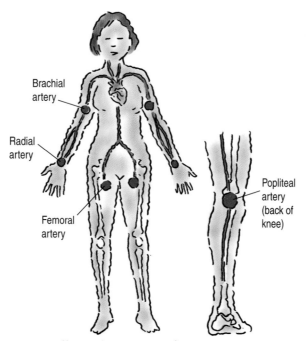

Here are the pressure points for major arteries.

BURNS

Burn injuries come from four main sources:

- *Thermal burns,* or heat burns, are caused by contact with hot liquids, solids, superheated gases, or flame.
- *Electrical burns* are caused by contact with low- or high-voltage electricity. Lightning injuries also are considered electrical burns.
- *Chemical burns* result when wet or dry corrosive substances come into contact with the skin or mucous membranes. The amount of injury with a chemical burn depends on the amount and concentration of the substance and how long it's in contact with the skin.
- *Radiation burns* are similar to thermal burns. They can result from overexposure to ultraviolet light or from any extreme exposure to radiation.

Burn injuries are classified according to their depth and the layers of tissue affected. The depth of the burn depends on three factors.

- the agent causing the burn
- the temperature
- the length of time exposed

Classifying Burn Injuries

There are four classifications of burn injuries.

- first-degree burn or **superficial burn**
- second-degree burn or **partial-thickness burn**
- third-degree burn or **full-thickness burn**
- fourth-degree burn

The table on page 473 describes causes, symptoms, and appearance of each classification of burn injury.

Body Surface Area and Burns

To treat burn patients, you need to assess how much of the body surface area (BSA) has been injured. The most common method for doing this is the **rule of nines.** This method uses percentages to calculate the total surface area of specific sections of the body.

- In an adult, nine percent of the skin is estimated to cover the head. Another nine percent covers each arm, including front and back. Twice as much, or 18 percent, of the total skin area covers the front of the trunk.

Characteristics of Burns According to Depth

Burn Depth	Causes	Skin Layers Involved	Symptoms	Wound Appearance	Recovery Course
First-degree or superficial	Sunburn, low intensity flash	Epidermis	Tingling, hyperesthesia (abnormal sensitivity to touch), pain soothed by cooling	Reddened; blanches (or turns white) with pressure; little or no edema	Complete recovery within a week; some peeling
Second-degree or partial thickness	Scalds, flash flame	Epidermis, dermis	Pain, hyperesthesia, sensitivity to cold air	Blistered, mottled red base; broken epidermis; weeping surface; edema	Recovery in 2–3 weeks; some scarring, depigmentation; infections may convert to third-degree
Third-degree or full thickness	Flame, long exposure to hot liquids, electric current	Epidermis, dermis, sometimes subcutaneous tissue	Pain-free; shock; hematuria (blood cells in urine); possible entrance and exit wounds if electrical	Dry, pale, white, leathery, or charred; broken skin with fat exposed; edema	May require escharotomy (incisions made through dead tissue to relieve pressure) and skin grafting; scarring; loss of function; loss of digits or extremity possible
Fourth-degree	Prolonged contact with flame, high-voltage electrical injury	Epidermis, dermis, subcutaneous tissue, sometimes muscle and bone	Pain-free; shock	Possibly black and depressed; exposed bones and ligaments	Skin grafting usually needed; scarring; loss of function; loss of digits or extremity possible; recovery time depends on severity

Another 18 percent of the skin area covers the back of the trunk, and 18 percent covers each lower extremity (including front and back). The area around the genitals, or the perineum, is one percent of the total body surface area.

- In infants and children, the percentages are the same as for adults, with two exceptions. The head is 18 percent of the total skin area, and the lower extremities are each 13.5 percent

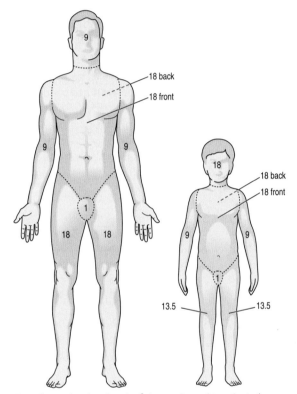

These figures show how the rule of nines can be used to estimate the burned area of an adult and a child.

Managing a Burn Patient

If you need to provide emergency treatment to a patient with burns, you can follow these guidelines. You should handle minor burns and major burns differently.

For minor burns that are second-degree and not larger than three inches in diameter, you should follow the following steps.

1. Cool the burn by holding the burned area under cool running water for about five minutes. If this is not possible, use cold compresses. You should never put ice on a burn.

2. Cover the burn with sterile gauze. Do not wrap the gauze too tightly.

For major burns, here are the steps you should follow.

1. Eliminate the source of the burn, if necessary. Be sure that the patient is not in contact with any smoldering materials or heat.

2. Have someone notify the physician and call EMS.

3. Assess the patient's airway, breathing, and circulation. Begin CPR if necessary.

4. Cover the area of the burn using a sterile bandage or sheet.

5. Administer oxygen as instructed by the physician.

6. Treat the patient for shock and accompanying low blood pressure.

7. Assist with necessary procedures for transporting the patient to the hospital.

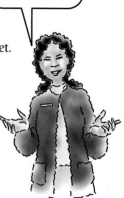

As with all serious emergencies, be sure to reassure a burn patient that EMS is on the way and that you'll stay until they arrive.

MUSCULOSKELETAL INJURIES

Injuries to muscles, bones, and joints are some of the most common problems you'll encounter. These injuries vary widely in their seriousness.

- Some injuries are simple, such as a fractured finger.
- Others may be life threatening, such as an open fracture to the femur, which can cause severe bleeding.

Injuries to muscles, tendons, and ligaments occur when a joint or muscle is torn or stretched beyond its normal limits. Fractures and dislocations usually result from external forces. However, they also can arise from diseases and bone degeneration.

Here are the major types of musculoskeletal injuries.

- **strain,** or an injury to a muscle and its supporting tendons
- **sprain,** or an injury to a joint capsule and its supporting ligaments
- dislocation
- fracture

Sprains and Strains

Strains and sprains both can cause the affected site to be unstable. If a ligament is torn, it can't stabilize the joint properly. Common symptoms of strains include:

- pain
- limited motion
- muscle spasms or weakness
- inflammation

Common symptoms of sprains are:

- inflammation
- pain
- bruising
- loss of ability to move the joint
- redness around the affected area

You can help reduce these symptoms by following *RICE*:

- *Rest* by reducing physical activity and keeping your weight off of the injured area for 48 hours.
- *Ice* the area for approximately 20 minutes about 4 to 8 times a day.
- *Compression* of the injury by a wrap or special cast or boot can help reduce swelling.
- *Elevation* above heart-level can reduce swelling.

Further treatment will depend on the severity of the injury.

- For mild injuries, treatment will include exercise to prevent joint stiffness and muscle atrophy.
- For moderate injuries, care must be taken to prevent further injury. For example, weakened ligaments can take up to eight weeks to heal.
- For severe injuries, surgery may be required.

Dislocations

A **dislocation,** or luxation, occurs when the end of a bone is displaced from its normal position in a joint. Dislocations often are caused by sudden impact to the joint in a fall, a blow, or other trauma. Common sites of dislocation are:

- shoulders
- elbows
- fingers
- hips
- ankles

Sometimes, a bone may be pulled from its socket, but all structures in the joint, such as ligaments and tendons, keep their proper relationships. This is called **partial dislocation,** or subluxation. Patients who have a dislocation or partial dislocation may have several symptoms, including:

- pain
- pressure

- limited movement
- deformity
- numbness or loss of pulse in the affected extremity

Dislocations usually are treated by realigning the bones and immobilizing the joint. The patient may require a program of exercises to strengthen the supporting muscles.

Fractures

A **fracture** is a break or disruption in a bone. Fractures often are caused by falls or other trauma. Other causes may be disease, tumors, and unusual stresses on a bone. Symptoms of fractures include:

- pain
- swelling
- lack of movement or unusual movement
- bruising
- deformity of the body part
- exposure of the bone through the skin
- numbness

Here are some types of fractures you might be most likely to see as emergencies in a medical office.

- *Simple or closed.* This is a fracture that doesn't protrude through the skin.
- *Compound or open.* In this case, the broken end of a bone protrudes through the skin. Infection is a major concern.
- *Greenstick.* This type of fracture is common in children. It is a partial or incomplete break. Only one side of a bone is broken.
- *Compression.* In this type of fracture, the damage results from applying a strong force against both ends of the bone. It often results from falls. Vertebrae are susceptible to compression fractures.
- *Pathological.* Fractures that result from disease processes are called pathological. Some diseases that may cause fractures are osteoporosis (brittle bones), Paget's disease (a skeletal disease noted by bowing of the long bones), bone cysts, tumors, or cancer.

Managing Musculoskeletal Injuries

It can be difficult in some emergencies to tell whether an injury is a strain, sprain, dislocation, or fracture. In most cases, it's best

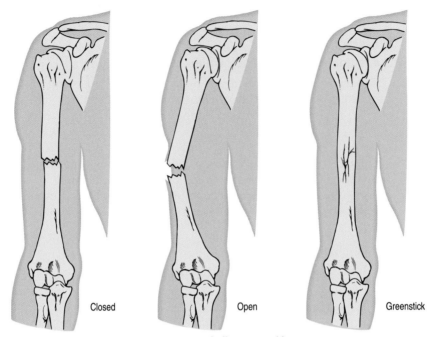

Closed   Open   Greenstick

These illustrations show examples of different kinds of fractures in the arm.

to treat the area as a fracture. This means you'll need to immobilize the joint above and below the injury site. Doing this helps the patient by:

- preventing further injury to soft tissues, blood vessels, and nerves
- relieving pain by stopping motion at the site

Also apply ice to the injured area as soon as possible. You should not apply the ice directly to the skin; instead, wrap the ice in a towel to avoid burning the skin. Ice will reduce the swelling that commonly occurs with this type of injury.

Types of Splints

Any device used to immobilize a sprain, strain, fracture, or dislocated limb is called a **splint**. Splinting material may be soft or rigid. Almost any object that will provide stability will do in an emergency. However, there are several types of commercial splints.

- traction
- air
- wire ladder
- padded board

> Never try to put a dislocated body part back into place.

SPLINT TIPS

With any type of splint, you need to check the injured extremity for signs of impaired circulation. Here are some tips for doing this check.

- Observe the extremity's skin color and the nail beds of the hand or foot. A pale or cyanotic color indicates that circulation is blocked.
- Locate a pulse in an artery away from the affected extremity. A weak or absent pulse indicates decreased circulation to the area.
- Watch for increased swelling of the extremity. While this may not indicate that the circulation is impaired, the swelling itself may reduce circulation.
- If the circulation is impaired with the splint in place, loosen or remove it immediately. Without adequate blood flow, tissue **ischemia** (decrease in oxygen) and **infarction** (death) may occur.

Slings

If the injured body part is an arm, a sling will help to immobilize the limb as well. A sling usually is applied after the arm has been splinted. If available, you can use a canvas triangular arm sling, or a triangular bandage. A sling also could be improvised from a large piece of cloth, such as a pillowcase or clothing.

APPLYING AN ARM SLING

Here are some key steps for applying an arm sling.

1. Position the injured limb across the patient's upper body. The hand should be at slightly less than a 90-degree angle. The fingers should be higher than the elbow. This helps to reduce swelling in the hand and fingers.
2. Place the triangle across the patient's upper body and under the injured arm.
   - The upper corner of the triangle is placed at the shoulder on the uninjured side of the body. Extend the corner across the nape of the neck.
   - The middle corner is placed under the elbow of the injured arm.
   - The third corner should be pointing at the foot on the uninjured side.

3. Bring up the third corner to meet the upper corner at the side of the neck.

4. Tie or use safety pins to secure the two corners together at the side of the neck. Never knot the sling at the back of the neck. It's uncomfortable for the patient.

5. Secure the elbow by fitting any extra fabric neatly around the injured limb and pinning.

6. Check the patient's comfort and the circulation to the distal part of the extremity.

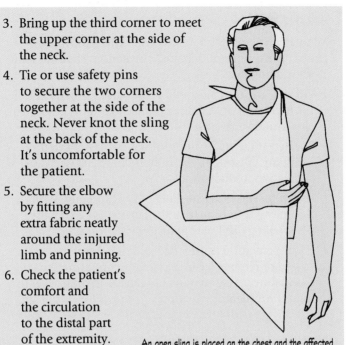

An open sling is placed on the chest and the affected arm is placed across the sling.

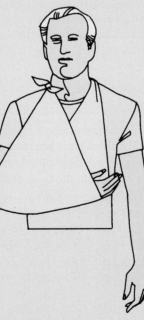

Tie the two corners together at the side of the neck.

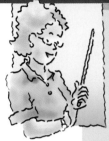

Your Turn to Teach

TEACHING PATIENTS ABOUT CRUTCHES

Crutches often are prescribed for conditions when the patient can't bear weight on one foot or leg. They may be wooden or aluminum. Medical assistants often are responsible for teaching patients how to use them safely. Here are the techniques to teach patients who must use crutches and can bear weight on one foot or leg.

Moving to a Standing Position

1. Move both crutches to the hand on the affected side.
2. Slide to the edge of the chair.
3. Push down on the chair with the arm on the unaffected side and stand up.
4. Rest on crutches until you get your balance.

Moving to a Sitting Position

1. Back up to the chair until its edge is against the back of the legs.
2. Move both crutches to the hand on the affected side.
3. Reach back for the chair with the hand on the unaffected side.
4. Lower yourself slowly into the chair.

Walking with Crutches

1. Move both crutches forward. The unaffected leg should bear your weight.
2. Support your weight on the hand grips of the crutches as you bring the unaffected leg forward.

Walking up Stairs

1. Hold on to the handrail and hold both crutches under the opposite arm. If there is no handrail to grasp, keep a crutch under each arm for balance.
2. Stand close to the bottom step.
3. Support the body's weight on your hands on the crutches. Step up to the first step with the unaffected leg. Remember that the good leg always goes up first.
4. Push down on the crutches, then step up with the weaker leg.
5. Get your balance before attempting the next step.

(continued)

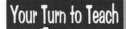

TEACHING PATIENTS ABOUT CRUTCHES (*continued*)

Walking down Stairs

1. Stand close to the edge of the top step.
2. Bend from the hips and knees to adjust to the height of the step below you. Don't lean forward! That can cause you to fall.
3. Carefully lower the crutches and the affected leg to the next step.
4. Then lower the unaffected leg to the lower step.
5. Get your balance before you attempt the next step.

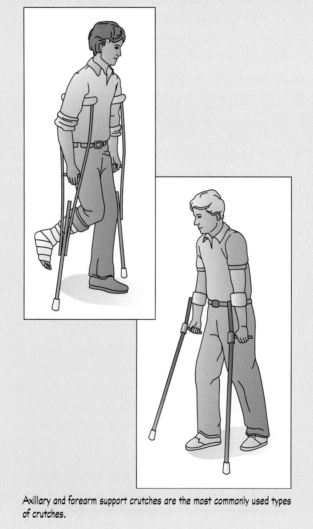

Axillary and forearm support crutches are the most commonly used types of crutches.

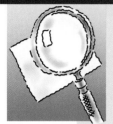

Closer Look   OTHER CRUTCH GAITS

Not all patients will be able to put weight on one leg. There are other types of crutch gaits that you should be familiar with.

- The four-point gait is used for patients who can put some weight on each foot. It is a slow gait, but one that provides stability and maximum support. The patient starts with the right foot and then advances the left crutch. Next the patient advances the left foot and then the right crutch. Once the patient is back to the beginning stance, the sequence starts again.

- The two-point gait is a bit faster than the four-point gait, but it requires more stability and offers less support. The sequence starts with moving the right foot and left crutch and then the left foot and right crutch. This is repeated again once more until back to the beginning position.

- The three-point gait requires good balance and good arm strength to support body weight. While it is a faster gait, it is not for everyone. The patient moves both crutches and the weaker leg forward at the same time. Then the stronger leg is moved forward while the arms support the body weight.

- The swing-to gait also requires good arm and upper body strength and a bit of practice, too. To begin, the patient lifts both feet and swings forward, landing the feet next to the crutches. Then he advances both crutches and repeats the same swinging move.

- The swing-through gait is similar to the swing-to gait. However, the main difference is that the body lands past the crutches during the swing movement. This is the fastest of all of the gaits.

CARDIOVASCULAR EMERGENCIES

Cardiovascular disease accounts for nearly a million deaths each year in the United States. The most common problem is coronary artery disease. As coronary artery disease progresses, less and less oxygen can get to the heart. This leads to tissue ischemia and eventual infarction of the cardiac tissue.

About two-thirds of sudden deaths from coronary artery disease occur out of the hospital. Most occur within two hours after symptoms begin. The early symptoms of myocardial infarction, or heart attack, include the following:

- chest pain not relieved by rest
- complaint of pressure in the chest or upper back
- nausea or indigestion
- chest pain that radiates up into the neck and jaw or down one arm
- anxiety
- shortness of breath
- cold sweats
- paleness

Early treatment can prevent many deaths related to heart attacks. This treatment may include:

- basic life support
- early defibrillation
- advanced life support

If CPR is started right away and the patient is quickly and successfully defibrillated, chances of survival improve greatly. If the patient has no pulse and you suspect a heart attack is the cause, the AED should be used as soon as possible, if one is available.

NEUROLOGICAL EMERGENCIES

Seizures are caused by abnormal electrical activity in the brain. During a seizure, several different behaviors can occur. Here are some typical examples.

- erratic muscle movements
- strange sensations
- complete loss of consciousness

A seizure is not a disease. It's a symptom of another disorder. Epilepsy, head injury, and drug toxicity all can cause seizures.

Assessing Seizure Patients

It's important to take a thorough history when assessing a seizure patient. The history should include:

- information about previous seizure disorders
- the frequency of the seizures, if they've happened before
- medications the patient is taking
- any history of head trauma

- any history of alcohol or drug abuse
- any recent fever
- any presence of a stiff neck (as seen in meningitis)
- any history of heart disease, diabetes, or stroke

Managing Seizure Patients

In managing a patient who's having a seizure, your first priority is to assess the patient's responsiveness, airway, breathing, and circulation. In some types of seizures, the patient loses consciousness and can't protect the airway.

During a seizure, the body's muscles will contract tightly, including the muscles of the face. Because of this, it's important that you don't try to put any object in the patient's mouth. If you try to force an object between the teeth to prevent the patient from biting his or her tongue, you may injure yourself or the patient.

Patients often vomit during a seizure and lose bowel and bladder control. You need to clear and maintain the patient's airway. You should never give the patient any food or water. Assisting the patient into the recovery position (on one side) will help secretions such as blood or vomit drain from the mouth. You also may remove secretions from the mouth using a suction machine, if one is available.

After gaining control of the airway, the most important thing you can do for a patient during a seizure is to protect the patient from injury. Don't hold the patient down at any time. Only move the patient if you are in a dangerous place, for example the top of a flight of stairs. Move items that could hurt the patient away from the area. If possible, you should put something soft under the patient's head to prevent injury. If the patient lost consciousness and fell at the beginning of the seizure, you will need to protect the neck and cervical spine until the spine can be immobilized.

ALLERGIC REACTIONS

An **allergen** is a substance that causes a person to have an allergic reaction. This is a general reaction that occurs after the body has been exposed to a substance to which it's sensitive. Common types of allergens include:

- drugs
- insect venom
- pollen
- foods

Allergens can enter the body in several ways. The most common ones are:

- by injection
- by inhalation
- by absorption through the skin or mucous membranes

> You need to ask patients about allergies at every visit. Note any allergies on the front of their chart and again in their chart's medication record.

In some cases, a person may have symptoms within seconds after exposure to the allergen. In other cases, the reaction may be delayed for several hours.

Signs and Symptoms

Always check the patient's medical record and ask about allergies before administering any medications in the office. This is critical to preventing reactions in patients with known allergies.

Repeated exposures to a substance that produces a simple allergic reaction eventually may lead to anaphylaxis. An anaphylactic reaction is much more severe than an ordinary allergic reaction.

You should know the signs and symptoms of allergic reactions and watch for them in your patients. A key rule to remember is that the sooner the symptoms occur after the exposure, the more severe the reaction is likely to be. Be observant and ready to treat any patient who shows any of these early symptoms.

- severe itching
- a feeling of warmth
- tightness in the throat or chest
- a rash

If these conditions are left untreated and the situation worsens, anaphylaxis could be the result.

Closer Look ALLERGY SHOTS

Patients with moderate to severe allergy symptoms often receive frequent injections of specific allergens. These can reduce the symptoms associated with certain allergies.

After an injection, the patient should be monitored closely for anaphylaxis. The patient should not be permitted to leave the office for a prescribed amount of time, usually 20 to 30 minutes after the injection. When documenting that an injection was given, you also should note the condition of the patient at discharge.

Anaphylaxis

Anaphylaxis occurs when the body's immune system recognizes a substance to which the person is extremely allergic. Most of the emergencies that result from allergic reactions are due to anaphylaxis. Anaphylactic reactions can lead to airway obstruction, cardiovascular collapse, shock, and even death.

The main cause of death in anaphylactic reactions is swelling of the tissues in the airway, leading to airway obstruction. You need to observe a patient having an allergic reaction closely for any signs of airway involvement. You should watch out for:

- wheezing
- shortness of breath
- coughing
- choking
- feelings of tightness in the neck and throat

Along with these signs of airway involvement, patients with severe allergic reactions may experience:

- tachycardia
- hypotension
- pale skin
- dryness of the mouth
- diaphoresis, or profuse sweating
- other signs of shock

Managing Allergic and Anaphylactic Reactions

Patient care will depend on the severity of the allergic reaction. Some allergic reactions are mild, without respiratory problems or signs of shock. These can be managed by administering oxygen or medications such as antihistamines to relieve symptoms (as directed by the physician). If respiratory involvement occurs without signs of shock, the physician may order epinephrine to be given subcutaneously.

The patient with a severe anaphylactic reaction who is in shock needs more aggressive treatment. This treatment will include:

- additional medications
- an intravenous line
- monitoring of the patient's cardiac rhythm

TREATING ANAPHYLACTIC REACTIONS

The main goal in treating a patient who's having an anaphylactic reaction is to restore respiratory and circulatory function. Here are the steps you should take.

- Don't leave the patient. Have another staff member call the physician immediately and bring the emergency kit or crash cart, including oxygen. Another staff member also should call EMS.

- Help the patient into a supine position.

- Assess the patient's respiratory and circulatory status by obtaining blood pressure, pulse, and respiratory rates.

- Observe the patient's skin color and warmth.

- If the patient complains of being cold or is shivering, cover her with a blanket.

- Start an intravenous line if the physician orders one (or assist with starting an intravenous line). Administer oxygen and other medications as ordered.

- Document vital signs and any medications and treatments.

- Communicate relevant information to the EMS personnel, including copies of the patient's progress notes or medication record as needed.

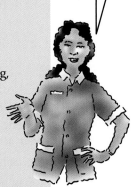

A patient who's having a severe allergic reaction often will be anxious. Reassure the patient and try to help the patient remain calm while you provide emergency care.

POISONING

There are many substances in the home and workplace that can lead to poisoning. Some examples are:

- over-the-counter and prescription medications
- household chemicals
- industrial chemicals

Most toxic exposures occur in the home. Almost half of these occur in children ages one to three. Household chemicals often are designed to have a pleasant odor and color. This may make them appealing to young children if not stored properly.

About 90 percent of reported poisonings are accidental. Intentional exposure usually involves adolescents and adults who are abusing these substances. They tend to have a higher death rate. Fortunately, deaths from drug overdoses and poisonings are rare. However, you need to know how to respond if a patient comes to the office or phones with a possible poisoning situation.

The Poison Control Center

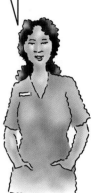

Your office's emergency action procedures should include directions on how and when poison control should be contacted.

The American Association of Poison Control Centers (AAPCC) has established standards and regional poison control centers throughout the country. Physicians, nurses, and pharmacists are on the staff at these centers. The poison control center is a valuable resource. Its phone number should be posted near all phones in the medical office.

The professionals at the poison control center will help in several ways.

- They will evaluate a potential or known toxic exposure.
- They will instruct the caller in the use of syrup of ipecac to induce vomiting, if that is medically indicated.
- They will check on the patient's progress by follow-up telephone calls.

Managing Poisoning Emergencies

Few toxic substances have specific **antidotes** or remedies to control or stop the effect of the poison. So managing a poisoning emergency involves treating the signs and symptoms and assessing the organ systems involved.

The patient may arrive at the medical office after the poisoning. More commonly, the patient or caregiver phones the office requesting information. In either case, you need to obtain the following information before calling a poison control center.

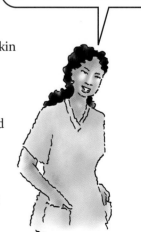

Never give a patient syrup of ipecac or try to induce vomiting unless the poison control center directs you to do so.

- the nature of the poisoning (ingested, inhaled, skin exposure)
- the age and weight of the patient
- the name of the substance
- an estimate of the amount of substance involved
- when the exposure occurred
- the patient's present signs and symptoms

Once the poison control center has been notified and given instructions, you must be prepared to treat the patient as directed. Also notify EMS to transport the patient to the hospital.

HEAT AND COLD-RELATED EMERGENCIES

Life depends on the body's ability to control its core temperature within a range of several degrees. Measured rectally, this core temperature is about 99.6°F (37.6°C). The peripheral temperature is usually lower (98.6°F orally). However, several conditions can disrupt the normal temperature-regulating mechanisms of the body. These conditions are grouped under two main categories.

- **Hyperthermia** is a general condition of excessive body heat.
- **Hypothermia** is an abnormally low body temperature.

Another cold-related condition that may require emergency care is frostbite.

Managing Hyperthermia

Correct management of hyperthermia depends on assessing its type. The three main types of hyperthermia are:

- heat cramps
- heat exhaustion
- heat stroke

Heat Cramps. Heat cramps are muscle cramps that follow a period of heavy exertion and profuse sweating in a hot environment. Sweat is mainly water, but it also contains sodium, a key **electrolyte** needed for muscle function. An electrolyte is a substance found in the body that includes dissolved minerals such as potassium, sodium, and calcium. Heavy sweating will result in a sodium deficit. This will impair muscle function and cause cramps.

- A patient with heat cramps often complains of cramping in the calves of the legs and in the abdomen.
- Cramping also may occur in the hands, arms, and feet.
- Mental status and blood pressure usually remain normal, although an increased pulse rate is common.

Heat cramps signal the need for cooling and rest. Treatment varies depending on the severity.

- In uncomplicated cases, the patient is encouraged to take fluids by mouth. Give the patient a commercial electrolyte solution such as Gatorade. If a commercial solution isn't available, you can add salt to water or fruit juice (one teaspoon per pint).
- In more severe cases, nausea may make intravenous infusion necessary.

Teach patients that they can sometimes prevent heat cramps by drinking an electrolyte solution before physical exertion on a hot day. They also should drink every 20 minutes during exercise. Salt tablets are not recommended because they cause nausea.

Heat Exhaustion. Physical exertion in a hot environment without adequate fluid replacement can result in **heat exhaustion.** Heat cramps may or may not occur before this stage is reached. Body temperature usually remains normal or slightly above normal. Patients have central nervous symptoms, such as:

- headache
- fatigue
- dizziness
- syncope (fainting)

Typically, the skin will be moist and the pulse rate will be high. However, skin color, blood pressure, and respiratory rate will vary with the degree to which the body is able to hold off the distress. The following signs indicate the patient is in a late stage of heat exhaustion:

- pale skin
- low blood pressure
- rapid respiration

A person with heat exhaustion does not usually need to see a physician unless the conditions worsen. Tell patients that the first step in managing heat exhaustion is to get out of the heat and get inside or to a shady location. The person should lie down with her legs elevated. She should also drink cool water or a sports drink with electrolytes.

The person must be monitored so the condition doesn't become more serious and turn into heatstroke. If there is a fever greater than 102°F, fainting, confusion, or seizures, the patient must seek emergency medical assistance immediately.

Heat Stroke. Heat stroke is a true emergency. In **heat stroke,** the body is no longer able to compensate for the rapid rise in body temperature (greater than 105°F). This can lead to brain damage or death. Patients with heat stroke can deteriorate quickly into coma. Many patients have seizures. Here are the signs and symptoms of heat stroke.

- The skin is classically hot, flushed, and dry. There's an absence of sweating.
- Vital signs are elevated at first, but may drop and cardiac arrest may follow.
- The patient may be confused, irritable, or unconscious.

To manage heat stroke, you need to cool the patient's body quickly. Alert the physician. Then, follow office policy for the management of hyperthermia and heat stroke. You should include these steps:

1. Move the patient to a cool area.
2. Remove clothing that may be holding in the heat.
3. Place a wet sheet on the body or cool wet cloths on these key surface areas, where the ability to cool its blood is greatest:
   - the scalp
   - the neck
   - the axilla (armpits)
   - the groin
4. Administer oxygen as directed by the physician. Apply a cardiac monitor.
5. Notify EMS for transporting the patient to the hospital.

You'll learn more about cooling treatments later in the chapter.

Hypothermia

The body can tolerate a drop in core temperature of three to four degrees fahrenheit without loss of normal body function. However, further drops due to internal metabolic factors and significant heat loss to the environment can lead to hypothermia. Hypothermia may result from very cold air or immersion in cold water. These are the signs and symptoms of hypothermia.

- cool, pale skin
- lethargy and mental confusion
- shallow, slow respirations
- slow, faint pulse rate

There are several steps involved in managing a patient with hypothermia. You should contact EMS so the patient can be taken to a hospital emergency room. Until the ambulance arrives, basic management includes:

- handling the patient gently
- removing wet clothing
- covering the patient to prevent further cooling

You should not massage or rub the patient's skin. And do not apply any direct heat. Wrapping the patient in a blanket is enough until he gets to the hospital.

If there's evidence of rewarming (warm skin, no shivering, and respirations approaching normal), and if the patient is alert and able to swallow, give warm fluids by mouth. Avoid drinks that constrict peripheral blood vessels, such as coffee, tea, or other drinks containing caffeine. Fluids that cause dilation of the blood vessels, such as alcohol, also should be avoided. Warm beverages with sugar, such as hot chocolate, can be given to begin replacement of fuel the body needs to restore normal heat production.

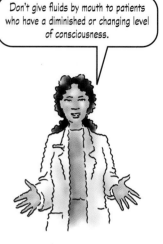

Don't give fluids by mouth to patients who have a diminished or changing level of consciousness.

Frostbite

The greatest risk of frostbite occurs in windy, sub-freezing weather. Body parts with a high ratio of surface area to tissue mass are the most vulnerable to frostbite. These areas are:

- fingers
- toes
- ears
- nose

Larger areas of the extremities are also vulnerable during profound cooling. The main factors that determine the extent of the frostbite are:

- the type of contact
- the duration of contact

For example, touching cold fabric is not as dangerous as coming into contact with cold metal, especially if the skin is wet or damp.

Types of Frostbite. There are two main categories of frostbite.

- *Superficial frostbite* appears as firm and waxy gray or yellow skin. The patient at first feels pain or tingling in the area and then a loss of sensation. No warning symptoms appear after the initial loss of sensation. But continued exposure can lead to blisters and deep frostbite.

- *Deep frostbite* most often affects the hands and feet. No warning symptoms appear after the initial loss of sensation. Once the nerve endings are numb, freezing progresses without pain. The skin becomes inelastic, and the entire area feels hard to the touch. The skin may appear white. Deep frostbite results in tissue death. The affected tissue must be removed surgically or amputated.

Managing Frostbite. Superficial frostbite can be managed by warming the affected part with another body surface. For example, placing an ungloved hand over the nose and ears can provide the necessary warmth.

For more severe cases of frostbite, rapid rewarming is necessary. First assess and treat the patient for hypothermia. After notifying EMS, you may be asked to do the following:

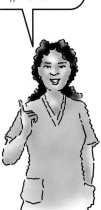

All patients with frostbite should be assessed for hypothermia.

- Immerse frozen tissue in lukewarm water (105°F or 41°C,) until the area becomes pliable and the color and sensation return. Never use hot water

- Don't apply dry heat.

- Don't massage the area. Massage may cause further tissue damage.

- Avoid breaking any blisters that may form.

Deep frostbite must be managed in a hospital to prevent further damage to the tissue. Bandage the frostbitten part with dry sterile dressings while waiting for EMS to transport the patient to the hospital. Frostbitten tissue is similar to burned tissue in that it's vulnerable to infection. Take care to keep the affected part as clean as possible.

BEHAVIORAL AND PSYCHIATRIC EMERGENCIES

Psychological distress may be mild, moderate, or severe. The type and amount of intervention necessary depends on the degree of intensity. It's important for you to know the difference between a **psychiatric emergency** and an **emotional crisis.**

- A psychiatric emergency is any situation in which the patient's moods, thoughts, or actions are so disordered or disturbed that harm or death may result for the patient or others if there is no intervention.

- An emotional crisis is a situation with much less intensity. It may be distressing to the patient. But it is not likely to end in danger, harm, or death. However, an emotional crisis can't be neglected. That's because it may turn into a full psychiatric emergency.

Like a medical emergency, a behavioral emergency can be very serious. Urgent situations usually require some form of professional intervention. They'll also probably require transportation to a hospital. The following guidelines are useful for handling a psychiatric emergency:

- Notify the physician and also EMS if you are directed to do so.

- Offer reassurance and general support to the patient and any caregivers or family members who may be present.

Secrets for Success

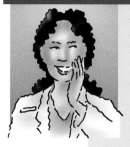

REMEMBERING WHAT TO DO

There's so much to remember in dealing with emergencies that it may seem overwhelming. Here's a study tip that may help.

Make a summary chart that shows what to do in different situations. On the left, list the different types of emergency situations that might occur, such as fracture, frostbite, heat emergencies, shock, poison, etc. On the right, list the key steps you need to follow.

Making the chart will help you organize and remember the information. Drill yourself on the steps by covering up the right side of the chart. Look at the heading you made on the left, and see if you can remember what you need to do.

- Accurately document information, including vital signs and the patient's behavior.
- Remain calm.

Other Urgent Situations

As a medical assistant, you may encounter many other situations that can lead to emergencies if first aid is not delivered promptly or if complications arise. In the medical office, the physician is usually available to treat these situations. However, it's important for you to know what to do in case the physician isn't available or so you can provide assistance.

FAINTING

Syncope, or fainting, is a sudden loss of consciousness due to insufficient oxygen or blood to the brain. Sometimes, fainting occurs without any warning signs. In other cases, one or more of these warning signs may be present.

- abnormally pale appearance
- feelings of dizziness
- nausea
- numbness or heaviness in extremities

Most fainting episodes last less than a couple of minutes. The main danger to the patient is from injuries that may occur as a result of falling when losing consciousness.

MANAGING FAINTING

If a patient shows signs of fainting, ask the patient to lower his or her head to increase the blood supply to the brain. You also may decide to ask the patient to lie down to avoid a potential fall. For a patient who has fainted, here's what you need to do.

1. Check the patient's airway and perform rescue breathing or CPR if necessary. Check the patient's vital signs.

2. Notify the physician of the patient's condition.

3. Loosen tight clothing. Cover the patient with a blanket for warmth.

4. Elevate the patient's feet above the level of the heart. This may help to relieve symptoms of fainting. But don't move the patient's legs if there is any chance of head or neck injuries or if the patient has heart problems.

5. Monitor vital signs.

6. Once the patient has recovered, slowly assist the patient into sitting position. Don't leave the patient alone until he has recovered.

The fainting episode should be documented in the patient's medical record, along with any care or treatment provided.

If the patient doesn't recover consciousness quickly or has other symptoms that may be life threatening (such as chest pain, loss of speech, or visual disturbances), it may be necessary to call EMS.

In rare cases, fainting may be a sign of a serious medical problem, such as heart disease or stroke. It also can be a complication of diabetes (low blood sugar) or medication use. Patients who don't regain consciousness may have slipped into a coma.

ASTHMA ATTACKS

Patients with asthma sometimes may experience an acute attack. The symptoms of an asthma attack are:

- wheezing
- coughing
- tightness in the chest
- shortness of breath

Patients often become frightened during an attack, because they're concerned about getting enough air.

MANAGING AN ASTHMA ATTACK

In managing an asthma attack, there are some key steps to follow.

1. Notify the physician that the patient is having breathing difficulties.

2. Assess the patient's airway, breathing, and circulation.

3. If the patient has an asthma inhaler, help the patient get out the device and use it, if necessary. Provide reassurance to keep the patient calm.

4. Administer asthma treatments with a nebulizer or medications to open up the patient's bronchi, as directed by the physician.

5. If there is little or no improvement, notify the doctor or call EMS.

DIARRHEA

Patients may develop diarrhea for any number of reasons. Some of the more serious causes for diarrhea include:

- food poisoning
- bowel diseases
- side effects of medication

Frequent or severe diarrhea can lead to more dangerous complications including:

- dehydration
- electrolyte imbalances
- shock

As you learned in Chapter 2, dehydration is an excessive loss of fluid from the body. Signs of dehydration include rapid heartbeat, extreme thirst, and possible confusion. You also must be alert for signs of shock when managing a patient with severe diarrhea.

Notify the physician of the patient's condition. Help the patient into a supine position, and elevate his or her legs. You may need to assist the physician in administering intravenous fluids to treat dehydration, if this is part of your scope of practice according to state laws.

VOMITING

Excessive vomiting is another condition that can lead to dehydration and imbalances in electrolyte levels. Although vomiting is associated commonly with influenza or food poisoning, it also may occur with various infections.

These patients are especially vulnerable to the fluid loss and electrolyte imbalances associated with severe vomiting.

- infants and young children
- elderly patients
- diabetic patients
- patients who also have diarrhea

> When providing emergency care to patients with vomiting, you need to use standard precautions to protect yourself from their body fluids.

MANAGING SEVERE VOMITING

Here are the steps for managing a patient experiencing severe vomiting.

1. Gather information about the patient's condition and when the problem began. Here are some key questions to ask.
   - When did the vomiting begin?
   - How often does it occur?
   - Is there pain associated with it?

2. Provide the patient with a basin to collect vomit. Inspect the contents for:
   - color
   - odor
   - consistency
   - blood, bile, undigested food, or feces

3. Make the patient comfortable by offering water and towels to clean her mouth and a cold compress for her forehead.

4. Check the patient's vital signs. Monitor the patient for dehydration and for signs of electrolyte imbalances (for example, an irregular pulse or leg cramps).

5. Assist the physician in giving intravenous fluids or anti-nausea medication, as directed and if permitted by state laws.

FEVER

As you read in Chapter 2, fever is a sign that the body is working to fight infection. The discomfort associated with a fever can usually be managed with acetaminophen or aspirin. However, a fever greater than 105°F (40°C) can lead to irreversible brain damage.

If a patient has an abnormally high temperature, you must provide treatment right away. Here's what to do.

1. Check the patient's responsiveness and other vital signs.
2. Notify the physician of the patient's condition.
3. Cool the patient by placing cool, damp towels on the axilla and groin.
4. Watch the patient carefully for signs of seizure, especially if the patient is a child. Continue to monitor vital signs.

EYE INJURIES

Injuries to the eye can be painful or irritating. Types of eye injuries include:

- burns to the eye
- foreign objects in the eye
- chemicals in the eye
- cuts or punctures of the eye or eyelid
- blows to the eye

Here are some tips for managing eye injuries.

- Have the patient wait for the physician in a darkened room. Patients with eye injuries are often sensitive to light.
- Remind the patient not to rub or touch the eye. An ophthalmic topical anesthetic may be applied to relieve pain or irritation, as directed by the physician.
- If there is swelling or contusion, apply cold, wet compresses.
- Don't try to remove any foreign object from the eye.

EYE IRRIGATION

If the injury is a result of a foreign object or substance, the physician may order that the eye be irrigated. In this procedure, sterile solution is used to wash out the eye.

Here are the steps for doing an eye irrigation.

1. Wash your hands and put on gloves for infection control.
2. Check the label for the solution three times, as you would for other medications. Make sure the solution label states it is for ophthalmic use.

3. Have the patient lie down with the affected eye down or sit with the head tilted so the affected eye is lower than the other eye. This helps to prevent contamination of the unaffected eye.

4. Drape the patient to protect the patient's clothing.

5. Place an emesis basin against the upper cheek near the eye. You may ask the patient to hold it.

6. Use clean gauze to wipe the eye from the inner canthus outward. This removes any debris from the lashes that might be washed into the eye.

7. Separate the patient's eyelids with the thumb and forefinger of your nondominant hand. Hold the syringe in your dominant hand. To steady the syringe, you may rest it lightly on the bridge of the patient's nose.

8. Keep the tip of the syringe about one inch from the eye. Gently irrigate from the inner to the outer canthus. Use gentle pressure. Don't touch the eye.

9. Use tissues to wipe away any excess solution from the patient's face.

EAR EMERGENCIES

Ear emergencies may involve the outer, middle, or inner ear. They have many different causes. For example, young children sometimes stick objects in their ears. Excessive buildup of cerumen (ear wax) also can cause problems.

Some signs and symptoms of ear emergencies include:

- dizziness
- loss of hearing
- nausea and vomiting
- earache
- bleeding or discharge from the ear
- swelling or redness
- an object visible in the ear

A common treatment for removing debris or foreign objects from the ear is irrigation. Irrigation also can be used to:

- remove discharge
- remove excessive or impacted cerumen
- treat an inflamed ear with antiseptic solution

Impacted wax can impair hearing, cause discomfort or even pain, and result in possible injury to the ear. Sometimes, before beginning the irrigation, medication must be instilled into the ear to soften the wax or relieve pain. You read about how to instill medicines into the ear in the Hands On procedures in Chapter 5.

EAR IRRIGATION

Here are the steps to follow if the physician asks you to irrigate a patient's ear. Ear irrigation is not a sterile procedure, but you should wash your hands before you begin to control infection and then apply gloves.

1. First, straighten the auditory canal. For an adult's ear, gently pull the ear up and back. In children, gently pull the ear slightly down and back. Then view the ear with an otoscope to locate the foreign matter or cerumen.

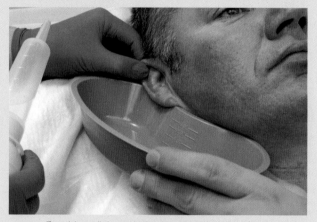

For adults, pull the ear back to straighten the auditory canal.

2. Drape the patient with a waterproof barrier or towel.
3. Tilt the patient's head toward the affected side.
4. Place an emesis basin under the patient's ear.
5. Fill an irrigating syringe or turn on an irrigating device.
6. With your nondominant hand, straighten the ear canal (as described above). With your dominant hand, place the tip of the syringe in the ear opening (auditory meatus). Direct the flow of the solution up toward the roof of the canal.

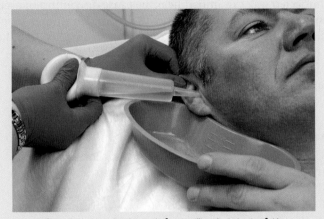

Place the basin under the ear before instilling the irrigation fluid.

7. Continue irrigating for the prescribed period or until the debris or cerumen has been removed.

8. Dry the patient's external ear with gauze. Have the patient sit for a while with the affected ear down. This allows the solution to drain.

9. Inspect the ear with the otoscope to see if the debris or cerumen has been removed. If the patient is experiencing any pain during this procedure stop and inform the physician.

Of course, you need to document the procedure.

Charting Example:
03/17/2007 3:30 P.M. Right ear irrigated with 500 mL sterile water; return clear with 2 2-mm pieces of yellow-brown cerumen noted. _____ S. Stark, RMA

NOSEBLEEDS

Nosebleeds, or epistaxis, can occur as a result of injury to the membranes in the nose. They also may result from another disease process, such as hypertension or cancer.

Most nosebleeds are not serious. They can be managed by following these steps.

1. Have the patient sit upright, with his or her head tilted slightly forward. This helps prevent nasal drainage down the throat, which can lead to nausea.

2. Compress the nostril (nares) against the septum using ice or a cold, wet compress. The nostril should remain compressed for five to ten minutes.

3. Remind the patient to sit still. The patient should not blow the nose until the physician advises it's okay.

If a nosebleed continues for more than ten minutes after treatment begins, it's considered severe. The patient may need to be transported to the hospital or the physician may perform additional treatment. Some additional treatments you may need to assist with are:

- inserting nasal packing material
- inflating a balloon catheter in the nose
- cautery treatment to seal off blood vessels

DISASTER EMERGENCIES

Your training and knowledge about medical emergencies may be useful in situations where large numbers of people are injured. Examples of such situations are:

- natural disasters such as tornados, floods, fires, hurricanes, or earthquakes
- terrorist acts, including acts of bioterrorism

Natural Disasters

In a natural disaster, medical personnel often are summoned to treat a wide range of emergency conditions. Some of the injuries you might have to deal with in a natural disaster include:

- shock
- muscular and soft tissue injuries
- musculoskeletal injuries
- burns

You can prepare yourself for a disaster situation by becoming familiar with standard protocols for responding to disasters. Here are some general tips for managing victims during or after a natural disaster.

- Make sure the scene is safe. You may need to wait for the scene to be secured by proper authorities (police, fire, civil defense) before you evaluate the patient.
- Practice standard precautions when caring for wounds. After some natural disasters, it may be difficult to find

running water. If water is not available, use an alcohol-based product to wash your hands.

- Watch carefully for the presence of other injuries that may not be obvious.
- Obtain a history from the patient, and perform a head-to-toe examination to rule out other injuries.

> There's a risk of tetanus for both victims and responders in a disaster. Tetanus is a nervous system disorder caused by bacteria that can enter the body through punctures and other cuts and wounds.

Acts of Terrorism

In an act of **bioterrorism,** toxic substances or biological agents are deliberately released to harm people in the community. Several substances have been identified as possible weapons.

- anthrax
- smallpox
- plague
- tularemia
- botulism

If bioterrorism occurs, medical offices will provide an important resource for health care. They are likely to be one of the places where unusual patterns of illness or behavior are first noticed. You should be alert to any unusual patterns. Here are some important events to watch for.

- an unexpected number of patients with a particular illness
- clusters of patients arriving from the same location
- clusters of patients with the same disease arriving within a short period of time
- an unusual age distribution for a disease
- a disease with an unusual exposure route
- a disease that occurs outside its normal transmission season
- disease that has an unusual pattern of resistance
- an unusual strain of a disease

> Medical responses to bombings and similar terrorist acts would be much like responses to natural disasters.

If you notice any unusual patterns, you should notify the physician.

Heat and Cold in Treating Emergencies

You may have noticed that heat and cold are used in treating many of the emergencies and urgent situations you've read

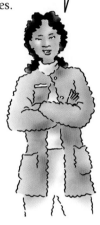

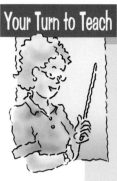

Your Turn to Teach

HELPING PATIENTS BE PREPARED

You can help teach your patients about how to be prepared for a large-scale emergency. Here are some tips to teach your patients about being prepared.

- *Create an emergency action plan.* Remind patients to make a plan about what to do should an emergency occur. For example, family members may not be together. They need a plan for how they will contact each other or where they will meet if disaster strikes.

- *Learn first aid and CPR.* These skills can become important for patients and their family members in the case of a large-scale emergency.

- *Keep emergency supplies at home and in your car.* When assembling first aid and other emergency supplies, patients should keep in mind the special needs of their family. For example, infants may need diapers or formula. The patients themselves may require certain medications.

about in this chapter. Here are some general guidelines for using such treatments.

- Heat may be used to relieve muscle spasms, to relieve pain, to provide local or systemic warming, or to promote healing by increasing blood flow to an area.

- Cold can be used to reduce swelling, to relieve pain, to provide local or systemic cooling, to decrease bleeding or hemorrhage, and to decrease inflammation.

Using heat and cold to treat symptoms involves some important considerations. For example, it's critical to check that the temperature of the treatment is correct. In general, treatment temperatures should be kept within the following limits:

- warm: tepid (95°F to 98°F) to very warm (115°F)
- cold: neutral (93°F to 95°F) to very cold (50°F)

You'll need to watch for **rebound** as well. Rebound is an effect in which the body responds to temperature extremes by producing the opposite effect of what was intended. For example, one reason for applying heat is to cause vasodilation. But if heat is applied for too long (usually 30 minutes is the maximum), the body will try to compensate. Vasoconstriction will occur—the opposite of the effect desired.

Several types of hot and cold treatments exist. They include:

- compresses
- soaks
- hot packs
- cold packs

APPLYING COMPRESSES

Warm or cold compresses may be used in the medical office. You can follow the same basic steps for either type. If the compress is being applied to an area with an open lesion, sterile technique is required.

1. Always check the physician's order first to determine the appropriate solution.
2. Pour the solution into a basin. For warm compresses, the solution should be warmed to 110 degrees F (or an ordered temperature). Check the temperature with a bath thermometer. If it's too hot, it will injure the patient.
3. The patient may need to remove clothing and/or put on a gown, depending on where the compresses will be applied. If necessary, drape the patient to protect privacy.
4. Protect the examination table or other surface with a waterproof barrier. Wet surfaces may be uncomfortable for the patient and cause chilling.
5. Place absorbent material or gauze in the prepared solution. Wring out excess moisture. Compresses should be moist, but not dripping.
6. Lightly place the compress on the patient's skin. Ask the patient whether the temperature of the compress is causing pain or discomfort. Observe the skin for changes in color.

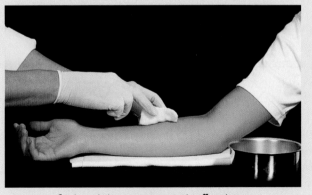

Gently touch the wet compress to the affected area.

7. Gently arrange the compress so it fits the contours of the area. The material must be against the skin for maximum benefits. Cover the compress with plastic or a waterproof barrier.

8. Check the compress frequently for moisture and temperature.

9. After the prescribed amount of time (usually 20 to 30 minutes), remove the compress and discard disposable materials. Disinfect reusable equipment when you have the opportunity to do so.

Don't forget to document the procedure.

Charting Example:
10/16/2007 10:45 a.m. Hot compress applied to left ankle × 20 min. Skin pink after treatment. No broken areas noted on skin. _____ B. Barth, CMA

> Hot water bottles or ice packs may be used to maintain the compress temperature.

USING SOAKS

Soaks can be used as a warm or cold treatment. Here are some basic steps for a soak.

1. Get a basin or container that is large enough to immerse the body area. A container that's too small may cause muscle spasms.

2. Fill the container with the appropriate cold or warm solution. For warm solutions, check the temperature with a bath thermometer. You want to avoid burning or injuring tissues.

3. The area to be soaked should be lowered slowly into the basin. Immersing too quickly can shock the patient. Add padding around the edges of the container as needed for comfort.

4. Check the solution's temperature every five to ten minutes.

5. Sometimes, more water or solution must be added to maintain the temperature. Remove some of the solution. Then add more warmed or cold solution as appropriate. Hold your hand between the patient and the added solution while it's being poured. Mix or swirl the soak to create an even temperature.

6. After the prescribed amount of time (usually 15 to 20 minutes), remove the body part from the solution. Carefully dry the area with a towel to prevent discomfort.

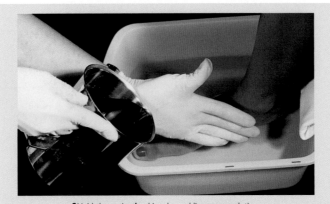

Shield the patient's skin when adding more solution.

7. As time allows, clean up and care for equipment.

8. Document the procedure, including the temperature, length of soak, skin color before and after treatment, and patient reaction.

Charting Example:
05/27/2007 9:43 a.m. Left foot placed in warm water for 20 min. per doctors orders. Skin checked every five minutes. Skin pink after treatment. No broken areas noted on skin. Patient stated, "My foot feels a lot better."_____
_____ B. Sutter, CMA

HOT PACKS AND HOT WATER BOTTLES

Always keep in mind that some patients are particularly sensitive to heat. This precaution especially applies to:

- infants
- elderly patients
- confused or disoriented patients
- patients with circulatory problems
- patients with diabetes

With this in mind, here are some guidelines for applying a commercial hot pack or hot water bottle:

1. If using a hot water bottle, check for leaks to avoid getting the patient wet.

2. Fill the hot water bottle about two-thirds full with warm water (110°F). Place the bottle on a flat surface with the opening up. Press out the excess air. If using a commercial hot pack, follow the manufacturer's directions to activate it.

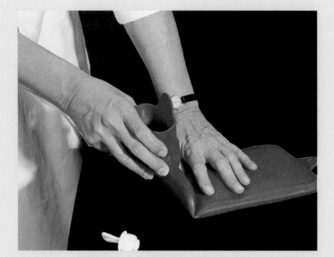

Press out air from the bottle before capping.

3. Wrap the pack or bottle securely with a towel. Doing this will make it more comfortable and help prevent burns.

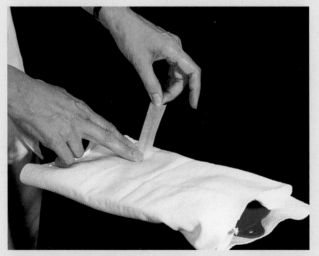

Wrap a towel around the bottle and secure the bottle before placing it on the patient's skin.

4. Assess the color of the patient's skin where the treatment is to be applied. You need to document its appearance before treatment.

5. Place the wrapped hot pack or bottle on the area. It must be securely against the skin for the greatest benefit.

6. Leave the treatment on the patient for the prescribed amount of time. This should be no longer than 30 minutes, to avoid adverse effects.

7. While the treatment is on the skin, assess the skin every five minutes. Remove the treatment immediately if you observe any of the following:
   - pallor, or an abnormally pale skin color, which may be a sign of rebound
   - excessive redness, which suggests the pack is too hot
   - swelling, which suggests tissue damage

Charting Example:
07/11/2007 3:00 p.m. Hot pack to left shoulder posterior upper back × 30 minutes as ordered. Skin pink before treatment, slightly reddened after treatment. Pt. stated pain in upper back and shoulder relieved. Oral and written instructions given for applications at home four times per day Pt. verbalized understanding. _____ M. Rose, RMA

USING COLD PACKS

Commonly used methods for applying cold are a commercial cold pack or an ice bag filled with ice chips. Here are the basic steps for treating a patient with a cold pack.

1. Before filling a reusable ice bag, check the bag for leaks. This will help avoid getting the patient wet. If you're using a commercial ice pack, read the manufacturer's directions.

2. Fill the ice bag about two-thirds full with ice. Press it flat on a surface to remove excess air. Then, seal the bag. If you're using a commercial ice pack, activate it.

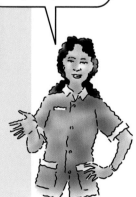

When filling an ice bag, small chips are better than large ones because they more easily fit body contours.

3. Cover the bag or pack with a towel or other material. The pack or bag should not be in direct contact with the skin.

4. Assess the skin for color and warmth. Place the covered ice pack or bag on the injured area.

5. Secure the pack or bag in place with gauze or tape.

6. Don't leave the treatment in place longer than 30 minutes. If it's in place too long, it may cause a rebound effect.

7. Assess the skin under the treatment frequently. Remove it immediately if these signs appear:
   - pallor
   - mottling
   - redness

When you document the procedure, include the site of the application, the results of the treatment, and the patient's response.

Charting Example:

11/22/2007 10:45 a.m. Ice bag applied to (L) anterior thigh as ordered × 20 minutes. Skin before treatment swollen, with large contusion noted, no break in skin. After treatment, area pale and cool to touch, swelling decreased. Verbal and written instructions given to pt. for application four times a day at home; pt. verbalized understanding. _____ B. Barry, CMA

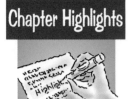

Chapter Highlights

- Emergencies in the medical office may involve staff, patients in the office, or patients who arrive seeking emergency treatment. For major emergencies, the patient is helped until EMS arrives. For minor emergencies, the patient is treated and sent home with follow-up instructions.

- Every medical office should have an emergency action plan and a crash cart or kit with emergency medical supplies and equipment. Emergency numbers should be displayed by all telephones. It's also important that staff be familiar with signs and symptoms that can indicate an emergency.

- In any emergency, there are three steps to follow: identify and treat any life-threatening problems, including rescue breathing or CPR; gather information by asking the patient questions and assessing general appearance, level of consciousness, vital signs, and skin; perform a physical examination for a head-to-toe assessment to identify problems not immediately known.

- Patient reassurance is a critical aspect of emergency care. Patients may be panicky, confused, or in pain. The medical assistant needs to remain calm and focus on the patient.

- All emergency care must be documented. Documentation should include the patient's symptoms, the nature of the emergency, and any treatment performed. Events should be recorded in chronological order.

- Major emergencies that may require immediate treatment include shock, soft tissue and musculoskeletal injuries, cardiovascular injuries, neurological injuries, severe allergic reactions, poisoning, and cold- and heat-related emergencies. Each of these has its own set of signs, symptoms, and procedures for management.

- Injuries to bones, muscles, and joints vary widely in their severity. In an emergency, it can be difficult to tell the difference between sprains, strains, dislocations, and fractures. In most cases, the injured area should be immobilized using splints.

- It's important to know the difference between a psychiatric emergency and an emotional crisis. A psychiatric emergency is life threatening for the patient or others without immediate intervention. An emotional crisis is not likely to result in danger or harm.

- Some of the minor emergencies medical assistants may need to deal with are fainting, asthma attacks, severe diarrhea or vomiting, high fevers, eye injuries, ear emergencies, or nosebleeds.

- Training and knowledge about medical emergencies may be useful in natural disasters or if acts of terrorism occur. Medical assistants need to be familiar with standard protocols for emergencies.

- Heat and cold are used to treat many different kinds of major and minor emergencies. Common treatments include compresses, soaks, hot packs or hot water bottles, and cold packs or ice bags.

GLOSSARY

accommodation   the ability of the pupils to adjust when focusing on objects at different distances [Chapter 3]

aerobe   microorganism that requires oxygen to survive; contrast with *anaerobe* [Chapter 1]

afebrile   the status of a patient whose temperature is within normal limits; contrast with *febrile* [Chapter 2]

allergen   substance that gives rise to hypersensitivity or allergy [Chapter 8]

allergy   reaction to a drug that results in hives, dyspnea, or wheezing [Chapter 5]

alternative medicine   unconventional methods of medical treatment such as acupuncture, acupressure, hypnosis, yoga, and herbal supplements [Chapter 7]

ampule   small glass container that must be broken at the neck so the solution can be aspirated into a syringe [Chapter 5]

anaerobe   microorganism that does not require oxygen to survive; contrast with *aerobe* [Chapter 1]

anaphylactic shock   acute general allergic reaction within minutes to hours after the body has been exposed to an offending foreign substance [Chapter 8]

anaphylaxis   type of potentially life-threatening allergic reaction [Chapter 5]

antagonism   type of drug interaction in which one drug decreases the effects of another; contrast with *potentiation* [Chapter 5]

anthropometric measurements   measurements that document the height and weight of a patient [Chapter 2]

antibiotics   type of drug that interferes with the growth of or destroys organisms [Chapter 1]

antibodies   proteins created by the body to destroy foreign antigens; also known as immune globulins or gamma globulins [Chapter 1]

antidote   substance that stops or reduces the effects of another, harmful substance [Chapter 8]

applicator   device for applying local treatments and tests [Chapter 3]

approximation   the process of bringing tissue surfaces as close as possible to their original positions [Chapter 4]

apothecary system of measurement   uncommon and inaccurate system of measurement; rarely used in doctor's offices [Chapter 5]

artifact   abnormal signal taken during an ECG that does not reflect electrical activity of the heart during the cardiac cycle [Chapter 6]

assessment   an established or possible diagnosis based on subjective and objective information provided and gathered during a report [Chapter 2]; the process of determining a patient's wellness, identifying any life-threatening problems, and providing necessary care [Chapter 7]

asymmetry   lack or absence of symmetry; inequality of size or shape on opposite sides of the body; contrast with *symmetry* [Chapter 3]

auscultation   act of listening for sounds within the body, usually with a stethoscope, such as to evaluate the heart, lungs, intestines, or fetal heart tones [Chapter 3]

autoclave   piece of equipment used to sterilize medical instruments [Chapter 4]

Babinski reflex   foot reflex that can be tested by stroking the sole of a patient's foot with a percussion hammer [Chapter 3]

bactericidal   ability of a substance to kill bacteria [Chapter 1]

bandage   *noun,* soft material applied to a body part to hold a dressing in place, immobilize a body part, or aid in controlling bleeding; *verb,* to apply a wrapping material for treatment [Chapter 4]

barium studies   examinations performed after administration of barium sulfate; generally given to patients with gastrointestinal (GI) symptoms [Chapter 6]

baseline data   original or initial measure with which other measurements will be compared [Chapter 2]

benign   not cancerous or malignant; contrast with *malignant* [Chapter 3]

bimanual examination   examination in which one gloved, lubricated hand is inserted into the vagina while the other hand is placed on the abdomen; allows the examiner to inspect internal structures of the pelvic cavity [Chapter 3]

biohazard   substance that is a risk to the health of living organisms [Chapter 1]

biopsy   removal and examination of a small amount of tissue for diagnostic purposes [Chapter 4]

bioterrorism   terrorist act that uses a biological agent, such as harmful bacteria or viruses, as a weapon [Chapter 8]

buccal medication medication administered between the cheek and gum of the mouth [Chapter 5]

carbohydrates prime energy source for the human body; turned into sugar in the body and then stored as fat [Chapter 7]

cardiac cycle period from the beginning of one heartbeat to the beginning of the next [Chapter 2]

cardinal signs measurements of bodily functions (weight, height, temperature) essential to maintaining life processes; also known as vital signs [Chapter 2]

cardiogenic shock extreme form of heart failure that occurs when the heart's left ventricle is so damaged that the heart can no longer adequately pump blood to body tissues; may follow death of cardiac tissue during a myocardial infarction (heart attack) [Chapter 8]

cardiologist doctor specializing in diagnosing and treating disorders of the cardiovascular system (heart, arteries, and veins) [Chapter 6]

cardiopulmonary resuscitation (CPR) manual process used to maintain breathing and/or blood circulation after cardiac arrest [Chapter 8]

carrier individual whose body serves as a source of nutrients and an incubator where pathogens can grow and reproduce; a reservoir of disease [Chapter 1]

cassette special holder used for the protection of unprocessed x-ray film [Chapter 6]

catheter sterile, flexible tube that is inserted directly into the urinary bladder, causing the patient to urinate [Chapter 5]

cerumen yellowish or brownish wax-like secretion found in the external ear canal; earwax [Chapter 3]

chemical name name initially given to every medication, which identifies the chemical components of that medication [Chapter 5]

chief complaint reason a patient is at a particular health care facility [Chapter 2]

cholesterol waxy, fat-like substance made in the liver, and found in the blood and in all cells of the body, that is needed for making cell walls, tissues, and hormones; too much cholesterol may be harmful to a person's health [Chapter 7]

closed-ended questions queries that often require only a *yes* or *no* answer and do not offer detailed information about a patient's conditions [Chapter 2]

closed wound wound in which the skin remains unbroken and severe damage to tissue and blood vessels may cause bleeding within a confined area [Chapter 8]

coagulation   process of changing from a liquid to a solid or semi-solid mass; the blood-clotting process [Chapter 4]

compliance   patient's willingness to accept treatment; contrast with *noncompliance* [Chapter 7]

computed tomography (CT)   diagnostic procedure in which x-rays are taken from a series of angles and then analyzed by a computer to create a series of cross-sectional pictures of the body structure; some images can be three-dimensional [Chapter 6]

contagious disease   infectious disease communicable by contact with someone who has it, with a bodily discharge of that person, or with an object touched by the person or the person's bodily discharges [Chapter 1]

contaminated   impure because of contact or mixture with an undesired substance [Chapter 1]

contraindication   condition or instance for which a particular drug or other treatment should not be used [Chapter 5]

contrast medium   substance that x-rays will not pass through that is introduced into the body to make the tissue being examined stand out in radiographic visualization [Chapter 6]

controlled substances   restricted medications and drugs that may be addictive and that are regulated by the Drug Enforcement Administration [Chapter 5]

contusion   type of closed wound resulting in a bruise, collection of blood under the skin, or damaged tissue [Chapter 8]

coordination   manner in which the muscles and groups of muscles work together during movement [Chapter 3]

coping skills   methods used by individuals to alleviate intense stressors; beyond our conscious ability to control; psychological defenses against unpleasant situations [Chapter 7]

cyst   sac of fluid or semisolid material under the skin [Chapter 4]

defibrillation   restoration by electric shock of the normal rhythm of a heart [Chapter 8]

dehiscence   unintended separation of the sutured edges of a surgical wound [Chapter 4]

dehydration   abnormal and excessive depletion of body fluids [Chapter 2]

demographic data   important information about a patient (i.e., address, phone number, date of birth) [Chapter 2]

deplete   to greatly reduce the quantity or amount of a thing [Chapter 1]

desiccate   to dry up or cause to dry up [Chapter 4]

detoxification   process of clearing drugs out of a person's body and treating withdrawal symptoms; varies with the type of substance, length of abusing the substance, and person's overall health [Chapter 7]

diagnosis identification of a disease or condition by evaluating physical signs and symptoms, health history, and laboratory tests; a disease or condition identified in a person [Chapter 2]

diaphoresis profuse sweating [Chapter 2]

diastole period during which the heart pauses briefly to rest and refill with blood; arterial pressure drops during this phase [Chapter 2]

digital examination palpation performed using only the fingers [Chapter 3]

diluent diluting agent; used when preparing injections [Chapter 5]

direct transmission direct contact between an infected reservoir host and the susceptible host resulting in the transmission of an infectious disease; contrast with *indirect transmission* [Chapter 1]

disinfection level of infection control in which a disinfectant, or germicide, inactivates virtually all recognizable pathogenic microorganisms, except spores on inanimate objects; bleach is an example of a disinfectant [Chapter 1]

dislocation displacement of a bone at a joint from its normal position; contrast with partial dislocation [Chapter 8]

dissect to separate during surgery different anatomical structures along natural lines by cutting the tissues that connect them [Chapter 4]

dormant not active or growing, although able to become active or grow at a later time, as in a *dormant* bacteria or virus [Chapter 1]

dosimeter device that records the amount of radiation to which a worker has been exposed [Chapter 6]

dressing covering applied directly to a wound to apply pressure, support, absorb secretion, protect from trauma or microorganisms, stop or slow bleeding, or hide disfigurement [Chapter 4]

drug any substance that may modify one or more of the functions of an organism [Chapter 5]

dyspnea difficult or labored breathing; contrast with *hyperventilation* [Chapter 6]

ecchymosis black and blue mark that accumulates under the skin in the area of a contusion [Chapter 8]

echocardiogram procedure that uses sound waves to visualize the shape, motion, and blood flow of the heart [Chapter 6]

edema accumulation of fluid within the tissues [Chapter 4]

electrocardiogram (ECG/EKG)   diagnostic tool used for evaluating the electrical pathway through the heart [Chapter 3]

electrodes   disposable adhesive items used by electrosurgical units; electrodes come in various shapes and sizes, which determine the amount of electric current delivered to the patient's tissue [Chapter 4]

electrolyte   chemical substance dissolved in the blood and having numerous basic functions such as conducting electrical currents; the principal electrolytes are sodium, potassium, chloride, and bicarbonate [Chapter 8]

emotional crisis   psychological situation that is unlikely to end in danger, harm, or death; contrast with *psychiatric emergency* [Chapter 8]

endoscope   soft, flexible tube that passes down a patient's esophagus into the stomach and small intestine or up into the colon for direct visualization of these organs [Chapter 4]

enema   injection of liquid into the lower intestine (bowel) by way of the anus to clean it before examination [Chapter 5]

enrich   to add an ingredient to a substance (especially to a food), or increase its proportion, in order to make it more healthful or effective [Chapter 7]

enteral   within or by way of the intestines, especially as a route for administering medications [Chapter 5]

ethylene oxide   sterilizing agent used to destroy microbial life, including spore forms [Chapter 4]

evaluation   process of indicating how well the patient is progressing toward a particular goal; to appraise; to determine the worth or quality of something or someone [Chapter 7]

excise   to remove something from the body, such as an organ or a tumor, by cutting [Chapter 4]

expiration   process of removing air from the lungs by exhaling it through the nose or mouth; contrast with *inspiration* [Chapter 2]

exposure control plan   written plan regarding exposure to biohazards; required by OSHA for offices with 10 or more employees [Chapter 1]

exposure risk factor   required written policy stating an employee's risk of exposure to communicable diseases [Chapter 1]

extension   act of straightening a flexed limb (contrast with *flexion*); also, the stretching of a fractured or dislocated limb to restore it to its natural position [Chapter 3]

extraocular "outside the eye" movement of the eye; normal eye movement is classified as "EOM (extraocular movement) intact" [Chapter 3]

extremity limb or appendage of the body; the end of a long or pointed structure [Chapter 2]

exudate drainage [Chapter 4]

familial disorders disorders that occur within a particular family [Chapter 2]

fatty acids long chains of molecules, found in fats and oils and in cell membranes, that come from fats [Chapter 7]

febrile status of a patient whose temperature is above normal limits; contrast with *afebrile* [Chapter 2]

fenestrated drapes sterile drapes used during surgery with an opening to expose the operative site while covering adjacent areas [Chapter 4]

fiber threadlike tissue or cell, such as a muscle cell or nerve or connective tissue [Chapter 7]

fibrin elastic whitish protein involved in the clotting of blood [Chapter 4]

flexion bending a limb at the joint to decrease the angle between the bones; contrast with *extension* [Chapter 3]

fluoroscopy special x-ray technique for examining a body part by immediate projection onto a fluorescent screen [Chapter 6]

forceps surgical instruments used to grasp, handle, compress, pull, or join tissue, equipment, or supplies [Chapter 4]

fracture break, rupture, or crack in a body tissue or structure, especially in bone or cartilage [Chapter 8]

fulguration electrosurgery process that destroys tissue with controlled electric sparks [Chapter 4]

full thickness burn third-degree burn resulting from extended exposure to hot liquid, electrical current, or flame [Chapter 8]

gait manner or style of walking [Chapter 3]

gauge diameter of a needle lumen; can vary from 18 (large) to 30 (small); the higher the number, the smaller the gauge [Chapter 4]

generic name name given to medications prior to commercial distribution and use [Chapter 5]

heat exhaustion condition often resulting from physical exertion in a hot environment without adequate fluid replacement; body temperature usually remains normal or slightly above normal; patients have central nervous system symptoms such as headache, fatigue, dizziness, or fainting [Chapter 8]

heat stroke   emergency condition in which the body is no longer able to compensate for the rapid rise in body temperature and may undergo brain damage or death; skin is hot, flushed, and dry; demands rapid cooling of the body [Chapter 8]

hematoma   swelling of tissue that is filled with blood as a result of a broken blood vessel [Chapter 8]

hemorrhage   escape of a large volume of blood from a blood vessel [Chapter 2]

hemostasis   blood cell production [Chapter 4]

hemostat   surgical instrument with slender jaws used for grasping blood vessels and establishing hemostasis [Chapter 4]

hereditary disorder   disorder transmitted from parent to offspring [Chapter 2]

hernia   protrusion of an organ, such as the intestines, through a weakened muscle wall [Chapter 3]

homeopathic medication   tiny doses of substances that, in normal doses, would produce the symptoms of the disease being treated [Chapter 2]

hyperpyrexia   dangerous state of extremely elevated body temperatures, between 105° and 107° Fahrenheit [Chapter 2]

hypertension   elevated blood pressure [Chapter 2]

hyperthermia   general condition of excessive body heat; contrast with *hypothermia* [Chapter 8]

hyperventilation   respiratory rate that greatly exceeds the body's oxygen demand; contrast with *dyspnea* [Chapter 8]

hypothermia   general condition of lowered body heat; contrast with *hyperthermia* [Chapter 8]

hypovolemic shock   caused by loss of blood or other body fluids; may also be caused by diarrhea, vomiting, or profuse sweating resulting from dehydration [Chapter 8]

immune system   body's defense against invading pathogens; examples of this system include the skin, digestive enzymes, mucus, and tears [Chapter 1]

immunity   body's ability to fight off a microorganism once infection has occurred; B and T cells play a major role in immunity [Chapter 1]

immunization   act or process of rendering an individual immune to a specific disease [Chapter 1]

implementation   process of initiating and carrying out an action such as a teaching plan or patient treatment [Chapter 7]

incise   to cut into a surface [Chapter 4]

incision   a cut into body tissue, usually occurring as part of a surgical procedure [Chapter 4]

indirect transmission transmission of disease that occurs through contact with a vector such as contaminated food or water, disease-carrying insects, inanimate objects, or improperly disinfected medical instruments; contrast with *direct transmission* [Chapter 1]

induration hardened area at the injection site after an intradermal screening test for tuberculosis [Chapter 5]

infarction death of tissues due to lack of oxygen [Chapter 8]

infectious disease disease caused by a pathogenic microbe, such as a virus or bacteria, that is capable of spreading from the infected person to others [Chapter 1]

infiltration occurs when IV fluid infuses into the tissues surrounding the vein during catheterization, usually because the catheter has been dislodged [Chapter 5]

informed consent consent given by a patient to a physician after explanation of procedures and risks has been communicated to the patient; required by federal law [Chapter 4]

inguinal lymph nodes lymph nodes of the groin [Chapter 3]

inspection looking at areas of the body to observe physical features; examiner inspects patient's general appearance, including movements, skin and membrane color, contour, and symmetry or asymmetry [Chapter 3]

inspiration inhaling of air into the lungs; contrast with *expiration* [Chapter 2]

instillation administration of a liquid drop-by-drop [Chapter 5]

interaction combined effect of two or more drugs taken by a patient; the positive or negative influence of one drug on the action of another [Chapter 5]

intermittent occurring at intervals [Chapter 2]

intradermal injections administered into the dermal layer of the skin by inserting a needle at a 10- to 15-degree angle [Chapter 5]

intramuscular injection administered directly into muscle; needle held at a 90-degree angle to the skin [Chapter 5]

irrigation process of flushing a wound, cavity, or medical instrument with water or other fluid to clean it [Chapter 5]

ischemia decrease in oxygen to tissues [Chapter 8]

keratosis skin condition characterized by growth and thickening [Chapter 4]

lacto-ovovegetarian vegetarian diet supplemented only with eggs, milk, and cheese [Chapter 7]

lactovegetarian vegetarian diet supplemented only with milk and cheese [Chapter 7]

larynx   modified upper part of the respiratory passage; also called a voice box [Chapter 3]

lead   electrode or electrical connection attached to the body to record electrical impulses in the body, especially the heart or brain [Chapter 6]

learning goals   description of what the patient should learn from implementation of the teaching plan [Chapter 7]

learning objectives   steps or procedures the patient must understand or demonstrate to accomplish the learning goal [Chapter 7]

lentigine   brown skin macule occurring after exposure to the sun; freckle [Chapter 4]

lesion   a localized abnormality in the structure of an organ or tissue (typically the skin) due to infection, injury, or disease [Chapter 4]

ligament   flexible band of tissue that holds joints together [Chapter 3]

local anesthetic   substance injected to numb an area prior to surgery [Chapter 4]

local effect   effect confined to a specific part of the body; contrast with *systemic effect* [Chapter 5]

lubricant   water-soluble gel used to reduce friction and provide easy insertion of an instrument in a physical examination [Chapter 3]

magnetic resonance imaging (MRI)   technique that uses a combination of high-intensity magnetic fields, radio waves, and computer analysis to create cross-section images of the body [Chapter 6]

malignant   cancerous; contrast with *benign* [Chapter 3]

manipulation   passive movement of joints to determine the extent of movement or range of motion [Chapter 3]

Mantoux test   test for past or present infection with tuberculosis in which a small amount of tuberculin is injected under the skin [Chapter 5]

medical asepsis   practices that render an object or area free from pathogenic microorganisms; commonly referred to as clean technique; prevents the transmission of microorganisms from one person or area to any other within the medical offices [Chapter 1]

medical history   record containing information about a patient's past and present health status, the health status of related family members, and relevant information about a patient's social habits [Chapter 2]

medication   substance administered to a person to treat a disease or other health condition [Chapter 5]

mensuration act or process of measuring [Chapter 3]

metabolism breakdown of food into usable units through physical and chemical changes [Chapter 2]

metric system system of measurement commonly used in doctors' offices; measured in increments of 10 [Chapter 5]

microbe organism, especially a bacterium, that's too small to be seen without the aid of a microscope; the nontechnical term for *microorganism* [Chapter 1]

microorganisms living organisms that can be seen only with a microscope; part of our normal environment; can be found on skin and throughout gastrointestinal, genitourinary, and respiratory systems; disease-producing microorganisms are referred to as pathogens and are classified as bacteria, viruses, fungi, or protozoa; also called *microbes* [Chapter 1]

microsurgery surgery performed on small body structures or cells with the aid of a microscope and other specialized instruments [Chapter 4]

mucosa membrane lining all body passages, such as the digestive tract and the urinary tract, that reach the exterior of the body, and which has cells and glands that secrete mucus; also called a mucous membrane [Chapter 3]

murmurs abnormal heart sounds created when blood courses through the heart valves; there are functional and organic murmurs; functional murmurs may occur as results of increased body temperature or elevated stress; organic murmurs are always present [Chapter 6]

nasal septum wall or partition dividing the nostrils [Chapter 3]

nebulizer device for administering respiratory medications as a fine inhaled spray [Chapter 5]

needle holder used to hold and pass a needle through tissue during suturing [Chapter 4]

neurogenic shock shock caused by a dysfunction of the nervous system following a spinal cord injury [Chapter 8]

neurological reflex uncontrolled and automatic response to stimulation that involves an impulse passing from a nerve receptor along a nerve to a nerve center and then from the nerve center to affect a muscle or a gland [Chapter 3]

nomogram graph displaying three curves, each measuring a different variable, in such a way that drawing a straight line across them will connect the related values of each variable [Chapter 5]

noncompliance when a patient is unwilling to accept treatment; contrast with *compliance* [Chapter 7]

normal flora healthy microorganisms that occur naturally in the human body [Chapter 1]

nuclear medicine diagnostic procedures using radionuclides and electromagnetic radiation; generally used in radiology departments [Chapter 6]

nutrition study of the body's food consumption and its ability to utilize food to maintain and repair itself [Chapter 7]

obturator smooth, rounded, removable inner portion of a hollow tube, such as an anoscope, that allows for easier insertion [Chapter 4]

occult type of blood examination in which a gloved finger is inserted into the rectum; a stool test may be obtained from any stool obtained from the finger [Chapter 3]

open-ended questions queries that encourage the patient to respond with more than one or two words and can lead to the identification of a patient's condition or complaint [Chapter 2]

open wound skin is broken and the patient is susceptible to external hemorrhage and wound contamination; may be the only surface evidence of a more serious injury; open wounds include abrasions, lacerations, major arterial lacerations, puncture wounds, avulsions, amputations, and impalements [Chapter 8]

ophthalmoscope medical tool used to inspect the interior structures of the eye [Chapter 3]

otorhinolaryngologist physician who specializes in treating disorders and disease of the ears, nose, and throat [Chapter 3]

over-the-counter medications medications that can be obtained without a prescription [Chapter 2]

palpation technique in which the examiner feels the texture, size, consistency, and location of parts of the body with the hands [Chapter 2]

panic sudden and overpowering feeling of terror or extreme anxiety [Chapter 7]

Papanicolaou (Pap) smear test in which cells obtained from the cervix or vagina are examined microscopically for abnormalities including cancer [Chapter 3]

parenteral route for medication administration by any method other than orally [Chapter 5]

partial dislocation incomplete displacement of a bone from a joint; also called a subluxation; contrast with *dislocation* [Chapter 8]

partial thickness burn second-degree burn to the epidermis or dermis [Chapter 8]

pathogens disease-producing microorganisms; classified as bacteria, viruses, fungi, or protozoa [Chapter 1]

percussion tapping or striking the body with the hand or an instrument to produce sounds; direct percussion is performed by striking the body with a finger; indirect percussion is performed by placing a finger on the area and then striking that finger with a finger from the other hand [Chapter 3]

perfusion   injection of fluid into a blood vessel, usually to supply nutrients and oxygen to tissues or an organ [Chapter 8]

peripheral   pertaining to or situated from the center [Chapter 3]

PERRLA   normal pupil reaction to light, which means that pupils are equal, round, and reactive to light and accommodation [Chapter 3]

personal protective equipment (PPE)   safety materials, such as gloves, goggles, and face shields [Chapter 1]

pharmacodynamics   study of the way drugs act on the body, including the actions on specific cells, tissues, and organs [Chapter 5]

pharmacokinetics   study of the action of drugs within the body based on the route of administration, rate of absorption, duration of action, and elimination from the body [Chapter 5]

pharmacology   study of drugs, their actions, dosages, and side effects [Chapter 5]

placebo effect   power of believing that something will make you better when there is no chemical reaction that warrants such improvement [Chapter 7]

planning   using the information gathered during assessment of a patient to determine how you will approach the patient's learning needs [Chapter 7]

plaque   elevated solid lesion on skin or mucosa; larger than 1 cm [Chapter 2]

polyp   a usually noncancerous tissue growth that protrudes from the mucous lining of an organ such as the nose or intestine, often causing an obstruction [Chapter 3]

postural hypotension   blood pressure that drops suddenly when a patient stands from a sitting or lying position; orthostatic hypertension [Chapter 2]

potentiation   when one drug prolongs or multiplies the effect of another drug; contrast with *antagonism* [Chapter 5]

present illness   problem or condition for which a patient is being seen in the medical office that day [Chapter 2]

pressure point   specific places on the body where you can press an artery against a bone to stop the flow of blood [Chapter 8]

preventive medicine   dedicated to deterring ailments and injury prior to onset; some common practices of preventive medicine include regular physical examinations, annual vaccinations, and regular breast examinations [Chapter 7]

preservative   substance that delays decomposition [Chapter 4]

projection   view of an object relative to the position of the person who is doing the viewing; for example, straight ahead, right, left, above, or below [Chapter 6]

psychiatric emergency   any situation in which the patient's moods, thoughts, or actions are so disordered or disturbed that harm or death may result for the patient or others if no intervention occurs [Chapter 8]

psychomotor skill   skill that requires a patient to physically perform a task [Chapter 7]

punch biopsy   used to remove a small piece of tissue via a small circular tube [Chapter 4]

purulent   wound drainage with any color other than pink; a sign of infection [Chapter 4]

pyrexia   a fever of 102° Fahrenheit or higher rectally or 101° Fahrenheit or higher orally [Chapter 2]

radiograph   processed x-ray film containing a visible image [Chapter 6]

radiography   art and science of producing diagnostic images with x-rays [Chapter 6]

radiologist   doctor who interprets x-rays and imaging studies and performs radiation therapy [Chapter 6]

radiology   branch of medicine concerned with diagnostic and therapeutic applications of x-rays [Chapter 6]

radiolucent   tissues in the body, such as those found in the lungs, that permit the passage of x-rays; contrast with *radiopaque* [Chapter 6]

radionuclides   radioactive materials with short life spans; designed to concentrate in specific areas of the body [Chapter 6]

radiopaque   tissues, such as bone, that do not permit the passage of x-rays; contrast with *radiolucent* [Chapter 6]

range of motion   the extent of a patient's joint movement [Chapter 3]

ratchet   notched mechanisms found in many forceps that click into position to maintain tension [Chapter 4]

rebound   body's response to extended periods of extreme temperature, exerting the opposite effect (for example, feeling cold when hyperthermic) [Chapter 8]

rectovaginal   examination in which the examiner places a gloved index finger in the vagina and the middle finger in the rectum at the same time; the rectum is usually inspected and palpated for lesions, hemorrhoids, and sphincter tone; a stool sample may be obtained to test for occult blood [Chapter 3]

relapsing   stage of fever in which fever returns after an extended period of normal readings [Chapter 2]

remittent   stage of fever in which fever fluctuates; contrast with *sustained* [Chapter 2]

rescue breathing   forcing of air into the lungs of a person who is not breathing on her own, usually by a mouth-to-mouth technique; usually performed as part of cardiopulmonary resuscitation (CPR) [Chapter 8]

resident flora   microorganisms living in the human body that are healthy and normal; also called normal flora; contrast with *pathogens* [Chapter 1]

resistance   body's natural ability to defend against pathogens; decreased with old age [Chapter 1]

respiration   exchange of gases between the atmosphere and the blood in the body [Chapter 2]

retract   to pull back layers of tissue to expose the areas beneath [Chapter 4]

rhythm strip   long strip of a certain lead or combination of leads that may be used to define certain cardiac arrhythmias [Chapter 6]

rule of nines   the most common method of determining the extent of burn injury; the body surface is divided into sections of nine percent or multiples of nine percent [Chapter 8]

sanitization   proper techniques for disposing of waste [Chapter 1]

sanitizing   the practice of lowering the number of microorganisms on a surface by use of low-level disinfectant practices [Chapter 4]

seizures   abnormal discharge of electrical activity in the brain; may cause erratic muscle movements, strange sensations, or a complete loss of consciousness [Chapter 8]

septic shock   shock caused by a general infection of the bloodstream in which the patient appears seriously ill; may be associated with infection such as pneumonia or meningitis, or may occur without an apparent source of infection [Chapter 8]

serrations   teeth found on forceps [Chapter 4]

serum   the watery fluid that remains after blood is coagulated or has had its solid parts separated by centrifuging [Chapter 4]

shock   lack of oxygen to the individual cells of the body, including the brain, as a result of a decrease in blood pressure [Chapter 8]

side effects   reactions to medications that are predictable and that occur in some patients who take the medications [Chapter 5]

signs   objective information that can be observed or perceived by someone other than the patient [Chapter 2]

sinus   any of the air-filled cavities in the bones of the skull, especially those connected to the nostrils; a narrow tract (also called a fistula) leading to a pus-filled cavity and serving for the discharge of pus [Chapter 3]

sound   long instrument for exploring or dilating body cavities or searching cavities for foreign bodies [Chapter 4]

speculum   instrument designed to allow examiners to investigate body cavities [Chapter 3]

sphygmomanometer   blood pressure cuff; used when assessing a patient's blood pressure [Chapter 2]

spirometer   instrument used to measure the air entering and leaving the lungs [Chapter 6]

splint   any device used to immobilize a sprain, strain, fracture, or dislocated limb [Chapter 8]

spore   bacterial life form that resists destruction by heat, drying, or chemicals; spore-producing bacteria include botulism and tetanus [Chapter 1]

sprain   injury to a ligament when a joint is extended beyond its normal range of motion, without dislocation or fracture [Chapter 8]

sterile field   surgical asepsis that must be maintained during surgery so as not to infect a patient [Chapter 4]

sterilization   process, act, or technique for destroying microorganisms using heat, water, chemicals, or gases [Chapter 4]

strain   injury to muscle tissue that can result from wrenching, twisting, overexertion, or overuse [Chapter 8]

stress   occurs when the sympathetic nervous system stimulates the release of the hormone epinephrine, which raises the pressure in the fight or flight response [Chapter 7]

subcutaneous injection   injection into the fatty layer of tissue below the skin; needle is positioned at a 45-degree angle to the skin [Chapter 5]

subcutaneous tissue   fatty layer of tissue below the skin [Chapter 4]

sublingual medication   medication placed under the patient's tongue; must not be swallowed [Chapter 5]

superficial burn   first-degree burn affecting the epidermis [Chapter 8]

surgical asepsis   sterile procedure used to free an item or area from all microorganisms; also known as sterile technique; prevents microbes from spreading to or from patients [Chapter 4]

sustained   stage of fever in which fever is constant; contrast with *remittent* [Chapter 2]

suture to close wounds and incisions in order to bring tissue layers into close approximation [Chapter 4]

sutures used to close wounds and incisions and to bring tissue layers into close approximation [Chapter 4]

swaged needle needle classified by eye; also called atraumatic [Chapter 4]

symmetry equality in size, shape, or position of parts on opposite sides of the body; contrast with *asymmetry* [Chapter 3]

symptoms subjective information that indicates diseases or changes in the body as sensed by the patient [Chapter 1]

synergism drug interaction in which two drugs work together; contrast with *antagonism* [Chapter 5]

systemic effect affecting the entire body or an entire body system, especially the nervous system; contrast with *local effect* [Chapter 5]

systole contraction of the heart by which the blood is forced onward and the circulation kept up [Chapter 2]

teleradiology radiology concerned with the transmission of digitized medical images over electronic networks and with the interpretation of the transmitted images for diagnostic purposes [Chapter 6]

tendon tough, flexible fibers that bind muscle to bone [Chapter 3]

topical medication medication applied directly to the skin or mucous membranes [Chapter 5]

trade name brand name of a given drug (for example, Valium is a trade name for diazepam) [Chapter 5]

transdermal medications medication applied to the skin [Chapter 5]

transient flora normal flora found in abnormal regions of the body; can become pathogens under the right conditions [Chapter 1]

transillumination during a paranasal sinus examination, the room is darkened and a penlight or flashlight is placed against the upper cheek or periorbital ridge [Chapter 3]

tympanic membrane thin, semitransparent membrane in the middle ear that transmits sound vibrations; the eardrum [Chapter 3]

ultrasound use of high-frequency sound waves, not x-rays, to create cross-sectional still or real-time (motion) images of the body [Chapter 6]

varicose veins occur when the superficial veins of the legs swell and distend; valves of the veins eventually fail to close properly, allowing blood to pool and stretch the walls of the veins; the most common circulatory disease of the lower extremities [Chapter 3]

vasoconstriction   following vascular damage, the vein constricts to reduce blood loss [Chapter 2]

vasodilation   opening the lumen of vessels, increasing blood supply to the heart [Chapter 2]

vector   organism that transmits a pathogen from one organism or source to another [Chapter 1]

vegetarian   an individual who eats only vegetables and excludes all foods of animal origin [Chapter 7]

vehicle   means by which a substance, such as a medicine or bacteria, is conveyed from one place to another [Chapter 1]

venipuncture   piercing of a vein by a needle, usually in order to withdraw blood or administer intravenous fluids or medication [Chapter 5]

viable   capable of growing and living [Chapter 1]

vial   glass or plastic container sealed at the top by a rubber stopper [Chapter 5]

virulent   highly pathogenic and disease producing; describes a microorganism [Chapter 1]

vital signs   values that indicate a person's rate of heart beat (pulse), breathing rate (respiration), body temperature, and blood pressure [Chapter 2]

wheal   transient elevation of the skin caused by edema of the dermis and surrounding capillary dilation [Chapter 5]

x-rays   high-energy waves that cannot be seen, heard, felt, tasted, or smelled and that can penetrate fairly dense objects, such as the human body [Chapter 6]

FIGURE CREDITS

Illustrations in *Medical Assisting Made Incredibly Easy: Clinical Competencies* have been borrowed from the following sources:

Anatomical Chart Company (chapter 3, unnumbered figure 14).
Bickley LS, Szilagyi PG. Bates' Guide to Physical Examination and History Taking. 9th ed. Philadelphia: Lippincott Williams & Wilkins, 2006 (chapter 2, unnumbered figure 26).
Caltech Industries, Midland, MI (chapter 1, unnumbered figures 24 and 26; chapter 3, unnumbered figure 20).
Carter PJ, Lewson S. Lippincott's Textbook for Nursing Assistants: A Humanistic Approach to Caregiving. Philadelphia: Lippincott Williams & Wilkins, 2004 (chapter 1, unnumbered figure 25; chapter 4, unnumbered figures 2, 66, and 67; chapter 5, unnumbered figure 37; chapter 7, unnumbered figure 3).
Cohen BJ. Medical Terminology: An Illustrated Guide. 4th ed. Baltimore: Lippincott Williams & Wilkins, 2003 (chapter 5, unnumbered figures 21 and 28).
Evans-Smith P. Taylor's Clinical Nursing Skills: A Nursing Process Approach. Philadelphia: Lippincott Williams & Wilkins, 2005 (chapter 1, unnumbered figures 28 and 29; chapter 2, unnumbered figures 22, 25, and 42; chapter 3, unnumbered figure 27; chapter 4, unnumbered figures 38, 45, and 62-64; chapter 5, unnumbered figures 41 and 47-57; chapter 6, unnumbered figures 42 and 44-46).
Katena Products, Denville, NJ (chapter 3, unnumbered figure 5).
LifeArt. Philadelphia: Lippincott Williams & Wilkins, 2004 (chapter 2, unnumbered figure 37; chapter 3, unnumbered figure 29-31).
Molle EA, Kronenberger J, Durham LS, West-Stack C. Lippincott Williams & Wilkins' Comprehensive Medical Assisting. 2nd ed. Baltimore: Lippincott Williams & Wilkins, 2005 (chapter 1, unnumbered figures 16, 17, 30, 31A, 31B, 32, and 33; chapter 2, unnumbered figures 2, 6, 8, 10, 11, 12, 15, 16, 18-21, 28, 31, 32, 36, and 38-42; chapter 3, unnumbered figures 2-4, 10, 11, 15-17, and 35-37; chapter 4, unnumbered figures 6, 7, 12-24, 37, 39, 41, 43, 44, 47, 50, 55-61, 65, 68, and 69; chapter 5,

unnumbered figures 5, 16, 18, 19, 23, 26, 27, 36, 40, 43-45, 46, and 59; chapter 6, unnumbered figures 2, 3, 5-12, 16, 17, 19, 20, 22, 24, 25, 29, 31-34, 41, 47, and 48; chapter 7, unnumbered figures 7 and 15; chapter 8, unnumbered figures 5-7, 11, 21, 23, 40, and 42-44).

Moore KL, Dalley AF. Clinically Oriented Anatomy. 5th ed. Baltimore: Lippincott Williams & Wilkins, 2005 (chapter 3, unnumbered figure 28).

Nettina SM. The Lippincott Manual of Nursing Practice. 8th ed. Philadelphia: Lippincott Williams & Wilkins, 2005 (chapter 3, unnumbered figure 9).

Protech, Palm Beach Gardens, FL (chapter 6, unnumbered figure 14).

Shils ME, Shike M, Ross AC, Caballero B, Cousins RJ. Modern Nutrition in Health and Disease. 10th ed. Baltimore: Lippincott Williams & Wilkins, 2006 (chapter 7, unnumbered figure 22).

Smeltzer SC, Bare BG. Textbook of Medical-Surgical Nursing. 9th ed. Philadelphia: Lippincott Williams & Wilkins, 2000 (chapter 3, unnumbered figures 32 and 38; chapter 4, unnumbered figure 29).

Taylor C, Lillis C, LeMone P. Fundamentals of Nursing: The Art and Science of Nursing Care. 5th ed. Philadelphia: Lippincott Williams & Wilkins, 2004 (chapter 3, unnumbered figures 7A and 8; chapter 4, unnumbered figures 28-35, 58, and 60; chapter 7, unnumbered figure 24; chapter 8, unnumbered figures 25-27, 36, and 37).

United States Department of Labor, Occupational Safety and Health Administration. OSHA's Form 300: Log of Work-Related Injuries and Illnesses, revised January 2004 (chapter 1, unnumbered figure 20).

United States Department of Agriculture, Center for Nutrition Policy and Promotion, April 2005 (chapter 7, unnumbered figure 20).

Welch Allyn, Skaneatels Falls, NY (chapter 3, unnumbered figure 7B).

Willis MC. Medical Terminology: A Programmed Learning Approach to the Language of Health Care. Baltimore: Lippincott Williams & Wilkins, 2002 (chapter 3, unnumbered figure 13).

INDEX

Page numbers in *italics* denote figures; those followed by a t denote tables.

A

Abbreviations, medical, 267t
Abdomen, physical examination, 135, 464–465
Abnormal breathing, 79
Absorbable sutures, 207
Absorption, pharmacokinetics, 271
Achilles tendon, 138
Active acquired artificial immunity, 10
Active acquired natural immunity, 10
Acts of terrorism, 504
Acupressure, 426
Acupuncture, 425–426, *426*
Acute stage, infectious disease, 12
Adapting teaching material, 409–410
  for patient education, 409–410
Adhesives, 205
Afebrile, 64
Affection, in Maslow's hierarchy of needs, 401
After surgical procedures, 213–254
Age, as obstacle to learning, 406
AHFS (*see* American Hospital Formulary Service)
AIDS, 15
Air bubbles, removing from medication, *320*
Airway, 453
  assessing/opening, 454–457
  opening, 454–455t
Alcohol abuse, 433
Allergen, 485
Allergic reactions, 274–276, 485–488
  anaphylactic reactions, 487–488
  anaphylaxis, 487
  signs, 486
  symptoms, 486
Allergy shots, 486

Alternative medicine, 425–426
  acupressure, 426
  acupuncture, 425–426
  hypnosis, 426
  yoga, 426
American Hospital Formulary Service, 276
Amphetamines, 435
Ampules, 292
  for injections, *292*
Amputations, 469–470
Anaerobes, 5
Anaphylactic reactions, 487–488
Anaphylactic shock, 467
Anaphylaxis, 274, 487
Aneroid sphygmomanometer, *80*
Anesthetic administration, 203
Angles of insertion, *298*
Animals, pathogen transmission, 14
Annual rectal examinations, 139
  and fecal occult blood test, 139
Answering patient's questions, 198–200
Antagonism, 273
  medications, 273
Anterior, 62
Anthropometric, defined, 56
Anthropometric measurements, 55–62
  balance beam scale, 56–58
  children, physical measurements, 59–62
    infant length, measurement of, 60
    infant weight, measurement of, 60–61
  dial scale, 58
  digital scale, 58
  height, 58–59
  weight, 55–58
Antibodies, 9
Antidotes, 489
Anxious patient, 51

Apgar score, 78
Apical pulse, *74*
Apothecary system, 278–280
Apothecary system of measurement, 278
Approximate equivalents, 281t
Apron, lead-lined, *348*
Arm fractures, *478*
Arm sling application, 479–480
Arms
    physical examination, 465
    scrubbing with sterile brush, *164*
Arteries as pulse points, *72*
Arteriosclerosis, 84
Artifacts, types of, 369–370t
Asepsis, 1–41, 162–165
    active acquired artificial immunity, 10
    active acquired natural immunity, 10
    anaerobes, 5
    antibodies, 9
    bacteria, 3
    bactericidal, 5
    body protection, 4–5
        darkness, 5
        eyes, 4–5
        gastrointestinal tract, 5
        genitourinary tract, 5
        moisture, 5
        mouth, 5
        neutral pH, 5
        nutrients, 5
        oxygen, 5
        respiratory tract, 5
        skin, 4
        temperature, 5
    carrier, 7
    chronic infections, 11
    contagious diseases, 2
    contamination, 27–30
        biohazard cleanup, 27–28
        biohazard waste, 30
        waste container, 28–29
            biohazard waste container, 29
            regular waste container, 29
            sharps waste container, 29
    control plan, 20–23
    dormant infection, 11
    exiting reservoir, 7
    fighting infection, 7–12
    fungi, 3
    germs, 2–3
    guidelines, medical office, 20–27

hepatitis B, 31–40
    exposure prevention, 31–32
    exposure response, 32–40
immune system, 8
immune system failure, 10
infection control, 15–19
    disinfection, 18–19
        complexity of object, 19
        length of exposure, 19
        prior cleaning, 18
        strength of disinfecting solution, 19
        temperature, 19
        type of microorganism, 18
        types of, 18
    levels, 17–19
    medical asepsis, 15–17
        clean hands, 15–16
        clean workplace, 17
    sanitization, 17
    sterilization, 19
infection process, 6–7
latent infections, 11–12
manual, 20–21
microbes, 2
microorganism survival, 5–6
microorganisms, 2
natural immunity, 9
normal flora, 4
passive acquired artificial immunity, 9–10
passive acquired natural immunity, 9
pathogens, 2
personal protective equipment, 24–25
portal of entry, 7
protozoa, 3
reservoir host, 6–7
resident flora, 4
risk factors, 20
safety equipment, 25–27
    eyewash station, 27
    immunization, 27
    MSDS binder, 25
    personal protective equipment, 27
    waste containers, 25–26
spores, 3
spread of infection, 13–15
    direct transmission, 13
    indirect transmission, 13
stages of infectious disease, 12
    acute stage, 12
    convalescent stage, 12
    declining stage, 12

Asepsis (*continued*)
  incubation stage, 12
  prodromal stage, 12
  standard precautions, 24
  susceptible host, 7
    identification of, 11
  symptoms, 10
  transmission of pathogens, 13–15
    animals, 14
    human hosts, 14
    insects, 15
  types of immunity, 9–10
  types of infections, 11–12
  vehicle of transmission, 7
  viruses, 3
Asking questions to patients, 48
Assessment in teaching, 393–394
Assisting physician, 122–126
  dorsal recumbent position, 123
  erect position, 123
  Fowler's position, 124
  helping patient, 122
  helping physician, 122
  knee-chest position, 124
  lithotomy position, 123
  moving patient, 122–123
  patient examination positions,
      123–126
  prone position, 123–124
  reverse Trendelenburg position, 124
  semi-Fowler's position, 124
  Sims' position, 123
  sitting position, 123
  standing position, 123
  supine position, 123
  Trendelenburg position, 124
Assisting with surgery, 202–213
  common medical office surgical
      procedures, 208–210
  electrosurgery, 210–212
  laser surgery, 212–213
  local anesthetics, 202–203
  passing instruments, 203–204
  wound closure, 204–208
Asthma attacks, 496–497
Atherosclerosis, 84
Atorvastatin, 274
Atraumatic needles, 206
Audiovisual material, in teaching, 396
Auditory canal, *501*
Augmented unipolar leads, 365
Auscultation, 118
Auscultatory gap, 82
Autoclave, 167–173, *169*

loading, 170–171
maintenance, 172–173
operation, 227–228–228
placement in, *171*
working, 171–172
wrapping instruments for steriliza-
    tion, 224–226
Autoclave indicator tape stripes, *170*
Autoclave pouches, *224*
Autoclave tape, 169
Autoclave wrapping material, 169
Autoclaved items, storing, 172–173
Automatic external defibrillator,
    459–460
Axillary, 65
Axillary temperature, measurement
    of, 93–94
Ayre spatula, 115
  use in pelvic exam, *115*

B
Babinski reflex, 108
Back, physical examination, 464–465
Bacteria, 3
Bactericidal, 5
Bag-mask valve, *457*
Balance beam scale, 56–58
Balance scale, *57*
Bandage application, 216–218
  circular turn, 216
  figure-eight turn, 217
  reverse spiral turn, 217
  spiral turn, 217
Bandage scissors, 178
Bandage types
  staple bandages, 218–219
  suture bandages, 218–219
Bandages, 213, 217–218
Barium, *351*
Barium studies, 350–352
Baseline data, 55
Beans, 415
Behavioral emergencies, 494–495
Belonging/affection, in Maslow's hier-
    archy of needs, 401
Biceps tendon, 138
Bimanual technique, palpation of
    pelvic organs, *157*
Biohazard cleanup, 27–28
Biohazard spill kit, 28
Biohazard spill supplies, 29
Biohazard waste, 30
Biohazard waste container, 29

Biohazardous, 20
Biohazardous spills, cleaning, 39
Biohazards, exposure to, 21
Biopsy, 208
Bioterrorism, 504
Blades, scalpel, *179*
Bleach, *18*
Bleeding, 468–471
Bleeding control, 471
Blocked airway, 455–456
Bloodborne pathogens, training
    regarding, 23
Blood gases, 378–379
Blood pressure, 63, 79–85, *100*
   activity, effect on, 84
   age, effect on, 84
   arteriosclerosis, 84
   atherosclerosis, 84
   auscultatory gap, 82
   body position, effect on, 84
   diastolic pressure, 80
   diseases affecting, 83
   getting reading, 81–82
   Korotkoff sounds, 82
   measurement, 80–81, 99–103
   medications, effect on, 84
   normal, 82–84
     pulse pressure, 83
   stress, effect on, 84
   systolic pressure, 79
   weight, effect on, 84
Blood pressure cuff, size, *81*
Blood sounds, called bruit, *129*
Body, examination of, 128–138
Body position, effect on blood pres-
    sure, 84
Books for patient education, 408
Brain, CT scan, *354*
Brand name, 257
Breast examination, 132, 141
Breast self-examination, 132–134
Breathing, 453
Breathing techniques, 431
Bronchoscopy, 378
BSA method, in dose calculation, 285
Burn injuries, classification of, 472
Burns, 472–475
   body surface area, 472–474
   burn injuries, classification, 472
   characteristics, 473t
   chemical burns, 472
   electrical burns, 472
   radiation burns, 472
   rule of nines to estimate, *474*
   thermal burns, 472

C

Carbohydrates, 419–420
Cardiac catheterization, 375
Cardiac cycle, 79, 367, *368*
Cardiac stress test, 373–374
Cardinal signs, 62
Cardiogenic shock, 466
Cardiologist, 360
Cardiopulmonary resuscitation, 446,
    457–458, 461–462
Cardiovascular disorders
   cardiac catheterization, 375
   cardiac stress test, 373–374
   coronary arteriography, 375–376
   diagnosing, 360–376
   echocardiography, 374–375
   electrocardiogram, 361–370
     electrodes, placing, 364
     interpreting, 367–370
       P-R interval, 367
       P wave, 367
       QRS complex, 367
       S-T segment, 367
       T wave, 368
       U wave, 368
     leads, 365–366
      augmented unipolar leads, 365
      standard bipolar leads, 365
      unipolar precordial leads, 366
   Holter monitors, 370–373
     continuous recording, 371
     incident recording, 372
   tests, 361
Cardiovascular emergencies, 483–484
Carotid arteries, physical examina-
    tion, 129
Carotid pulse, palpating, *453*
Carrier, 7
Cassette, 342
Cell collection, 115
Celsius scale, *67*
Celsius thermometer, 66
Cervical biopsies, 209, 241–242
Cervical fractures, 464
Cervical scraper, 115
Changing sterile dressings, 214
Charting sample, for patient educa-
    tion, 398–399
Chemical burns, 472

Chemical name, prescription, 257
Chemical sterilization, 174, 229–230
Chest, physical examination,
  131–135, 464–465
Chest electrode placement, for elec-
  trocardiogram recording, *365*
Chest lead application, *382*
Chicken pox, 15
Chief complaint, 52
  determination, 52–53
Children, 406
  calculating doses, 285–287
  cardiopulmonary resuscitation,
    461–462
  physical measurements, 59–62
    infant length, measurement of,
      60
    infant weight, measurement of,
      60–61
Cholesterol, 420–421
Chronic infections, 11
Chronology of present illness, 54
Circulation, 453
Clark's rule, in dose calculation, 286
Cleaning by hand, 166
Cleaning of examination room, 128
Cleaning surgical instruments,
  responsibility for, 185–188
Closed wound, 468–469
Coagulation, 211
Cocaine, 434–435
Cold chemical sterilization, 173–174
Cold/heat in treating emergencies,
  504–511
  cold packs, 510–511
  compresses, application, 506–507
  hot packs, 508–510
  hot water bottles, 508–510
  soaks, 507–508
Cold packs, 510–511
Colon cancer, screening, 139
Colonoscopy, 139
Color perception, measurement of,
  153–154
Colostomy, 178
Colposcopy, 241–242
Common medical office surgical pro-
  cedures, 208–210
Common surgical instruments,
  175–185
Communication barriers, 50
Communication skills, 48–49
  asking questions, 48
  examples, asking, 48

paraphrasing, 48
reflecting, 48
silence, allowing, 48
summarizing, 48
Community resources, 439
Compendium of Drug Therapy, 276
Compresses, *506*
  application, 506–507
Compression, 476
Compression fracture, 477
Computed tomography, 354
Conditions needed for patient educa-
  tion, 399–404
Conduction, 64
Conjunctival sac, *333*
Consent form, *199*
Contagious diseases, 2
Contaminated glove removal, 35–37
Contamination, 27–30
  biohazard cleanup, 27–28
  biohazard waste, 30
  waste container, 28–29
    biohazard waste container, 29
    regular waste container, 29
    sharps waste container, 29
Continuous recording, Holter moni-
  tors, 371
Contrast examinations
  preparing patients, 353
  scheduling, 352
Contrast medium, 351–352
Contrast medium examinations,
  349–352
Control of temperature, 68–71
Control plan, 21–23
Control plan for infection, 21–23
Controlled substances, 258, 262
  disposal, 264
  inventory monitoring, 263–264
  physical dependence, 262
  prescribing, 264–265
  psychological dependence, 262
Controlled Substances Act, 261
Controlled substances inventory
  form, *263*
Contusion, 468
Convalescent stage, infectious disease,
  12
Convection, 64
Converting between measurement
  systems, 280–281
Coordination, 138
Coping skills, 430
Coronary arteriography, 375–376

Cotton-tipped applicator, 115
  for physical examination, *107*, 108
  use in pelvic exam, *115*
Coumadin, 274
CPR, 505
Crack, 434–435
Crutch gaits, 483
Crutches, 481–482, *482*
Cryosurgery, 209
CT (*see* Computed tomography)
Cultural differences, 120
Culture tests, 170
Curved scissors, 176
Cystectomy, 178

D

Darkness, 5
Date, prescriptions, 265
DEA number, prescriptions, 266
Declining stage, infectious disease, 12
Defibrillation, 458–460
Dehiscence, 205
Demographic data, 44
Demonstration, in teaching, 396
Depressants, 435
Depth of respiration, 78
Dermatology instruments, 181
Desiccated, 209
Determination of chief complaint,
  52–53
Diagnosing, 360–376
Diagnosis, 43, 347–355
Diagnostic testing, 340–391
  cardiovascular disorders
    cardiac catheterization, 375
    cardiac stress test, 373–374
    coronary arteriography, 375–376
    diagnosing, 360–376
    echocardiography, 374–375
    electrocardiogram, 361–370
      electrodes, placing, 364
      interpreting, 367–370
        P-R interval, 367
        P wave, 367
        QRS complex, 367
        S-T segment, 367
        T wave, 368
        U wave, 368
      leads, 365–366
        augmented unipolar leads,
          365
        standard bipolar leads, 365
        unipolar precordial leads, 366

Holter monitors, 370–373
  continuous recording, 371
  incident recording, 372
  tests, 361
follow-up, 380–391
radiology, 341–360
  barium studies, 350–352
  computed tomography, 354
  contrast medium examinations,
    349–352
  diagnosis, 347–355
  fluoroscopy, 352–353
  magnetic resonance imaging,
    354–355
  medical assistant's role, 357–360
    educating patients, 358
    film handling/storing, 359
    transfer of study information,
      359–360
  nuclear medicine, 355
  patient positions, 343–344
  positron emission tomography,
    355
  radiation, side effects of, 357
  radiation safety for clinical staff,
    346–347
  radiation safety for patients,
    344–346
  radiation therapy, 356–357
  scheduling x-rays, 352
  single photon emission computed
    tomography, 355
  sonography, 354
  treatment, 355–357
    embolization, 356
    laser angioplasty, 356
    percutaneous transluminal
      coronary angioplasty, 356
    vascular stents, 356
  x-rays, 342–347
respiratory testing, 376–379
  blood gases, 378–379
  bronchoscopy, 378
  oximetry, 376–377
  pulmonary function tests, 376
    forced expiration volume, 376
    tidal volume, 376
Dial scale, *57*
Diaphoresis, 71
Diarrhea, 497
Diastole, 80
Diastolic pressure, 80
Diet modification for medical conditions, 423

Dietary guidelines, 416–418
Diets for medical conditions, 423t
Digital scale, *57, 58*
Direct percussion, 117
Director, 180
  for knife, scalpel, *180*
Disaster emergencies, 503–504
  acts of terrorism, 504
  natural disasters, 503–504
Discussion, in teaching, 396
Disease prevention, patient education, 437–438
Diseases affecting blood pressure, 83
Disinfectants, *18*
Disinfection, 17–19
  length of exposure, 19
  prior cleaning, 18
  strength of disinfecting solution, 19
  temperature, 19
  type of microorganism, 18
Dislocation, 476–477
Disposable paper thermometer, *69*
Disposable sterile supplies, *19*
Disposable surgical packs, 189
Disposable suture removal kit, *219*
Disposable thermometers, 68
Disposal of controlled substances, 264
Distal, 62
Distance visual acuity, measurement of, 151–152
Distribution, pharmacokinetics, 271
Documentation in teaching, 398–399
Documentation of complaint, 87
Documentation of emergency, 450–451
Documentation of patient education, 398t
Doppler device, *76*
Doppler unit, 75–76
Dormant infection, 11
Dorsal recumbent position, 123, *125*
Dorsalis pedis pulse, *76*
Dose calculation, 282–287
  BSA method, 285
  Clark's rule, 286
  formula method, 284–285
  Fried's rule, 287
  ratio method, 283–284
  Young's rule, 285–286
Dosimeter, 347
Drainage, incision, 209
Drapes, types of, 200–201
Draping patient, *91*, 201, *201*
Dressing, changing, 247–248

Dressings, 213
Dropper tip insertion, *335*
Drug Enforcement Agency, 258
Drugs (*see* Medications)
Duration of present illness, 54
Dyspnea, 378

E

Ear, instruments for examination of, 113–114
Ear emergencies, 500–502
Ear medications, instilling, 335–336
Ears
  medication via, 306
  physical examination, 130
Ecchymosis, 468
ECG (*see* Electrocardiogram)
Echocardiography, 374–375
-Ectomy, 178
Edema, 223
Education of patient, 392–442 (*see also* Patient education; Teaching)
Educational background, as obstacle to learning, 407
EKG (*see* Electrocardiogram)
Elastic bandages, 215–216
Electrical burns, 472
Electrocardiogram, 139, 361–370
  electrodes, placing, 364
  interpreting, 367–370
    P-R interval, 367
    P wave, 367
    QRS complex, 367
    S-T segment, 367
    T wave, 368
    U wave, 368
  leads, 365–366
    augmented unipolar leads, 365
    standard bipolar leads, 365
    unipolar precordial leads, 366
  safety, 371
Electrocardiogram hook-up, chest leads, 366
Electrocardiogram leads, coding, 367t
Electrocautery, 211
Electrode maintenance, 370
Electrodes, 210
  placing, 364
Electrodesiccation, 211
Electrolyte, 490
Electronic thermometer, 67, 95
  placement, *68*
Electrosection, 211

Electrosurgery, 208, 210–212
  electrocautery, 211
  electrodesiccation, 211
  electrosection, 211
  electrosurgical unit, maintenance,
    212
  fulguration, 211
  safety, 211–212
Electrosurgical unit, maintenance of,
  212
Elements of teaching plan, 408–409
  evaluation, 408
  learning goal, 408
  learning objectives, 408
  material to be covered, 408
Elevation, 476
Embolization, 356
Emergencies, 443–513
  action plan, 445–451
  allergic reactions, 485–488
    anaphylactic reactions, 487–488
    anaphylaxis, 487
    signs, 486
    symptoms, 486
  asthma attacks, 496–497
  behavioral, 494–495
  bleeding, 468–471
  burns, 472–475
    body surface area, 472–474
    burn injuries, classification of,
      472
    chemical burns, 472
    electrical burns, 472
    radiation burns, 472
    thermal burns, 472
  cardiovascular emergencies,
    483–484
  diarrhea, 497
  disaster emergencies, 503–504
    acts of terrorism, 504
    natural disasters, 503–504
  documentation of emergency,
    450–451
  ear emergencies, 500–502
  emergency care, 444–445
    steps for handling, 445
  emergency medical kit, 447–448
  eye injuries, 499–500
  fainting, 495–496
  fever, 498–499
  heat/cold in treating, 504–511
    cold packs, 510–511
    compresses, application of,
      506–507

    hot packs, 508–510
    hot water bottles, 508–510
    soaks, 507–508
  medical emergency, 449–450
  musculoskeletal injuries, 475–483
    dislocations, 476–477
    fractures, 477
    slings, 479–483
    sprains, 475–476
    strains, 475–476
    types of splints, 478–479
  neurological emergencies, 484–485
    seizure, 485
    seizure patients, assessing,
      484–485
  nosebleeds, 502–503
  physical examination, 462–465
    abdomen, 464–465
    arms, 465
    back, 464–465
    chest, 464–465
    head, 463–464
    legs, 465
    neck, 463–464
  poisoning, 488–489
    Poison Control Center, 489
    poisoning emergencies, 489
  primary assessment, 452–460
    airway, 453
      assessing/opening, 454–457
    breathing, 453
    cardiopulmonary resuscitation,
      457–458
    circulation, 453
    defibrillation, 458–460
    rescue breathing, 457
    responsiveness, 453
  psychiatric, 494–495
  recognizing emergency, 449
  secondary assessment, 460–462
    general appearance, 460
    level of consciousness, 460–462
    skin, 462
    vital signs, 462
  shock, 466–468
    anaphylactic shock, 467
    neurogenic shock, 467
    septic shock, 467
    types, 466–467
  soft tissue injuries, 468–471
    closed wounds, 468–469
    open wounds, 469–471
      amputations, 469–470
      impaled objects, 470–471

Emergencies (*continued*)
temperature-related emergencies, 490–494
frostbite, 493–494
managing, 493–494
types of, 493
heat cramps, 490–491
heat exhaustion, 491
heat stroke, 491–492
hyperthermia, 490–492
hypothermia, 492–493
types of emergencies, 466–495
vomiting, 497–498
Emergency call, 452
Emergency medical kit contents, 447–448
Emergency medical services system, 448
Emergency supplies, 505
Emotional crisis, 494
Endoscope, 173
Endoscopy, 3
Enema, 306
Equipment, use of, in teaching, 402–403
Equivalents, 280
Erect position, 123, *125*
Esteem/self-respect, in Maslow's hierarchy of needs, 401
Ethylene oxide, 165
Evaluation in teaching, 397–398, 408
Evaporation, 64
Examination positions, 126t
Examination room cleaning, 128, 142–143
Examination room preparation, 119
equipment, 119
examination table, 119
supplies, 119
Examination tables, 142
cleaning, 38, 143
Examples, asking for, 48
Excise, 208
Excision of lesion, 208–209
cryosurgery, 209
electrosurgery, 208
laser surgery, 208
standard method, 208
Excisional surgery, 239–240
Excretion, pharmacokinetics, 271
Exercise, 423–425
Exiting reservoir, 7
Expiration, 77
Exposure control plan, 21–23
External respiration, 76

Extraocular, 130
Exudate, 210
Eye injuries, 499–500
Eye irrigation, 499–500
Eye medications, instilling, 333–334
Eye movement, physical examination, 129
Eyes, 4–5
medication in, 306
physical examination, 129–130
Eyewash station, 27, *27*

F

Factors affecting pulse rates, 73–76
blood volume, 74
body type, size, 74
exercise, 74
fever, 74
gender, 74
medications, 74
stress, 74
time of day, 73
Factors influencing temperature, 69–70
age, 70
emotions, 70
exercise, 70
fever, 70–71
gender, 70
heat, 70
illness, 70
time of day, 70
Fahrenheit scale, thermometer calibration, *67*
Fahrenheit thermometer, 66
Fainting, 495–496
Falls, prevention of, 412–413
Familial disorder, 45
Family history, 45
Fats, 419, 421
Febrile, 64
Fecal occult blood test, 139
Female genitalia, physical examination, 137–138
Fenestrated drapes, 200
Fetus, ultrasound of, *354*
Fever, 71, 498–499
stages, 70
Fibrin, 223
Fighting infection, 7–12
First impressions, 50
Flexible sigmoidoscopy, 139
Fluoroscopy, 352–353
Follow-up tests, 127t

Follow-up to diagnostic testing, 380–391
Follow-up to patient examination, 127
Food and Drug Administration, 258
Food group categories, 418t
   patient education, 418t
Food guide, 415–416
   beans, 415
   grains, 415
   meats, 415
   milk/milk products, 415
   oils, 415
   vegetables, 415
Food labels, *420*, 440
Food-medication interactions, 273–274
Food preparation, 422
Food pyramid, 416, *417*
Forced expiration volume, 376
Forceps, 174–176, *177, 196*
   storing, 195
Fowler's position, 124, *125*
Fractures, 477
   arm, *478*
   vertebrae, *478*
Fried's rule, in dose calculation, 287
Frostbite, 493–494
   managing, 493–494
   types, 493
Fulguration, 211
Full thickness burn, 472
Fungi, 3

G

Gait, 138
Gastrointestinal tract, 5
Gauge, 206
Generic name, prescription, 257
Generic prescriptions, 266
Genitalia
   female, physical examination, 137–138
   male, physical examination, 135–137
Genitourinary tract, 5
Germs, 2–3
GI tract (*see* Gastrointestinal)
Glass thermometer, 65–66, *66*, 88–90
   calibration, *67*
   reading, *66*
Gloves
   lead-lined, *348*
   for physical examination, *107*
   sterile, *191–193*

Good samaritan laws, 450
Gooseneck lamp, 112, *112*
Grains, 415–416
Graph paper, ECG, *363*
Greenstick fracture, 477
Groin, physical examination, 135
Guidelines for physical examination, 139–160
Gynecology instruments, 182

H

Hair removal, 237–238
Hallucinogens, 435–436
Handling radiology film, 359
Hands
   cleaning, 15–16, 32–34
   scrubbing with sterile brush, *164*
Head, physical examination, 128–138, 463–464
Head lamp, *113*
Healing process, 219–223
   healing by primary intention, 219–221
   healing by secondary intention, 221
   healing by tertiary intention, 221–223
Health care, patient education, 411–442
Health care topics, 411–442
Heat/cold in treating emergencies, 504–511
   cold packs, 510–511
   compresses, application, 506–507
   hot packs, 508–510
   hot water bottles, 508–510
   soaks, 507–508
Heat cramps, 490–491
Heat exhaustion, 491
Heat loss, production, factors affecting, *70*
Heat stroke, 491–492
Heat transfer, 64
   mechanisms, 64t
Heat transfer mechanisms, *64*
Height, 58–59
Height measurement, 58–59
Helping patient, 122
Helping physician, 122
Hematoma, 469
Hemostasis, 176
Hemostat use, *250*
Hemostats, 176
Hepatitis B, 15, 31–40
   exposure prevention, 31–32
   exposure response, 32–40

Herbal supplements, 427–428, 427t, 428
Hereditary disorders, 45
Hernia, 135
HIPAA, 48
Histobrush, 115, *115*
Holter diaries, 372–373
Holter monitor, 370–373, *371*
   application, 385–386
   continuous recording, 371
   incident recording, 372
Homeopathic medications, 53
Hot packs, 508–510
Hot places, 64–65
Hot water bottles, 508–510
Human hosts, pathogen transmission, 14
Hyperpyrexia, 70
Hyperthermia, 490–492
Hyperventilation, 453
Hypnosis, 426
Hypothermia, 490, 492–493
Hypovolemic shock, 466

I

Ice, 476
Illegal drugs, 265, 434–436
   amphetamines, 435
   cocaine, 434–435
   crack, 434–435
   depressants, 435
   hallucinogens, 435–436
   marijuana, 434
   narcotics, 436
Illness, as obstacle to learning, 405–406
Immune system, 8
   failure, 10
Immunity, 9
Immunization, 9, 27, 139–141
Impaled objects, 470–471
Incident recording, Holter monitors, 372
Incision, 179
   drainage, 209
Incubation stage, infectious disease, 12
Indirect percussion, 117, *117*
Individualized patient education, 438
Infants
   calculating doses, 285–287
   cardiopulmonary resuscitation, 461–462

length measurement, 60
   weighing, 60–61, *61*
Infection control, 1–41
   active acquired artificial immunity, 10
   active acquired natural immunity, 10
   anaerobes, 5
   antibodies, 9
   bacteria, 3
   bactericidal, 5
   biohazard equipment, 25–27
   body protection, 4–5
      darkness, 5
      eyes, 4–5
      gastrointestinal tract, 5
      genitourinary tract, 5
      moisture, 5
      mouth, 5
      neutral pH, 5
      nutrients, 5
      oxygen, 5
      respiratory tract, 5
      skin, 4
      temperature, 5
   carrier, 7
   chronic infections, 11
   contagious diseases, 2
   contamination, 27–30
      biohazard cleanup, 27–28
      biohazard waste, 30
      waste container, 28–29
         biohazard waste container, 29
         regular waste container, 29
         sharps waste container, 29
   control plan, 20–23
   disinfection, 18–19
      complexity of object, 19
      length of exposure, 19
      prior cleaning, 18
      strength of disinfecting solution, 19
      temperature, 19
      type of microorganism, 18
      types of, 18
   dormant infection, 11
   exiting reservoir, 7
   fighting infection, 7–12
   fungi, 3
   germs, 2–3
   guidelines, medical office, 20–27
   hepatitis B, 31–40
      exposure prevention, 31–32
      exposure response, 32–40

HIV, 31–40
  exposure prevention, 31–32
  exposure response, 32–40
immune system, 8
immune system failure, 10
infection control, 15–19
  disinfection, 18–19
    complexity of object, 19
    length of exposure, 19
    prior cleaning, 18
    strength of disinfecting solution, 19
    temperature, 19
    type of microorganism, 18
    types of, 18
  levels, 17–19
  medical asepsis, 15–17
    clean hands, 15–16
    clean workplace, 17
  sanitization, 17
  sterilization, 19
infection process, 6–7
latent infections, 11–12
levels, 17–19, 17t
manual, 20–21
medical asepsis, 15–17
  clean hands, 15–16
  clean workplace, 17
microbes, 2
microorganism survival, 5–6
microorganisms, 2
natural immunity, 9
normal flora, 4
passive acquired artificial immunity, 9–10
passive acquired natural immunity, 9
pathogens, 2
personal protective equipment, 24–25
portal of entry, 7
protozoa, 3
reservoir host, 6–7
resident flora, 4
risk factors, 20
safety equipment, 25–27
  eyewash station, 27
  immunization, 27
  MSDS binder, 25
  personal protective equipment, 27
  waste containers, 25–26
sanitization, 17
spores, 3
spread of infection, 13–15

direct transmission, 13
indirect transmission, 13
stages of infectious disease, 12
  acute stage, 12
  convalescent stage, 12
  declining stage, 12
  incubation stage, 12
  prodromal stage, 12
standard precautions, 24
sterilization, 19
susceptible host, 7
  identification of, 11
symptoms, 10
transmission of pathogens, 13–15
  animals, 14
  human hosts, 14
  insects, 15
types of immunity, 9–10
types of infections, 11–12
vehicle of transmission, 7
viruses, 3
Infection control plan, 20
Infection process, 6–7
Infectious disease, spread, 15t
Infectious waste, disposing of, 30
Inferior, 62
Influenza, 15
Informed consent, 197–198
  inability of patient to give, 468
Inhalation, medication by, 305
Injection types, 295–298
  intradermal injections, 295–297
  intramuscular injections, 297–298
  subcutaneous injections, 297
  Z-track method, 298
Injections, 292–298
  equipment, *292*
  insulin syringes, 294
  needle selection, 294
  needles, 293–295
  syringes, 293–295
    types of, 294–295
  tuberculin syringes, 294
  vials, 292–293
Inscription, prescription, 265
Insects, pathogen transmission, 15
Inspection, 116
Inspiration, 77
Instruments, 106–116, 181–185t
Instruments for physical exam, 106–111
Instruments for specialized examinations, 111–116
Insulin syringe, 294, *296*

Interactions of medications, 269–276
Internal respiration, 76
Internet resources for patient educa-
    tion, 436–437t
Interpreting electrocardiogram,
    367–370
    P-R interval, 367
    P wave, 367
    QRS complex, 367
    S-T segment, 367
    T wave, 368
    U wave, 368
Interviewing patients, 45–52
    communication barriers, 50
    communication skills, 48–49
        asking questions, 48
        examples, asking for, 48
        paraphrasing, 48
        reflecting, 48
        silence, allowing, 48
        summarizing, 48
    fist impressions, 50
    before interview, 49
        location, 49
        preparation, 49
Intradermal injection, 295–297,
    321–323
Intramuscular injection, 294,
    297–298, 328
    recommended sites, 299–301t
    Z-track method, 330–331
Intravenous (IV) medication route,
    298–304
    setting rate, 303
    starting IV, 301–302
    TKO/KVO rates, 304
Inventory monitoring, controlled sub-
    stances, 263–264
Iodine, 351–352
Irrigation fluid, basin placement, 502
IV (intravenous), 298–304
    equipment, 302
    fluid, 302
    problems with, 304
    setting rate, 303
    starting, 301–302
    TKO/KVO rates, 304

K

Kelly hemostats, 176
Keratosis, 208
Knee-chest position, 124, 125
Korotkoff sounds, 82

L

Labels, food, 418–422, 420
    carbohydrates, 419–420
    cholesterol, 420
    fats, 419
    minerals, 420–422
    protein, 420
    sodium, 420
    vitamins, 420–422
Lacto-ovovegetarian, 423
Lactovegetarian, 423
Laryngeal mirror, 114
Laryngoscope, 114
Larynx, 113
Laser angioplasty, 356
Laser surgery, 208, 212–213
Latent infections, 11–12
Lateral, 62
Latex allergy, 26
Lead-lined apron, gloves, 348
Leads, 365–366
    augmented unipolar leads, 365
    standard bipolar leads, 365
    unipolar precordial leads, 366
Learning goal, in teaching plan, 408
Learning objectives, in teaching plan,
    408
Lecture, in teaching, 396
Legal regulations regarding medica-
    tions, 258–265
Legs, physical examination, 138, 465
Lentigine, 208
Lesion excision, 208–209
    cryosurgery, 209
    electrosurgery, 208
    laser surgery, 208
    standard method, 208
Level of consciousness, 460–462
Levels of disinfection, 18t
Ligaments, 138
Lights, 112
Limb lead application, 382
Lipitor, 274
Listening skills, 49
Lithotomy position, 123, 125
Local anesthetics, 202–203
Location of present illness, 54
Log of work-related injuries, illnesses,
    22
Lubricant, 116
Lung radiograph, chest x-ray, 343
Lymph nodes, glands, physical exami-
    nation, 129

M

Magnetic resonance imaging, 354–355, *355*
Male genitalia, physical examination, 135–137
Malignancy, 130
Mammogram, 141
  positioning, *350*
Mammography, 350
Manipulation, 117
Mantoux test, 296
  needle insertion, *298*
Manual for infection control, 20–21
MAO inhibitors, 274
Marijuana, 434
Maslow's hierarchy of needs, 399–401, *400*, 402
  belonging/affection, 401
  esteem/self-respect, 401
  physiological needs, 400
  safety/security, 400
  self-actualization, 401
Mastectomy, 83
Measles, 15
Measurement of blood pressure, 80–81
Measurement systems, converting between, 280–281
Meats, 415
Mechanical washing, 166
Medial, 62
Medical abbreviations, 267t
Medical asepsis, 1–41
  active acquired artificial immunity, 10
  active acquired natural immunity, 10
  anaerobes, 5
  antibodies, 9
  bacteria, 3
  bactericidal, 5
  body protection, 4–5
    darkness, 5
    eyes, 4–5
    gastrointestinal tract, 5
    genitourinary tract, 5
    moisture, 5
    mouth, 5
    neutral pH, 5
    nutrients, 5
    oxygen, 5
    respiratory tract, 5
    skin, 4
    temperature, 5
  carrier, 7

chronic infections, 11
contagious diseases, 2
contamination, 27–30
  biohazard cleanup, 27–28
  biohazard waste, 30
  waste container, 28–29
    biohazard waste container, 29
    regular waste container, 29
    sharps waste container, 29
control plan, 20–23
dormant infection, 11
exiting reservoir, 7
fighting infection, 7–12
fungi, 3
germs, 2–3
guidelines, medical office, 20–27
hepatitis B, 31–40
  exposure prevention, 31–32
  exposure response, 32–40
immune system, 8
immune system failure, 10
infection control, 15–19
  disinfection, 18–19
    complexity of object, 19
    length of exposure, 19
    prior cleaning, 18
    strength of disinfecting solution, 19
    temperature, 19
    type of microorganism, 18
    types of, 18
  levels, 17–19
  medical asepsis, 15–17
    clean hands, 15–16
    clean workplace, 17
  sanitization, 17
  sterilization, 19
infection process, 6–7
latent infections, 11–12
manual, 20–21
microbes, 2
microorganism survival, 5–6
microorganisms, 2
natural immunity, 9
normal flora, 4
passive acquired artificial immunity, 9–10
passive acquired natural immunity, 9
pathogens, 2
personal protective equipment, 24–25
portal of entry, 7
protozoa, 3
reservoir host, 6–7
resident flora, 4

Medical asepsis (*continued*)
  risk factors, 20
  safety equipment, 25–27
    eyewash station, 27
    immunization, 27
    MSDS binder, 25
    personal protective equipment, 27
    waste containers, 25–26
  spores, 3
  spread of infection, 13–15
    direct transmission, 13
    indirect transmission, 13
  stages of infectious disease, 12
    acute stage, 12
    convalescent stage, 12
    declining stage, 12
    incubation stage, 12
    prodromal stage, 12
  standard precautions, 24
  susceptible host, 7
    identification of, 11
  symptoms, 10
  transmission of pathogens, 13–15
    animals, 14
    human hosts, 14
    insects, 15
  types of immunity, 9–10
  types of infections, 11–12
  vehicle of transmission, 7
  viruses, 3
Medical assistant's role in physical
    exam, 118–128
  assisting physician, 122–126
  examination room, preparation, 119
  examination room cleaning, 128
  follow-up procedures, 127
  patient preparation, 119–122
Medical conditions affecting patient
    education, 405t
Medical emergency, 449–450 (*see also*
    Emergencies)
Medical history, 42–104
  demographic data, 44
  family history, 45
  interviewing patients, 45–52
    communication skills, 48–49
      asking questions, 48
      examples, asking for, 48
      paraphrasing, 48
      reflecting, 48
      silence, allowing, 48
      summarizing, 48
    before interview, 49
      location, 49
    medical history, 44–45

past history, 44
patient interview, 86
review of systems, 44–45
social history, 45
Medical kit, emergency, 447–448
Medical office
  biohazard equipment, 25–27
  biohazard waste, 30
  contamination, handling, 27–30
  controlled substances in, 262
  emergencies, 443–513
  emergency care in, 444–445
  guidelines, 20–27
  packs prepared in, 189
  prescriptions in, 265–269
  safety equipment, 25–27
  scales used in, *57*
  surgery, 161–254
  suture removal kit, *219*
Medication action, 269–276
  factors influencing, 271–272
  pharmacodynamics, 270
  pharmacokinetics, 271–272
    absorption, 271
    distribution, 271
    excretion, 271
    metabolism, 271
Medication administration, 276–287
  apothecary system, 278–280
  dose calculation, 282–287
    BSA method, 285
    Clark's rule, 286
    formula method, 284–285
    Fried's rule, 287
    ratio method, 283–284
    Young's rule, 285–286
  household system, 280
  measurement systems, converting
    between, 280–281
  metric system, 278
    converting within, 281–282
  systems for measuring, 278–282
Medication errors, 307–308
Medication interactions, 272–276
  allergic reactions, 274–276
  antagonism, 273
  atorvastatin, 274
  food-medication interactions,
    273–274
  MAO inhibitors, 274
  potentiation, 273
  side effects, 274–276
  synergism, 273
  tetracycline, 274
  warfarin, 274

Medication-related terms, 273–274t
Medication routes, 287–339
  ears, 306
  eyes, 306
  inhalation, 305
  injection types, 295–298
    intradermal injections, 295–297
    intramuscular injections, 297–298
    subcutaneous injections, 297
    Z-track method, 298
  injections, 292–298
    insulin syringes, 294
    needle selection, 294
    needles, 293–295
    syringes, 293–295
      types of, 294–295
    tuberculin syringes, 294
    vials, 292–293
  intravenous route, 298–304
    setting rate, 303
    starting IV, 301–302
    TKO/KVO rates, 304
  mouth, 288–292
  nose, 306
  rectal administration, 306–307
  skin medications, 305
  topical medications, 305
  transdermal medications, 305
  vaginal administration, 307
Medication types, 257–258
  over-the-counter medications, 257
  prescription-only medications, 257
    chemical name, 257
    generic name, 257
    trade name, 257
Medications, 256, 259–261t, 413–414
  Drug Enforcement Agency, 258
  effect on blood pressure, 84
  Food and Drug Administration, 258
  legal regulations, 258–265
  sources, 258
Meniscus on mercury-free column, *102*
Mensuration, 118
Mercury-free column sphygmo-
    manometer, *80*
Mercury-free glass thermometer, 88–90
Metabolism, 63
  pharmacokinetics, 271
Methods of sterilization, 166t
Metric prefixes, 279t
Metric system, 278
  converting within, 281–282
Microbes, 2
Microorganism survival, 5–6
Microorganisms, 2–3

Microscope, 3
Microsurgery, 207
Mid-line, 62
Milk/milk products, 415
Minerals, 420–422
Minor medical office surgery, 161–254
  after surgical procedures, 213–254
  asepsis, 162–165
  assisting with surgery, 202–213
    common medical office surgical
      procedures, 208–210
    electrosurgery, 210–212
    laser surgery, 212–213
    local anesthetics, 202–203
    passing instruments, 203–204
    wound closure, 204–208
  healing process, 219–223
  preparing patient for surgery,
    196–202
    answering patient's questions,
      198–200
    informed consent, 197–198
    positioning patient, 200–201
    skin preparation, 201–202
  sterilization techniques, equipment,
    165–174
    autoclave, 167–173
    cold chemical sterilization,
      173–174
    sanitizing, 166–167
  surgery preparation, 188–196
    peel-back packages, solutions,
      194–196
    sterile surgical packs, 189–194
    sterile transfer forceps, 194
  surgical instruments, 174–188
    care/cleaning, responsibility for,
      185–188
  surgical scrub, 163–165
  wound care, 213–219
Minor surgery, 161–254
Moisture, 5
Mononucleosis, 15
Mouth, 5
  medication by, 288–292
  physical examination, 131
Moving patient, 122–123
MRI (*see* Magnetic resonance imaging)
MSDS binder, 25
Mucosa, 130
Musculoskeletal injuries, 475–483
  dislocations, 476–477
  fractures, 477
  slings, 479–483
  sprains, 475–476

Musculoskeletal injuries (*continued*)
strains, 475–476
types of splints, 478–479

N

Narcotics, 436
Nasal medications, instilling, 337
Nasal septum, physical examination, 130
Nasal speculum, 109, *109*
Natural disasters, 503–504
Natural immunity, 9
Nebulizer, 305
Neck, physical examination, 128–138, 463–464
Need to learn, 399
Needle assembly, *293*
Needle gauges, *294*
Needle holder, 176
Needle selection, 294
Needles, 293–295
Negative stress, 429–430
Neurogenic shock, 467
Neurological emergencies, 484–485
seizure, 485
seizure patients, assessing, 484–485
Neurological reflexes, 108
Neutral pH, 5
Nomogram, 285
Nomogram use, *286*
Nonabsorbable sutures, 207
Noncompliance, 397
Normal blood pressure, 82–84
Normal flora, 4
Normal respiration rates, 77
Nose
instruments for examination, 113–114
medication via, 306
physical examination, 130–131
Nosebleeds, 502–503
Nostrils, physical examination, 130
Nuclear medicine, 355
Nutrition, 415–423
food guide, 415–416
beans, 415
grains, 415
meats, 415
milk/milk products, 415
oils, 415
vegetables, 415
food labels, 418–422
carbohydrates, 419–420
cholesterol, 420
fats, 419
minerals, 420–422
protein, 420
sodium, 420
vitamins, 420–422
general dietary guidelines, 416–418
personal food pyramid, 416

O

Obstacles to learning, 405–407
age, 406
educational background, 407
illness, 405–406
pain, 405–406
physical impairments, 407
Obturator, 184
Office surgery, 161–254
after surgical procedures, 213–254
asepsis, 162–165
assisting with surgery, 202–213
common medical office surgical procedures, 208–210
electrosurgery, 210–212
laser surgery, 212–213
local anesthetics, 202–203
passing instruments, 203–204
wound closure, 204–208
healing process, 219–223
preparing patient for surgery, 196–202
answering patient's questions, 198–200
informed consent, 197–198
positioning patient, 200–201
skin preparation, 201–202
sterilization techniques, equipment, 165–174
autoclave, 167–173
cold chemical sterilization, 173–174
sanitizing, 166–167
surgery preparation, 188–196
peel-back packages, solutions, 194–196
sterile surgical packs, 189–194
sterile transfer forceps, 194
surgical instruments, 174–188
care/cleaning, responsibility for, 185–188
surgical scrub, 163–165
wound care, 213–219
Oils, 415

Open wounds, 468–471
  amputations, 469–470
  impaled objects, 470–471
  types, 470t
Opening airway, 454–455t, 454–457
Ophthalmic medical assistants, 114
Ophthalmology instruments, 183
Ophthalmoscope, 110–111
Oral, 64
Oral medications
  administration, 313–315
  forms, 290t
Oral temperature, measurement of,
    88–90
Oral thermometer, *68*
Orientation, using correct words for, 62
Orthopedic instruments, 183
OSHA (Occupational Safety and
    Health Administration)
  Form 300, log of work-related
    injuries, illnesses, *22*
  reporting to, 23
-Ostomy, 178
Otology instruments, 184
-Otomy, 178
Otorhinolaryngologist, 113
Otoscope, 109–110, *110*
Outside emergency training, 446
Over-the-counter medications, 53, 257
Overhead examination light, 112
Oximetry, 376–377
Oxygen, 5

P

Pain, as obstacle to learning, 405–406
Palpation, 117
Pap smear, 141
Paraphrasing, 48
Partial dislocation, 476
Partial thickness burn, 472
Passing instruments during surgery,
    203–204
Passive acquired artificial immunity,
    9–10
Passive acquired natural immunity, 9
Past history, 44
Patellar tendon, 138
Pathogen transmission, 13–15
  animals, 14
  human hosts, 14
  insects, 15
Pathogens, 2
Patient assessment, 50–52
  chief complaint, 52

present illness, 52
signs, 50
symptoms, 50–51
Patient education, 392–442
  adapting teaching material, 409–410
  alternative medicine, 425–426
    acupressure, 426
    acupuncture, 425–426
    hypnosis, 426
    yoga, 426
  assessment, 393–394
  charting sample, 398–399
  conditions needed, 399–404
    Maslow's hierarchy of needs,
        399–401
      belonging/affection, 401
      esteem/self-respect, 401
      physiological needs, 400
      safety/security, 400
      self-actualization, 401
    need to learn, 399
  disease prevention, 437–438
  documentation, 398–399, 398t
  elements of teaching plan, 408–409
    evaluation, 408
    learning goal, 408
    learning objectives, 408
    material to be covered, 408
  with equipment, 402–403
  evaluation, 397–398
  exercise, 423–425
  food group categories, 418t
  health care, 411–442
  health care topics, 411–442
  herbal supplements, 427–428
  implementation, 395–397
  individualized, 438
  Internet resources, 436–437t
  medical conditions affecting, 405t
  medications, 413–414
  nutrition, 415–423
    food guide, 415–416
      beans, 415
      grains, 415
      meats, 415
      milk/milk products, 415
      oils, 415
      vegetables, 415
    food labels, 418–422
      carbohydrates, 419–420
      cholesterol, 420
      fats, 419
      minerals, 420–422
      protein, 420

Patient education (*continued*)
    sodium, 420
      vitamins, 420–422
    general dietary guidelines, 416–418
    personal food pyramid, 416
  obstacles to, 405–407
    age, 406
    educational background, 407
    illness, 405–406
    pain, 405–406
    physical impairments, 407
  planning, 394–395
  preventive medicine, 411–412
  process, 393–404
  resources books, 408
  safety tips, 412–413
  strategies, 404
  stress management, 428–432
    negative stress, 429–430
    positive stress, 429–430
    relaxation techniques, 431–432
      breathing techniques, 431
      physical exercise, 431–432
      visualization, 431
  substance abuse, 432–437
    alcohol, 433
    illegal drugs, 434–436
      amphetamines, 435
      cocaine, 434–435
      crack, 434–435
      depressants, 435
      hallucinogens, 435–436
      marijuana, 434
      narcotics, 436
    smoking cessation, 432–433
  teaching aids, 396–397
  teaching environment, 401–402
  teaching methods, 396
    audiovisual material, 396
    demonstration, 396
    discussion, 396
    lecture, 396
    printed material, 396
    programmed instructions, 396
    role playing, 396
  teaching plan, 408–410
    elements of, 408–409
    example of, *409*
  teaching plans, 408–410
Patient examination positions,
    123–126
Patient history form, 46–47
Patient instructions, prescription,
    268–269

Patient positions, 343–344
Patient preparation, 119–122
  examination, preparation, 121
  information gathering, 119–121
  patients with special needs,
    121–122
Peel-back packages, solutions,
    194–196
Pelvic exam, *115*
Pelvic examination, 155–158
Penlight, 112, *112*
Percussion, 117
  direct percussion, 117
  indirect percussion, 117
Percussion hammer, 108
Percutaneous transluminal coronary
    angioplasty (PTCA), 356
Perfusion, 453
Peripheral, 130
Peripheral vision, physical examina-
    tion, 130
PERRLA, 129
Personal protective equipment, 20,
    24–27, 174
Personality changes, 434
PET (*see* Positron emission
    tomography)
Pharmacodynamics, 270
Pharmacokinetics, 270–272
  absorption, 271
  distribution, 271
  excretion, 271
  metabolism, 271
Pharmacology, 255–339 (*see also*
    Medication)
  administering, 256
  dispensing, 256
Phone, prescriptions by, 267–268
Physical dependence, controlled sub-
    stances, 262
Physical examination, 105–160,
    462–465
  abdomen, 464–465
  arms, 465
  back, 464–465
  body examination, 128–138
  chest, 464–465
  colon cancer, screening, 139
  gait, 138
  guidelines, 139–160
  head, 463–464
  immunizations for adults, 139–141
  instruments, 106–116

legs, 465
    medical assistant's role, 118–128
        assisting physician, 122–126
        examination room, 119
        examination room cleaning, 128
        follow-up procedures, 127
        patient preparation, 119–122
    neck, 463–464
    posture, 138
    preparing adult patient, 144
    rectal cancer, screening, 139
    reflexes, 138
    responsibilities, 106
    supplies, 106–111
    techniques, 116–118
Physical examination techniques,
        116–118
    auscultation, 118
    inspection, 116
    manipulation, 117
    mensuration, 118
    palpation, 117
    percussion, 117
        direct percussion, 117
        indirect percussion, 117
Physical exercise, 431–432
Physical impairments, as obstacle to
        learning, 407
Physician's Desk Reference, 276, 308
Physician's signature, prescription, 266
Physiological needs, in Maslow's hier-
        archy of needs, 400
Planning in teaching, 394–395
Plantar tendons, 138
-Plasty, 178
Pneumonia, 15
Podiatric medical assistants, 114
Poison Control Center, 489
Poisoning, 488–489
    Poison Control Center, 489
    poisoning emergencies, 489
Poisoning emergencies, 489
Polyps, 130
Portable ophthalmoscope, *111*
Portable otoscope, *110*
Portal of entry, 7
Portions, 419
Positioning patient for surgery,
        200–201
Positron emission tomography, 355
Posterior, 62
Postoperative instructions, 220–221
Postsurgical procedures, 213–254
Postural hypotension, 82

Posture, 138
Potentiation, 273
    medications, 273
PPE (*see* Personal protective
        equipment)
Prefilled cartridges, 295–296
    for injections, *292*
Prefilled medication cartridges, injec-
        tor devices, *297*
Prefixes in medical terminology, 3
Pregnant patients, 147
Preparation for patient interview, 49
Preparation for surgery, 188–202
    answering patient's questions,
        198–200
    informed consent, 197–198
    peel-back packages, solutions,
        194–196
    positioning patient, 200–201
    skin preparation, 201–202
    sterile surgical packs, 189–194
    sterile transfer forceps, 194
Prescription form, *311*
Prescription medications, 257, 291,
        311–312
    chemical name, 257
    generic name, 257
    trade name, 257
Prescriptions, 265–269
    date, 265
    DEA number, 266
    generic, 266
    inscription, 265
    patient instructions, 268–269
    patient's name, address, 265
    by phone, 267–268
    physician's signature, 266
    refills, 266
    signature, 266
    subscription, 266
Present illness, 52
    detailing, 53–55
        chronology, 54
        duration, 54
        location, 54
        quality, 54
        self-treatment, 54
        severity, 54
Preservative, 210
Pressure points, major arteries, *471*
Preventive medicine, 411–412
Primary intention, healing by,
        219–221
Printed material, in teaching, 396

Prior cleaning, 18
Privacy of patient, 122
Probe, 180
Process of learning, 393–404
Process of patient education, 393–404
Proctology instruments, 185
Prodromal stage, infectious disease, 12
Programmed instructions, in teaching, 396
Progress notes, *53*
Projections, x-ray exams, 343, 345–346t
Prone position, 123–124, *125*
Protein, 420
Protozoa, 3
Proximal, 62
Psychiatric, 494–495
Psychiatric emergency, 494
Psychological dependence, controlled substances, 262
Psychomotor skill, 403
PTCA (*see* Percutaneous transluminal coronary angioplasty)
Pulmonary function testing, 376, 387–388
  forced expiration volume, 376
  tidal volume, 376
Pulmonary function testing machine, *377*
Pulse, 72–76
  difficulty in finding, 75–76
  taking, 72–73
Pulse characteristics, 73
  rate, 73
  rhythm, 73
  volume, 73
Pulse oximeter, *378*
Pulse pressure, 83
Pulse rates, 63, 74
  age variations, 75
  factors affecting, 73–76
    blood volume, 74
    body type, size, 74
    exercise, 74
    fever, 74
    gender, 74
    medications, 74
    stress, 74
    time of day, 73
Punch biopsy, 209
Pupil, physical examination, 129
Purulent, 214
Pyrexia, 70

Q

Question-asking skills, 55

R

Rabies, 15
Radial pulse
  finger position for finding, *73*
  measurement, 97
Radiation, 64
  side effects, 357
Radiation burns, 472
Radiation safety
  for clinical staff, 346–347
  for patients, 344–346
Radiation therapy, 356–357
Radiographs, 341, 343, *359* (*see also* X-rays)
Radiography, 341
Radiography unit, *342*
Radiological procedures, assisting with, 358
Radiologists, 341
Radiology, 341–360
  barium studies, 350–352
  computed tomography, 354
  contrast examinations, scheduling, 352
  contrast medium examinations, 349–352
  diagnosis, 347–355
  fluoroscopy, 352–353
  magnetic resonance imaging (MRI), 354–355
  medical assistant's role, 357–360
    educating patients, 358
    film handling/storing, 359
    transfer of study information, 359–360
  nuclear medicine, 355
  patient positions, 343–344
  positron emission tomography (PET), 355
  radiation, side effects, 357
  radiation safety for clinical staff, 346–347
  radiation safety for patients, 344–346
  radiation therapy, 356–357
  scheduling x-rays, 352
  single photon emission computed tomography, 355

sonography, 354
treatment, 355–357
    embolization, 356
    laser angioplasty, 356
    percutaneous transluminal coronary angioplasty, 356
    vascular stents, 356
  x-ray machines, 342–347
  x-rays, 342–347
Radiolucent, 343
Radiopaque, 343
Range of motion, 117
Range-of-motion exercises, 424–425
Ratchets, 175
Rate of respiration, 78
Ratio method, in dose calculation, 283–284
Reassurance to patient, 124
Recognizing emergency, 449
Reconstituting dry medication, 293
Record-keeping, controlled substances, 309–310
Rectal cancer, screening, 139
Rectal drug administration, 306–307
Rectal examinations, 139
Rectal suppository placement, *307*
Rectal temperature, measurement of, 90–92
Rectovaginal, 137
Rectum, male, physical examination, 135–137
Refills, prescriptions, 266
Refined grains, 416
Reflecting, 48
Reflex hammer, *108*
Reflexes, 138
Regular waste container, 29
Relaxation techniques, 431–432
  breathing techniques, 431
  physical exercise, 431–432
  visualization, 431
Reporting to OSHA, 23
Rescue breathing, 453, 457
Reservoir filling, 171
Reservoir host, 6–7
Resident flora, 4
Resources books for patient education, 408
Respiration, 63, 76–79
  characteristics, 77–79
  depth, 78
  external respiration, 76
  internal respiration, 76
  measurement, 77, 98

normal respiration rates, 77
  rate, 78
  rhythm, 78
Respiratory disorders, 376
Respiratory rate, 63
Respiratory testing, 376–379
  blood gases, 378–379
  bronchoscopy, 378
  oximetry, 376–377
  pulmonary function tests, 376
    forced expiration volume, 376
    tidal volume, 376
Respiratory tract, 5
Responsiveness, 453
Rest, 476
Retina, physical examination, 130
Retractor, 180
Retractors, *180*
Reverse Trendelenburg position, 124, *125*
Review of systems, 44–45
Rhinology instruments, 184
Rhinoplasty, 178
Rhythm, pulse, 73
Rhythm of respiration, 78
Rhythm strip, 368
RICE, 476
Right to refuse care, 398
Risk factors, infection, 20
Role playing, in teaching, 396
Roles for clinical medical assistants, 114
Roller bandages, 215
ROM (*see* Range of motion)
Root words in medical terminology, 5
Routine test exam, 348
Rule of nines, 472, *474*

S

Safety, radiation
  for clinical staff, 346–347
  for patients, 344–346
Safety equipment, 25–27
  eyewash station, 27
  immunization, 27
  MSDS binder, 25
  personal protective equipment, 27
  waste containers, 25–26
Safety guidelines, 276–277
Safety of electrosurgery, 211–212
Safety/security, in Maslow's hierarchy of needs, 400

Safety tips, 412–413
  patient education, 412–413
Sanitizing, 17, 165–167
  in surgery, 166–167
Saturated fats, 421
Scales, *57*
Scalpels, 175, 178–179
  handles, *179*
Schedule of controlled substances, 262t
Scheduling, 414
Scheduling contrast examinations, 352
Scheduling x-rays, 352
Scissors, 175–178
  bandage scissors, 178
  curved scissors, 176
  straight scissors, 176
  suture scissors, 176
Sclera, physical examination, 129
Scrubbing hands, arms, with sterile brush, *164*
Secondary intention, healing by, 221
Seizure, 485
Seizure patients, assessing, 484–485
Self-actualization, in Maslow's hierarchy of needs, 401
Self-examination, breast, 132–134
Self-respect, in Maslow's hierarchy of needs, 401
Self-treatment of present illness, 54
Semi-Fowler's position, 124, *125*
Septic shock, 467
Serrations, 175
Serum, 213
Severity of present illness, 54
Sharps disposal, *28*
Sharps waste container, 29
Shock, 466–468
  anaphylactic shock, 467
  neurogenic shock, 467
  septic shock, 467
  types, 466–467
Shunts, 83
Side effects
  medications, 274–276
  radiation, 357
Signs, 50
Silence, allowing, 48
Sims' position, 123, *125*
Single photon emission computed tomography, 355
Sinuses, 131
  physical examination, 130–131

Sitting position, 123, *125*
Skin, 4, 462
  preparation for surgery, 201–202
Skin colors, abnormal, causes, 463t
Skin medications, 305
Skin preparation for surgery, 201–202
Sling, 479–483, *480*
Smears, *156*
Smoking cessation, 432–433
Soaks, 507–508
Social history, 45
Sodium, 420
Soft tissue injuries, 468–471
  closed wounds, 468–469
  open wounds, 469–471
    amputations, 469–470
    impaled objects, 470–471
Sonography, 354
Sources of medications, 258
Special indicators, 169–170
Specialized examinations, instruments, supplies for, 111–116
Specimen collection, 210
SPECT (*see* Single photon emission computed tomography)
Speculum, 109
  vaginal, *115*
Sphygmomanometer, 80, *80*
Splinting, 479
Splints, 478
  types, 478–479
Spores, 3
Sprains, 475–476
Spread of infection, 13–15
  direct transmission, 13
  indirect transmission, 13
Spring forceps, 176
Stages of infectious disease, 12
Standard bipolar leads, 365
Standard precautions, 24
Standing position, *125*
Staple bandages, 218–219
Staple remover, positioning, *251*
Staples, 205
  removing, 251–252
Sterile dressings, 214
  application, 244–246
Sterile field, 176, *243*
  flipping contents on to, 195
  maintaining, 197
Sterile gloves, *191–193*, 195, *245*
  application, 190–194
Sterile packs, opening, 231–233
Sterile solution, 235–236

Sterile surgical packs, 189–194
Sterile technique, *244*
Sterile transfer forceps, 176, 194–195, *195*, 234, *245*
Sterilization, 17, 19, 165–174
    autoclave, 167–173
    cold chemical sterilization, 173–174
    sanitizing, 166–167
    used instruments, *156*
Sterilization indicators, 170
Stethoscope, 110–111, *111*
Stethoscope diaphragm positioning, *101*
Storage, records, 188
Storing radiology film, 359
Straight scissors, 176
Strain, 475
Strategies for, 404
Strength of disinfecting solution, 19
Stress, effect on blood pressure, 84
Stress management, 428–432
    negative stress, 429–430
    positive stress, 429–430
    relaxation techniques, 431–432
        breathing techniques, 431
        physical exercise, 431–432
        visualization, 431
Subcutaneous injection, 294, 297
    administration, 324–326
Subcutaneous tissue, 206
Substance abuse, 432–437
    alcohol, 433
    illegal drugs, 434–436
        amphetamines, 435
        cocaine, 434–435
        crack, 434–435
        depressants, 435
        hallucinogens, 435–436
        marijuana, 434
        narcotics, 436
    smoking cessation, 432–433
Superficial burn, 472
Superficial frostbite, 493
Superior, 62
Supine position, 123, *125*
Supplies, 106–111
Supplies for physical exam, 106–111
Supplies for specialized examinations, 111–116
Surgery, 161–254
    after surgical procedures, 213–254
    asepsis, 162–165
    assisting with, 202–213

    assisting with surgery, 202–213
        common medical office surgical procedures, 208–210
        electrosurgery, 210–212
        laser surgery, 212–213
        local anesthetics, 202–203
        passing instruments, 203–204
        wound closure, 204–208
    healing process, 219–223
    preparing patient for surgery, 196–202
        answering patient's questions, 198–200
        informed consent, 197–198
        positioning patient, 200–201
        skin preparation, 201–202
    sterilization techniques, equipment, 165–174
        autoclave, 167–173
        cold chemical sterilization, 173–174
        sanitizing, 166–167
    surgery preparation, 188–196
        peel-back packages, solutions, 194–196
        sterile surgical packs, 189–194
        sterile transfer forceps, 194
    surgical instruments, 174–188
        care/cleaning, responsibility for, 185–188
    surgical scrub, 163–165
    wound care, 213–219
Surgical asepsis, 162–165
Surgical equipment, maintenance of, 186–187
Surgical instruments, 174–188
    care/cleaning, responsibility, 185–188
    clamps, 175–176
    forceps, 175–176
    hemostats, 176
    Kelly hemostats, 176
    needle holder, 176
    reducing damage to, 187
    scalpel, 175
    scissors, 175
    spring, thumb forceps, 176
    sterile transfer forceps, 176
    towel clamps, 176
Surgical packs, opening, 189–190
Surgical scissors, design of, *179*
Surgical scrub, 163–165
Surgical supplies, maintenance of, 187–188
Surgical terms, 178

Susceptible host, 7
  identification, 11
Suture bandages, 218–219
Suture material, *207*
Suture needles, 205–208
  classified by eye, 206
  classified by point, 206
  classified by shape, 206
  needle selection, 206
  suture material, 207–208
Suture removal kit, *219*
Suture scissors, 176
Sutures, 205
  removing, 249–250
  types, 207–208
Suturing, 175
Swaged needles, 206
Symptoms, 10, 50–51
Synergism, 273
  medications, 273
Syringe assembly, *293*
Syringes, 293–295
  types, 294–295
Systemic effect, 270
Systems for drug measuring, 278–282
Systole, 79
Systolic pressure, 79

T

Tape measure
  use in physical exam, 107, *107*
Teaching aids, 396–397
Teaching environment, 401–402
Teaching methods, 396
  audiovisual material, 396
  demonstration, 396
  discussion, 396
  lecture, 396
  printed material, 396
  programmed instructions, 396
  role playing, 396
Teaching plan, 408–410
  elements, 408–409
  example, *409*
Techniques, 116–118
Teleradiology, 356
Temperature, 5, 63–68
  axillary, 65
  control, 68–71
  disposable thermometers, 68
  electronic thermometers, 67
  factors influencing, 69–70
    age, 70

emotions, 70
exercise, 70
fever, 70–71
gender, 70
heat, 70
illness, 70
time of day, 70
  glass thermometers, 65–66
  hot places, 64–65
  oral, 64
  rectal, 65
  temporal scanner, 65
  tympanic, 65
  tympanic thermometers, 67–68
Temperature comparisons, 65t
Temperature control, factors influenc-
    ing, cold, 70
Temperature recording, 69
Temperature-related emergencies,
    490–494
  frostbite, 493–494
    managing, 493–494
    types of, 493
  heat cramps, 490–491
  heat exhaustion, 491
  heat stroke, 491–492
  hyperthermia, 490–492
  hypothermia, 492–493
Temporal scanner, 65
Tendons, 108
Tertiary intention, healing by, 221–223
Test results, follow-up to, 389
Testicular self-examination, 136–137
Tetracycline, 274
Thermal burns, 472
Thermometer placement, *94*
Throat
  instruments for examination,
    113–114
  physical examination, 131
Thumb forceps, 176, *250*
Thyroid, physical examination, 129
Tidal volume, 376
Tissue biopsy, 209
Tissue samples, preservative place-
    ment, *211*
Tongue depressors, 108
  for physical examination, *107*
Topical medications, 305
Towel clamps, 176, *178*
Trachea, physical examination, 128
Tracheotomy, 178
Trade name, prescription medica-
    tions, 257

Trans fats, 421
Transdermal medications, 305
  application, 332
Transfer forceps, 176, *195, 245*
Transillumination, 131
Transmission of pathogens, 13–15
  animals, 14
  human hosts, 14
  insects, 15
Traumatic needles, 206
Treadmill use, *374*
Trendelenburg position, 124, *125*
Triceps tendon, 138
Tuberculin syringe, 294, *296*
Tubular gauze bandages, 216
Tuning fork, 108–109
  in auditory test, *108*
Twelve-lead electrocardiogram,
    381–384
  completed application, *383*
Tympanic, 65
Tympanic membrane, 109
  viewed through otoscope, *130*
Tympanic thermometer, 67–68,
    68, 96
Types of disinfectants, 18
Types of emergencies, 466–495
Types of immunity, 9–10
Types of infection control, 17
Types of infections, 11–12

U

Ultrasonic cleaning, 168
Ultrasound, 354, *354*
Unipolar precordial leads, 366
Unit dose packages, *289*
  oral medications, *289*
United States Pharmacopeia Dispensing
    Information, 276
Unsaturated fats, 421
Urology instruments, 185

V

Vaginal cream, insertion of, *307*
Vaginal drug administration, 307
Vaginal speculum, 115, *115*
Varicose veins, 138
Vascular stents, 356
Vasoconstriction, 69
Vasodilation, 68
Vegetables, 415
Vegetarian, 423

Vehicle of disease transmission, 7
Venipuncture, 301
Vent hood, 174
Vertebrae, fractures in, *478*
Vials, 292–293
  holding, *204*
  for injections, *292*
Viruses, 3
Visualization, 431
Vital signs, 62–85, 462
  normal ranges, 63t
Vitamins, 420–422
Volume, pulse, 73
Vomiting, 497–498

W

Waiting for physician, 121
Waiting room, pathogens in, 14
Walking with crutches, 481
Wall-mounted ruler, *59*
Warfarin, 274
Waste container, 25–26, 28–29
Waste disposal guidelines, 40
Weight, 55–58
  effect on blood pressure, 84
Wheal, *322*
Wheel chairs, assisting patients in,
    145–146
Whole grains, 416
Withdrawing medicine, *317*
Women
  instruments for physical exam,
      114–116
    Ayre spatula, 115
    cell collection, 115
    cervical scraper, 115
    cotton-tipped applicator, 115
    histobrush, 115
    lubricant, 116
    vaginal speculum, 115
  physical examination, 141
    breast examination, 141
    guidelines for, 141
    mammogram, 141
    pap smear, 141
Work-related injuries, illnesses, log of,
    22
Workplace, cleaning, 17
Wound care, 213–219
  bandage application, 216–218
    circular turn, 216
    figure-eight turn, 217
    reverse spiral turn, 217

Wound care (*continued*)
  spiral turn, 217
 bandage types, 214–216
   elastic bandages, 215–216
   roller bandages, 215
   staple bandages, 218–219
   suture bandages, 218–219
   tubular gauze bandages, 216
 changing sterile dressings, 214
 sterile dressings, 214
Wound cleaning, *219*
Wound closure, 204–208
 adhesives, 205
 staples, 205
 suture needles, 205–208
   classified by eye, 206
   classified by point, 206
   classified by shape, 206
   needle selection, 206
   suture material, 207–208
 sutures, 205
Wound drainage, 215

Wound healing, *222*
 phases, 223

X

X-ray envelope, for processed radiographs, *359*
X-ray machines, 342–347
X-rays, 341–347
 fears regarding, 347
 patient preparation, 349t
 protection during, *348*

Y

Yoga, 426
Young's rule, in dose calculation,
  285–286

Z

Z-track injection method, 298